PERSON-CENTRED PRACTICES
A HOLISTIC AND INTEGRATED APPROACH

PERSON-CENTRED PRACTICES

A HOLISTIC AND INTEGRATED APPROACH

Mark Jukes and John Aldridge

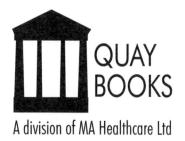

QUAY
BOOKS

A division of MA Healthcare Ltd

Quay Books Division, MA Healthcare Ltd, St Jude's Church, Dulwich Road, London SE24 0PB

British Library Cataloguing-in-Publication Data
A catalogue record is available for this book

© MA Healthcare Limited 2007
ISBN-10: 1-85642-330-1; ISBN-13: 1-85642-330-4

Printed by Athenaeum Press Ltd, Dukes Way, Team Valley, Gateshead, NE11 OPZ

Contents

Introduction

Mark Jukes and John Aldridge

Over the last 25 years or so, services for people who have learning disabilities have changed beyond all recognition. Almost everything about the service that we knew in the early 1970s has been swept away in an organisational and cultural revolution. The nature of the people we support, where we provide that support and how we provide that support are all radically different, and rightly so. Possibly the greatest change has been in the way we think about our clients and the nature of our relationship with them. We have moved from a paternalistic, controlling relationship based on the medical model towards one of partnership and empowerment, based on humanistic principles and a more holistic view of the person in a social model of care. Person-centredness is fundamental to this new way of working, in that it prompts us to build services from the person's perspective, to attend to issues that are important to the person and to provide support in ways that maximise involvement and choice (Department of Health 2002).

Most services for people who have learning disabilities have enthusiastically embraced person-centred approaches and, in accord with *Valuing People* (DH 2001) have promoted person-centred planning, health action planning and health facilitation as central building blocks. However, there does seem to be a paradoxical tension between old and new ways of working. Sanderson (2003) comments that:

'Person-centred planning is a different approach rooted in the values of the new paradigm [a developmental, rather than a medical model]. Instead of trying to "fix" people, the aim of person-centred planning is to discover what an individual's chosen lifestyle is and how this can be achieved'

What, then, is the role of the professional health worker in this process? Should we forget our expertise and skills in favour of an entirely developmental perspective? Although health work is not about attempting to 'fix' people (in terms of trying make them become what we want them to be), it arguably is about trying to fix health problems – helping people become healthier. The challenge here is about how we help people to improve their health in person-centred ways. We would argue that health-focused work and person-centred work are not incompatible. It is entirely possible to approach health-focused work through a process that meets the Five Key Features of Person-centred Planning (Sweeney & Sanderson 2002).

- **The person is at the centre**. We need to listen carefully to peoples' perspectives on their health and to attend to health issues that are worrying the person, not those that we think need 'fixing'.
- **Family members and friends are full partners**. Family members and friends often know a great deal about the person and this can be very helpful when we are working with people who have communication difficulties or difficulty in remembering. However, family involvement must be with the person's agreement or we are in danger of addressing the family's needs rather than the person's. That said, many health issues are whole family issues and we need to involve all members in deciding what approach should be taken.
- **Person-centred planning reflects a person's capacities, what is important to a person (now and for the future) and specifies the support they require**. We need to build health support services around the person and not try to 'shoehorn' the person into existing approaches. This requires a great deal of flexibility and innovative thought on the part of specialist services and considerable change on the part of generic health services. The recent reports from Mencap (2004; 2007) suggest that generic health services still have a long way to go in terms of meeting the needs of people who have severe learning disabilities. Specialist nurses could do much to help develop a person-centred response by generic services.
- **Person-centred planning builds a shared commitment to action that recognises a person's rights**. We would argue that this involves a partnership approach to identifying, meeting and evaluating a person's health needs. Peoples' rights include the right to services that help them improve their health. Equally, we need to recognise that people may choose not to attend to a particular health need (just as any other person has the right not to adopt a healthy lifestyle).
- **Person-centred planning leads to continual listening, learning and action and helps the person get what they want out of life**. This is about using our communication skills to listen carefully to what people say about their health, listening to their concerns and responding to the things they think are important. It is clearly not about prescribing health care because we think that it is 'in the person's best interests'.

This book is divided into four sections. **Section 1** focuses on conceptual models for practice. Three chapters represent established models of nursing, and learning disability nurses have adapted each model's ethos for application in the field of learning disability nursing practice.

The models' suitability for assessing and planning care needs with people is acknowledged and appraised in terms of contemporary issues. The practitioners identify the discrete focus and concepts where health is assessed and the loci for appropriate intervention is claimed. In the remaining two chapters in this section, established practitioners and learning disability nurse theorists develop their own innovative and original models from their extensive nursing practice and experience.

Section 2 deals with relatively new emergent areas which represent how, in specialist areas, the learning disability nurse can further influence the support for people with regard to supplementary nurse prescribing and acute liaison work across the health and social care sectors.

In **Section 3**, for the first time in a text on learning disability, the integrated nature of services for people with a learning disability across the United Kingdom and Éire-Ireland is discussed. Each chapter in this section is written by leading learning disability nurses who identify with the unique configuration of services, priorities and reforms in each country.

Readers will be able to digest each country's discrete and contemporary health and social care reforms and priorities as they impact on people with a learning/ intellectual disability.

In **Section 4**, three chapters identify fundamental concepts of self-awareness, reflection, leadership, management of change and safety planning. In the first two chapters, nurses are encouraged to acknowledge and recognise their own potential for leading and managing change.

Bringing about innovations in practice and sustaining practices which are person-centred is not an easy task. Learning disability nurses work across seamless services, and as a result relate with a large number of professionals, carers and families on and outside familiar or not-so-familiar boundaries. Sometimes change is viewed suspiciously or negatively, so attempting to work in a person-centred way requires unique skills for taking people along in person-centred directions.

The final chapter in this section, about safety planning, revisits risk assessment and management with people with a learning disability from a new perspective and considers such planning in person-centred ways.

This text is also a first from the perspective that original and adapted conceptual models and theories have been pursued by learning disability nurses and applied across the health and social care sectors.

In our first text on *Person-centred Practices – A Therapeutic Perspective* (2006), we focused attention on the therapeutic role and value of nurses in learning disability. This companion text concentrates on how learning disability nurses can address person-centred practices through the adoption of holistic frameworks for addressing the needs of people across a broad spectrum of complex needs in learning disability.

While we share the vision enshrined in *Shaping the Future* (United Kingdom Learning Disability Consultant Nurse Network 2006), this report did not quite go the distance in articulating how learning disability nurses can draw on theoretical conceptual models to help them illuminate and direct professional holistic practice.

We believe our text goes some way in addressing how nurses can embrace theories and frameworks, not only to delineate and evaluate practice, but for transforming practice through holistic engagement with the person with a learning disability. The ultimate goal and aspiration for learning disability nurses is to influence and shape individualised services through personal and professional self-awareness, reflection and leadership, and by managing change.

Mark Jukes
Birmingham City University, England

John Aldridge
University of Northampton, England
June 2007

References

Department of Health (2001) *Valuing People*: a new strategy for Learning Disability for the 21st Century, London, DH

Department of Health (2002) *Planning with People: Towards Person-centred Approaches*, guidance for implementation groups, London, DH

Jukes M, Aldridge J (2006) *Person-Centred Practices – A Therapeutic Perspective.* London, Quay Books

Mencap (2004) *Treat Me Right!* London, Mencap

Mencap (2007) *Death by Indifference.* London, Mencap

Sanderson H (2003) *Person-centred planning*, in Gates B (ed) *Learning Disabilities: Towards Inclusion* (4th edn). Edinburgh, Churchill Livingstone

Sweeney C, Sanderson H (2002) Person-Centred Planning: BILD Factsheet No. 007, Kidderminster, British Institute of Learning disabilities

United Kingdom Learning Disability Consultant Nurse Network (2006) *Shaping The Future: A Vision for Learning Disability Nursing*

Contributors

Editors

Mark Jukes Reader in Learning Disabilities, Birmingham City University, Birmingham, England

John Aldridge Senior Lecturer in Nursing (Learning Disabilities), University of Northampton, England

Contributors

Dr Owen Barr Senior Lecturer in Nursing, Institute of Nursing Research and School of Nursing, Magee Campus, University of Ulster, Northern Ireland

John Boarder Lecturer in Learning Disabilities, School of Healthcare Sciences, University of Wales (Bangor), Wales

Michael Brown Nurse Consultant and Lecturer, NHS Lothian, Primary Care Organisation, Edinburgh, Scotland

Maurice Devine Nurse Consultant (Learning Disability), Down Lisburn South Eastern Trust, Northern Ireland

Dave Ferguson Consultant Nurse (Mental Health in Learning Disabilities) Hampshire Partnership NHS Trust, Southampton, England

Anne-Marie Glasby Acute Liaison Nurse, South Birmingham Primary Care Trust, Birmingham, England

Brian Jones Lecturer in Learning Disabilities, School of Healthcare Sciences, University of Wales (Bangor), Wales

Paul Keenan Lecturer in Intellectual Disabilities Nursing, School of Nursing and Midwifery, The University of Dublin, Trinity College, Dublin, Éire Ireland

Premchuniall Mohabeersingh Principal Lecturer, Health Policy and Public Health Division, Faculty of Health, Birmingham City University, Birmingham, England

Neville Parkes Senior Lecturer (Learning Disabilities) University of Worcester, England

Penny Spencer Community Services Learning Disabilities Manager, Chy Govenek, Truro, Cornwall, England

Caron Thomas Nurse Consultant in Learning Disabilities, South Staffordshire Healthcare Foundation NHS Trust, Stafford, England

Judi Thorley Senior Nurse/Lecturer in Learning Disabilities, North Staffordshire Combined Healthcare NHS Trust and Keele University, Keele, England

Dr John Turnbull Director of Nursing, Ridgeway Partnership (Formerly Oxfordshire Learning Disability NHS Trust) and Visiting Professor in Learning Disability Nursing, University of Northampton, Northampton, England

Maureen Turner Principal Lecturer, Head of Adult Centred Care Division, Faculty of Life Sciences, School of Nursing and Midwifery, De Montfort University, Leicester, England

Abbreviations

A2A	Access to Acute
ABA/IRB	An Bord Altranais/Irish Nursing Board
ADR	adverse drug reaction
AIMS	Abnormal Involuntary Movement Scale
ANP	advanced nurse practitioner
APLD	Association of Practitioners in Learning Disability
APN	advanced practice nurse
AWHONN	Association of Women's Health, Obstetric and Neonatal Nurses
AWS	All Wales Strategy
AWSNAG	All Wales Senior Nurse Advisory group
CAMHS	Child and adolescent mental health services
CHP	community health partnership
CLDN	community learning disability nurse
CMHT	community mental health team
CNLD	community nurse for learning disability
CNS	clinical nurse specialist
CPA	care programme approach
CSCI	Commission for Social Care Inspection
CSPD	Commission on the Status of People with Disabilities
DH	Department of Health
DHSS	[former]Department of Health and Social Security
DHSSPS	Department of Health, Social Services and Public Safety Northern Ireland
DOHC	Department of Health and Children Eire Ireland
DRO	differential reinforcer of other [behaviours]
EE	expressed emotion
FedVol	National Federation of Voluntary Bodies
GOI	Government of Ireland
GSL	General Sales List
HAP	health action plan
HIQA	Health Information and Quality Authority
HIW	Healthcare Inspectorate Wales
HRB	Health Research Board
HSE	Health Service Executive
HSE	Health and Safety Executive
IDMHS	Intellectual Disability Mental Health Service

IM	intramuscular
LDIAG	Learning Disability Implementation Advisory Group Wales
LDN	learning disability nurse
LUNSERS	Liverpool University Neuroleptics Rating Scale
MHId	mental health of intellectual disability
MHRA	National Disability Authority Eire
NDG	National Development Group
NHO	National Hospitals Office Eire
NIDD	National Intellectual Disability Database
NPC	National Prescribing Centre
NPSA	National Patient Safety Agency
NSF	national service framework
OCISS	Office of the Chief Inspector of Social Services (Éire)
PALS	patient advice and liaison service
PAMIS	Profound and Multiple Impairment Service
PCCC	Primary, Community and Continuing Care (Éire)
PCT	primary care trust
PDF	professional development forum
PiP	partnership-in-practice agreement
POM	prescription-only medicine
RCN	Royal College of Nursing
RMHLDNI	Review of Mental Health and Learning Disability (NI)
RNMS	Registered Nurse Mental Subnormality
RPANI	Review of Public Administration northern Ireland
S4C	Sianel Pedwar Cymru (Channel Four Wales)
SAYIG	The 'same as you' implementation group
SCLD	Scottish Consortium for Learning Disability
SCOVO	Standing Conference of Voluntary Organisations for People with Learning Disability in Wales (now Learning Disability Wales)
SLA	service level agreement
SOP	Special Olympics Ireland SOP
SRV	social role valorisation
SUPLS	'service user priority-led service'
UDID	Unit for Development in Intellectual Disabilities
UKCC	United Kingdom Central Council
UKLDCNN	United Kingdom Learning Disability Consultant Nurse Network
WAG	Welsh Assembly Government
WTE	whole time equivalent

Models for practice in learning disability nursing

Models for practice
The Elements of Nursing

Mark Jukes

Introduction

This chapter describes the Elements of Nursing, a model for nursing devised by Roper, Logan and Tierney (1986).

Adaptation of the model for learning disability nursing practice will then be pursued, as the conception and development of the model was originally located in an era and context for the provision of community care policy and services.

Examining the literature in the application of Roper et al's model reveals a varied critical and – at times – simplistic and naïve response to the introduction of this model into nursing practice across different specialisms.

The adapted model for learning disability nursing will be illustrated and applied using a case study which presents a rationale and justification for the contemporary relevance of the model in the context of person-centredness and health facilitation. The case study identifies a person who presents with a myriad of complex health and social care needs.

A person-centred and holistic approach

In learning disability nursing, person-centred planning and person-centred care approaches initially require clarification, as claims to be person-centred emanate from a variety of different theoretical sources.

Person-centred planning (PCP) refers to a cluster of concepts and approaches which include:
- Essential lifestyle planning
- Personal futures planning
- Making action plans
- Planning Alternative Tomorrows with Hope (PATH)

All share a value which is based on inclusion. PCP aims to consider the:

> '...aspirations and capacities expressed by the service user or those speaking on their behalf, rather than needs and deficiencies'

> (Mansell & Beadle-Brown 2004, p1)

Sanderson et al (2002) identify the processes that epitomise PCP approaches:

- Find out what is important to the person, in their everyday life and in the future
- Identify what support they require
- Develop an action plan to facilitate the above
- Continue to reflect and act on the actions and the plan

In learning disability nursing, an important value-based concept to consider – for the adoption of any theoretical person-centred care approach for assessment in health or social care – is to perceive people as individuals. People may sometimes be able, other times disabled; sometimes independent, other times dependent. The broad spectrum of people defined as having a learning disability extends from complex physical and multiple profound disability through to borderline learning disability, and where the extent of communication is also extremely variable along the non-verbal/verbal continuum.

As McNally (2006) asserts, intellectual disability nurses are in a particularly strong position to implement and refine PCP, due to their specialist training and professional academic knowledge, and the high proportion of time they spend with people who have an intellectual disability. From this contact and the development of intensive relationships with people directly and with their families, learning disability nurses are concerned with a person-centred and holistic approach that aims to explore the physiological, biological, behavioural, social and spiritual dimensions pertaining to each person. This process is achieved and facilitated through the person, the learning disability nurse and other significant people including other professionals, and is fundamental in person-centred assessments and development of care plans.

People with a learning disability may also require assistance to moderate behaviours that might be seen as antisocial, to develop social and daily living skills and identify and achieve work, leisure and lifestyle interests. Nurses in learning disability need to be sensitive not only to the key principles of rights, independence, choice and inclusion (Department of Health 2001), but also in balancing a person's freedom with the professional, ethical 'duty of care'.

Traditionally, both in learning disabilities and mental health, the contemporary popularity of 'psychosocial' and other cognitive-behavioural interventions often support the biomedical construction in 'problems of living'. The emphasis is on identifying the problem rather than honouring the person and their potential.

In learning disability services, traditionally assessments have been used to classify or determine a person's suitability for a placement either for living or some form of day placement that involves occupation. In psychological terms we have predominantly used functional assessments to determine planned teaching goals so that we can teach the person new skills or new behaviours.

Barker (2004) refers to what may be considered a more preferred notion of a person's identity in that we are trying to study 'the whole person' in terms of levels of living. Barker proposes that we function on a number of levels:

- Physiology
- Biology
- Behaviour
- Beliefs
- Cognition
- Affect

Physiological Self: Although we are not sensitive to this level of functioning, the essence of our biochemical level of existence is critical to the stability of our lives. What constitutes our molecular/biochemical level of being a functional human is the most fundamental.

Biological Self: On occasions in experiencing pain on exertion can we acknowledge the exercising of various organs such as the heart, muscles and skeletal system, where the interaction of such systems gives us a clear indication that we are living and feel alive.

Behavioural Self: How we feel, think and act are constant transitions on a moment-to-moment basis in how we respond and behave to others.

Social Self: Where we are in relationship with others, whether close – such as family and friends – or generally in the broad spectrum of humanity

Spiritual Self: Where we live in the hope of fulfilment in our dreams, hopes and ultimately our beliefs. This is a subjective level where the views of self-and the world and others around us are perhaps symbolic, obscure and ill defined. These levels cumulatively add up to a whole lived experience that represents the 'whole self'.

Why nursing models?

Nursing models have evolved and developed since the 1950s as a means of attempting to think conceptually about 'what is nursing?'

Reilly (1975) provides an earlier insight into what nurse theorists were doing by observing that:

> *'We all have a private image (concept) of nursing practice. In turn, this private image influences our interpretation of data, our decisions, and our actions. But can a discipline continue to develop when its members hold so many differing private images? The proponents of conceptual models of practice are seeking to make us aware of these private images, so that we can begin to identify commonalities in our perceptions of the nature of practice and move towards a well ordered concept'*

McAllister (2007, p3) offers a contemporary view where:

> *'Nursing models help to articulate what nursing is, what nursing does, what nursing values are and that good nursing models illuminate the path ahead, helping nurses to imagine and forge ahead to what nursing might become'*

There are a variety of nursing models that represent different theoretical perspectives and contain shared assumptions as well as individual points of difference. They are usually classified into theories:

- Systems
- Developmental
- Interactional

Systems theory and models emphasise that the human body is made up of several interrelated subsystems, and systems models focus on physiological systems in addition to psychological and social systems in the person as a whole.

Systems interact with each other, have boundaries, need to be in a state of equilibrium (homeostasis), are affected by stress and conflict, and have feedback potentials to maintain the systems equilibrium. Examples of systems models are Roper et al (1986) Roy (1976) and Neuman (2002).

Developmental theories focus on human development whereby the process of development is affected by illness or accident. Current circumstances might be inhibiting growth or causing regression. The focus therefore is on growth and directional change. Peplau (1952) has been of predominant influence as a developmental model.

Interactional theories focus on the interaction between nurse and patient, and assume that interaction is meaningful, leading to adaptation of roles or behaviour. The assessment is likely to focus on the development of rapport between nurse and patient, their current roles and the person's perception of the situation. An example of such a model is Travelbee (1971).

Early nursing theories emphasised interpersonal relationships. For example, Peplau (1952) described psychodynamic nursing as the structural concepts of the interpersonal process which are the phases of the nurse–patient relationship – orientation, identification, exploitation and resolution.

Orlando (1961) emphasised the reciprocal relationship between patient and nurse, which comprises:

- The behaviour of the patient
- The reaction of the nurse
- The actions that the nurse designs for the patient's benefit.

The interaction of these elements with each other is *nursing process*.

Travelbee defined nursing as an interpersonal process – an experience that occurs between the nurse and an individual or group of individuals.

Philosophies emphasising the 'Art' of nursing came next. They include Henderson (1961;1969) whose definition was adopted and adapted as an introduction to the National Boards for England and Wales National Syllabus of Training for the Professional Register Part 5 Registered Nurse for the Mentally Handicapped 1982, and cited below [in brackets – my substitution of terms to reflect current terminology]:

> *'The function of the nurse for people with [learning disability] is*
> *directly and skilfully to assist the individual and his family, whatever*

the [disability], in the acquisition, development and maintenance
of those skills that, given the necessary ability, would be performed
unaided; and to do this in such a way as to enable independence to
be gained as rapidly and fully as possible, in an environment that
maintains a quality of life that would be acceptable to fellow citizens
of the same age' (Henderson (1961)

The Syllabus was based on a philosophy of care that recognises and accepts that people with a learning disability have the same human value as anyone else in society and embraces three fundamental principles.

1. People with a learning disability have the same rights and – as far as possible – the same responsibilities as other members of the community.

2. People with a learning disability have a right and a need to live like others in the community, and to receive services that meet their changing needs.

3. People with a learning disability should receive additional help from professional services to allow the full recognition and expression of their individuality.

(ENB & WNB 1988)

This overarching philosophy and principles still echo and resonate with the four key themes of *Valuing People* (DH 2001) – rights, choice, inclusion and independence.

Following on from nursing philosophies came conceptual models that reflect adaptation, behavioural field theory and systems approaches, as well as having an emphasis on science.

Here, theorists such as Neuman, Roy and Roper, Logan and Tierney developed their unique world views on the development of models for practice.

It is perhaps appropriate to commence this book with a chapter that focuses on the most well known – but at the same time excessively berated – nursing model in Britain today. The Elements of Nursing by Roper, Logan and Tierney (1986), is perceived by many as 'medically orientated, materialistic, and of a reductionism approach' and as Parker (1997, p2) continues to claim:

'We too easily discard something which is easy to comprehend,
straightforward and actually works in conjunction with medical
practice'

Origins of the Elements of Nursing

Elements of Nursing as a model for living and a model for nursing came out of a challenge for Nancy Roper while teaching nursing students to identify 'nursing', and initiated an extensive literature review and a research project to investigate whether there was a 'core' of nursing (Marriner Tomey & Alligood 1998).

As stated in the preface to the first edition, it was a way to assist learning to develop a way of thinking about nursing across the boundaries of different patient groups and health care settings. The model was seen as a meaningful framework for the nursing process, which was accelerating in preoccupation terms in British nursing. However, in the absence of a theoretical framework, it could not be applied congruently to practice (Tierney 1998).

In learning disability nursing services and practice, the nursing process was fast becoming a vehicle for psychologists to promote skills teaching educational programme planning, (Chamberlain 1986) with an emphasis on psychological functional assessment as opposed to a more holistic focus on what represents the whole person and total experience of living.

Nursing models can be classified into four major concepts:

- Nature of the individual
- Health and illness
- The role of the nurse
- Environment

The nature of the individual

The Elements of Nursing is seen in this concept as engaging in a process of living from conception to death, and continually changing and developing through this lifespan. During his or her lifespan a person carries out different types of activities, described as 'Activities of Living' (ALs). Each activity overlaps and cannot be isolated, and each is influenced by physical, emotional, sociocultural and economic factors, and each person's uniqueness is expressed in the individual way in which they carry out each living activity.

Health and illness

According to Roper, Logan and Tierney, health is difficult to define, and they provide no clear expressed definition. Rather, they suggest that it has a different meaning for each person and believe that it can only be defined in relation to the individual, taking into consideration personal expectation and level of functioning in ordinary living. However, in terms of the model's principles, health is viewed as the ability to carry out the ALs in a manner acceptable to the person and the society in which they live, without causing harm to themselves or others. The person copes successfully with the difficulties of living, or with the subsequent needs to adapt to differing degrees of dependence.

The role of the nurse

Nursing is described as helping people to prevent, solve, alleviate or cope with actual or potential problems related to the Activities of Living.

In addition, Roper defines nursing as an independent practitioner working in an organisation:

> 'Nursing is directly or indirectly enabling each person in a health
> care system to acquire, maintain or restore his/her maximum level
> of self-care/independence: or to cope with being dependent in any of
> their activities of daily living...Nursing incorporates co-ordination of
> help from other healthcare professions and at patient level it entails
> the performance of nursing activities from one of four groups of
> components of Nursing'   (Roper 1979)

Environment
The environment is referred to in terms of influences on each AL, but Roper et al do not define it specifically. Although no distinction is made between the internal and external environment, they do describe the physiological, psychological, social, economic and political factors that indicate that the ALs are influenced by an internal and external environment.

Major concepts
Figure 1.1 shows the Elements of Nursing where four major concepts are common. These are:
- Activities of living (ALs)
- Lifespan
- Dependence/independence continuum
- Five influencing factors:
  - Biological
  - Psychological
  - Sociocultural (including spiritual/religious/ethical)
  - Environmental
  - Politicoeconomic (including legal)

The interpretation of these four concepts produces the fifth main concept, 'individuality in living'.

Activities of living
Activities of living were a further refinement of ideas generated and contained in Henderson's (1969) original definition of nursing, which was later cited in the 1982 syllabus for learning disability nursing (ENB 1988).

The Elements of Nursing are defined as:

> *'Helping people to prevent, alleviate, solve or cope with problems*
> *(actual or potential) related to the Activities of Living'*

> (Roper et al 1990, p37)

The emphasis in this model is on prevention and health promotion much as helping people with existing problems (Tierney 1998). The person at the centre of the model is shown in Figure 1.1 by 12 activities of living.

ALs have many dimensions and their interconnectivity and complexity mean that we have to prioritise them in our daily living. Personality traits can influence how we do this.

For example, basic physiological motivational forces can focus our mind on being satisfied from our thirst, hunger or safety – or from a psychological perspective, we may be focused on our work, recreation or sexual satisfiers.

The relevance of the ALs need to be considered in particular where people who have a learning disability live and interact in a variety of settings – at home, in specialised NHS facilities, short-stay centres, assessment centres, day or respite care, social care or in supported living.

Figure 1.1 Representation of the Roper, Logan & Tierney model for nursing assisted by adoption of CARE to support the nursing process

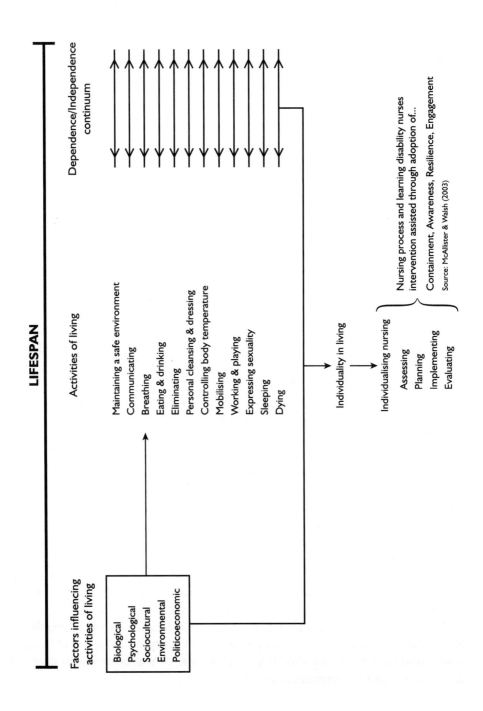

Lifespan

The Lifespan is defined as the temporal span of life on this earth from birth to death. Most countries have registry offices where births, deaths and causes of death must be recorded, and from these data several predictions can be made about the population. According to the National Patient Safety Agency (NPSA 2004) the literature suggests that the health care needs of people with intellectual disabilities are converging with those of the general population as improved care has fed into increased life expectancy (Moss & Turner 1995; Holland 2000). The relevance of the lifespan to nursing and the ALs is critical for appropriateness, relevance and prioritising of care.

Dependence/independence continuum

The Dependence/independence continuum acknowledges that there are stages when a person cannot yet (or no longer) perform certain ALs independently. It ranges from total dependence to total independence, and is bidirectional, which is important in learning disability nursing for recognition in stages of health/illness and maturational development.

Factors influencing ALs

Many factors have influenced or continue to influence the way in which a person enacts the activities of living. They are grouped under five headings – biological, psychological, sociocultural, environmental and politicoeconomic – and are applied to each particular AL. We use this holistic perspective to understand how a person can/cannot enact each AL.

Contextually, the importance of environmental and politicoeconomic factors due to community care policies are indispensable factors for analysis as assessment criteria for each AL. A myriad of lifestyle options impact on – and are available to – people with learning disabilities and their families.

Individuality in living

To individualise nursing, nurses need to know about the person's individuality in living, which is accomplished by using the phases of the nursing process through a dynamic and interactive process of engagement with the person. This refers to the style in which people attend to each of their ALs according to the achieved stage on the lifespan and place on the independence/dependence continuum, which have all been – and still are being – influenced by the interacting five groups of factors.

Individualising nursing

The nursing process individualises nursing through the phases of assessment, planning, implementation and evaluation. This is not incompatible with the process of 'caring' and the ideals of empowerment. The relationship between the nurse and person is a partnership to develop mutual goals – potential or actual.

Critical perspectives on the Elements of Nursing

The Elements of Nursing is popular in adult nursing and generally across the nursing profession (Clark & Gates 2006); is perceived by some as the archetypal model (Beech 2002); and has its roots in general nursing (Murphy et al 2000). In learning disabilities, Elliot-Cannon (1990) has further supported the model because as a model it perceives human beings who seek fulfilment, and focuses on the concepts of the 'independence continuum' and the 'lifespan' approach to long-term care and relationships. However, Elliot-Cannon (1990) has highlighted that due to little being defined as to what constitutes the person, the Activities for Living approach to assessment could be seen as mechanistic and as a 'checklist' approach for assessment (Reed & Robbins 1991). A further overemphasis on physical aspects of care has been observed (Minshull et al 1986; Walsh 1989) with simplistic use of the model in nursing practice. Additional criticism of nurses is a lack of understanding, coupled with the need for more adequate educational preparation (Murphy et al 2000).

From a simplicity and checklist perspective this is by no means due to the model's neglect of these factors, as it clearly delineates the need to address the psychological, sociocultural, environmental, politicoeconomic and physical factors that influence the activities of living. These factors are cited throughout Roper et al (1990) and Newton (1992).

McCann (2003) identified that although nurses adopted Roper et al (1981) in developing plans of care, nurses tended to underuse or even ignore the category 'expressing sexuality'. This claim was based on the notion that nurses needed to be more knowledgeable about the biological, psychological and social aspects of sexuality.

Criticisms in mental health nursing contend that the Roper et al (1990) model, along with Orem's (1980) self-care model and Roy's (1980) adaptation model, make no specific reference to forming nurse–patient relationships, and that there is clearly no indication in these models that relationship-centred activity is primary (Cutliffe & Goward 2000).

This is worthy criticism, and the intention of nursing models is to reflect practice and develop appropriate nurse–patient interactions for the development of a holistic assessment. Roper et al's model is not explicit in how an interaction or intervention is to be applied. The nurse in the role of assessor is required to develop purposeful communications, but can be open to individual application and interpretation.

Certainly in learning disability nursing, a humanistic approach to assessment and intervention in the form of developing relationships of a person-centred nature is critical, and where a psychosocial model could be adopted as a complementary adjunct to the Elements of Nursing. Questions and dialogue to further ascertain how a person perceives their current health status, are further necessities for being person-centred when individualising care needs. For those people with more complex needs, amplification needs to be reflected in more creative methods and needs for expression.

According to Cutliffe and Goward (2000), the centrality of communication is the essential component of mental health orientated models and theories. While one agrees that this perspective should resonate across other nursing specialties, it becomes one of many components in most other models and theories. As explored earlier, nursing models draw on a variety of theories and concepts, and include systems, developmental and interactionist theories. These theories can interrelate concepts in such a way as to create a different emphasis and perspective, or an alternative focus for the nurse practitioner to pursue to explore a variety of health care priorities and phenomenon.

As an example, a nurse working in an acute learning disability or mental health setting with a person who has anxiety related needs, may consider an attraction towards a developmental or interactionist perspective. In this case the nurse would focus on role relationship theory, and a growth potential focus with the person when embarking on and developing a person-centred assessment and care plan.

A systems approach may be appropriate to pursue with a person in a mental health setting who is admitted in a state of acute psychosis whereby his/her interrelated physiological, psychological and sociocultural systems are in a process of shutdown. The nurse here would assess the person's total system so that they can work with the person towards achieving homeostasis. As the person progresses along the independence continuum, a more growth promoting or interactionist perspective could then be adopted. The crucial point is that the nurse has knowledge of those theories and models for practice and can access them on initial assessment and introduction to the person who presents with a diverse and complex range of health phenomena.

In learning disability practice, this diversity and differing emphasis in nursing models is also highly relevant, due to the broad spectrum of needs identified across a diverse population, and where, for example, nurses must pursue the application of multidimensional perspectives in a variety of models and theories. Cognitive appraisal and synthesis are problematic in learning disability where communication is a high variable for levels of responsiveness across the non-verbal–verbal continuum in the population of people who have a learning disability. The versatility and differing focus in models is of particular necessity therefore, in such a diverse population.

Green (1988) identified that one of the major difficulties in selecting a conceptual model applicable to learning disability nursing, is that the needs of people with learning disabilities vary considerably. Nevertheless, Green acknowledges that Roper et al's focus on nursing intervention through the person's activities of living and normal routines is highly applicable to learning disability nursing. It is relevant partly because people with a learning disability live for extended periods in established settings, where staffing fluctuates, where the goal is to ascertain consistency in care standards and approaches. People with variable cognitive capacities, who cannot communicate their personal needs, require a learning disability nurse to pursue a robust model to support their potential and aspirations for quality in living experiences. Assessments of a holistic nature and focus are critical where nurse practitioners can assist in a holistic translation into care practices. Organisations have also attempted to organise the assessment of individual needs in such a framework as the activities of living, The Subscriber Network (2006), Taggart & McConkey (2001).

Northway & Jenkins (2003) claim that nursing models act as guides for nurses to meet the needs of individuals, and cite Roper et al (1996) as a popular example where activities such as expressing sexuality, working and playing offer the opportunity to enhance a person's quality of life.

Criticisms from nurses in learning disability follow the assumption that Roper et al reflects a medical model that is not compatible with current philosophies of care. Parley (2001) found in one learning disability service that when adopting Roper et al's (1986) model, although the focus on a dependence–independence continuum of health was pursued, there still remained a problem -solving focus that was at odds with person-centred outcomes. This perspective could once again be the result of inadequate interpretation of the model – Tierney (1998) refutes this criticism on the basis that conceptualisation of problems are identified as potential as well as actual, and should therefore be fully exploited with the person.

Person-centred care

Contemporary nursing practice promotes a person-centred philosophy throughout healthcare services, and reforms such as *The NHS Plan* (DH 2000) insist that professional practice relationships endorse this perspective. In learning disability services, person-centred planning is a central tenet, and has been given its seal of approval in *Valuing People* (DH 2001) as the focus for effective person-centred action. The emphasis is to ensure that the person is central to any needs-led service developments.

As stated by Aldridge (2003, p93) what people with a learning disability want may include health and well being as part of a person-centred plan. Kitson (1999) asserts that the most important jobs and skills of the nurse are:

- To put the person in the right environment to ensure optimal quality of life and recovery
- Monitoring and observation skills
- Interpersonal skills supported by the ability to communicate, inform, educate patients, relatives and carers
- To provide a continuous uninterrupted package of care, co-ordinated across geographical and service boundaries as well as between members of the health care team and the person's own family

Such elements are fundamental to person-centred care. To organise person-centred care, Kitson (1999) proposes that the nurse needs to ask these questions:

- How can I ensure the immediate environment is conducive to optimal care?
- How stable and predictable are the person's physiological functions?
- How stable and predictable are their psychological and emotional states?
- What do they need to know and learn about their condition or situation?
- How can I ensure the person has care that is uninterrupted and co-ordinated?

These questions are fundamental for the learning disability nurse to consider and adopt in their relationships and work with people who have a learning disability in a variety of settings. The adoption of a theoretical model of nursing such as the Elements of Nursing can provide the holistic overview and contribution towards developing and maintaining a quality of care and life that Kitson (1999) proposes for sustaining person-centred care. For the Elements of Nursing or other conceptual models to be implemented appropriately, it is critical that a humanistic and person-centred approach is adopted when applying a nurse–patient relationship and when teaching the concepts of assessment and planning of care to learning disability nurses. This is not just a classroom activity, but an intervention and interactionist approach in the practice arena of care, and an integral part of nursing curriculum for practice (Barr 2006).

For implementation purposes, a humanistic solution orientation approach could be adopted as opposed to a traditional problem-solving methodology. Parley (2001) identified this when implementing the Elements of Nursing.

Solution-focused nursing is rapidly gaining popularity and, as McAllister (2007, p2) points out:

> '...is interested in exploring and developing with clients their
> strengths and abilities rather than focusing solely on their weaknesses
> and disabilities [and which] supports not only person-centred care
> but the ethos behind person-centred planning'

As nurses in learning disability, our practice depends on sound therapeutic and interpersonal relationships that centre on developing inner growth for the people we engage with, and our assessments of need to be based on promoting growth and solutions.

Musker (2007) adopts a solution-focused approach to learning disabilities, which applies the CARE framework (containment, awareness, resilience and engagement) originally developed by McAllister and Walsh (2003) for mental health care settings.

This framework could be usefully applied in David's case study (see below) where its benefits with people who present with complex health and social care needs can be acknowledged. The CARE framework is an interpersonal and therapeutic approach to person-centred collaborative work, where the Elements of Nursing is seen as the core model for assessment.

It has already been established that criticisms of the Elements of Nursing are derived from the way the model has been poorly implemented. This has been observed to be due to a lack of knowledge and education about what constitutes a person-centred relationship.

In *Learning to use the Process of Nursing*, Roper et al (1981) suggest a series of questions the nurse can adopt for eliciting information about the activities of living from people as part of the assessment process.

The use of questions alone does not allow for an in-depth understanding or for a therapeutic or communication encounter to be pursued within a nurse–patient relationship. What is required from the nurse is an approach which acknowledges and internalises both a process and skills engagement as part of an interactional framework.

The CARE framework outlines approaches that nurse practitioners can internalise through educational exposure, and adopt to respond not only to the client's needs, but also to their own emergent needs as humans engaged in a person-centred relationship. The nurse remains therapeutic and can continue to care.

Clark and Gates (2006) adopt the Elements of Nursing when applying the model to people with profound intellectual disabilities and complex needs, and suggest that:

> '...the model be put into practice using the nursing process, and that
> the emphasis is on the person and nurse working together towards the
> goals' (Clark & Gates 2006, p.285)

However, no engagement process is offered to suggest how this framework and relationship between nurse and patient may be therapeutically pursued. The nursing process is a systematic approach, which allows for broad interpretation in how needs are identified and resolved.

CARE was originally developed for taking up practice in mental health care practice, and purports to offer benefits for clients, clinicians and mental health.

Box1.1 CARE framework

McAllister & Walsh (2003)

Containment
The challenge for the nurse is to:

- Promote accurate, helpful diagnosis
- Provide inner calm and relief of symptoms
- Provide a safe, secure environment
- Provide control when clients may be currently unable to provide for their own safety or be self-reliant

Containment as a word is deliberately selected as a move beyond the connotations that 'control' has in relationship to power and coercion (McAllister & Walsh 2003, p41). Containment work involves facilitation and a balance between paternalism and duty of care. People with complex needs often require a temporary dependency on the nurse, and to contain distress may involve use of medications. Limit setting – which may involve managing and controlling the behaviour of clients – promotes the client's use of self-control.

For David: Containment would be useful in his management of epilepsy, tuberous sclerosis, and inappropriate behaviours and expression of sexuality.

Awareness
The challenge for the nurse is to:

- Facilitate greater self-awareness and insight through learning and self-reflection

- Empower individuals, who become resilient and proud of who they are, and can speak up
- Bring about conscious awareness to those aspects of the person that negatively affect their ability to live a happy and healthy life

For David: Awareness relates to his personal identity, his complex health needs, and what he is capable of becoming in terms of his personal strengths and capabilities.

Resilience

Resilience describes those individuals who adapt to extraordinary circumstances.

The challenge for the nurse is to facilitate inner and external resources that help the patient/client to build their resilience and help them to:

- Adapt to – and accept – the illness or condition
- Cope well with the present and future
- Realise and enhance their inner strengths
- Make further social meaning and connections through problem solving

For David: The learning disability nurse can help David build up resilience in areas of his complex and chronic health needs, and maintain and promote what motivates him in life.

Engagement

The challenge for the nurse is to:

- Build a trusting partnership through active listening and empathising
- Convey hope and concern
- Engage with clients by being there both physically and emotionally
- Empower and support the client with practical and psychological supports
- Motivate the person to pursue the work necessary to achieve further self-understanding
- Facilitate a sense of meaning and manageability in the illness or recovery experience

For David: Engagement means attending to the broad spectrum of needs and where the nurse acts practically and therapeutically to support him.

These four elements exist together non-hierarchically and non-sequentially, and are vital when attempting to bring about therapeutic change with clients. The reader is encouraged to access the full paper by McAllister and Walsh (2003). See also Sheppard & McAllister (2003) in how the CARE framework has also been applied with a client who self-harms.

When applied to David, these elements can be seen to make a coherent therapeutic nurse interactional framework using an Elements of Nursing model for assessment. The nurse needs to be individually structured and apply sound clinical judgments and creativity in a person-centred way.

Adaptation of the Elements of Nursing

The author (Jukes 1987) adapted the Elements of Nursing model (Roper et al 1986) during an era of accelerated community integration for people with a learning disability from a hospital to a community 'ordinary living' model before the NHS Community Care Act (DH 1990).

This was an attempt by nurses in learning disability to implement the nursing process through assessment, planning, implementation and evaluation of nursing care for people with a learning disability. The early 1980s saw the development of the 1982 syllabus for nursing in learning disability with the emphasis on the nursing process. This led to the development of conceptual models of nursing specific to learning disability nursing by learning disability practitioners such as Hodges (1989), Aldridge (1987) with a seminal text published on models by Barber (1987).

It was through my practice and role as a senior nurse for continuing education where an initial stage was to conduct a survey into the educational needs of nurses, in the learning disability service (Jukes 1988a). This identified the nursing process as an educational need, combined with a second survey which identified that the Elements of Nursing was a preferred model of choice for practitioners to apply Jukes (1988b), Tierney (1998).

While working alongside nurse practitioners in the hospital and community homes in the learning disability service, we became increasingly dissatisfied with the wide range of psychological functional assessments such as Pathways to Independence (Jeffree & Cheseldine 1982) as a means to assess people's needs. In particular, we identified that such assessments could not assess 'total' personal needs. This applied when working with – and relating to – people with profound and multiple complex needs, and when relating with people with fewer complex needs. What nurses felt they required was an assessment model with the focus and potential to accommodate the broad spectrum of needs in learning disability.

The rationale for incorporating this adapted model into a chapter for this book is to celebrate the adapted model on its 20th year in adoption as a holistic model for practice. The model is still incorporated into services today and applied by learning disability nurses. It is also worth noting that the past 20 years for learning disability nurses has seen the development of contemporary models that reflect practice across seamless services, after an era of institutional social policy.

Wimpenny (2002) identified that in many cases theoretical models are put into use by a surrogate version, which is a functional version of the original theoretical model, and is invariably used as a guide, and – in this case –in a variety of environments, and which represents a framework or structure around which nurses collect data. This reflects the process and culture through which adaptation of the Elements of Nursing was conceived and developed. Wimpenny suggests that the subsequent writing that accompanies many case studies may not necessarily be congruent with the theoretical model but more of a reflection of the personal pattern of the individual nurse, built through personal experience and knowledge and represented in the way nursing is described by the individual.

The adaptation of the model came about through initial discussions with nurses about the relevance of the ALs and in particular how the five factors influencing the ALs (biological, psychological, sociocultural, environmental and politicoeconomic) directly impacted on and influenced people with a learning disability in a variety of settings.

Table 1.1 shows the Adapted model from a result of these consultations and piloting across the learning disability service.

Table 1.1 Adapted Elements of Nursing

Physical profile	Psychosocial profile
• Physical nature of self	• Psychological expression of self
• Normal health/appearance	• Communication
• Maintaining a safe environment	• Social network (family contacts, etc.)
• Elimination	• Holidays
• Vision	• Recreational activities
• Hearing	• Expression of sexuality
• Mobility	• Specific behaviour that challenges
• Dexterity	• Known likes and dislikes
• Dressing	• Choices to be offered
• Personal hygiene	• Spiritual and cultural needs
• Eating and drinking	• Social interactional skills
• Sleep pattern	• Specialised assessments and
• Menstruation	activities
• Additional information	

Occupational and educational profile		
• Occupational therapy	• School	• Housekeeping
• Social education centre	• Adult literacy/	• Personal laundry
• Employment	literacy skills	• Awareness and knowledge of money, time, days of the week

Jukes (2007)

ALs such as breathing, controlling body temperature and dying have been omitted as Roper et al (1981 p2) state:

> *'ALs need not be collected in any particular order, and in some circumstances not all ALs need to be considered'*

Nurses felt that the adapted Elements of Nursing model consists of not only the core ALs but also elaborations that embraced the life setting and lived environment in and across mainly residential 'ordinary life' settings. They further allowed nurses to make decisions about priorities, relatedness and relevance with people when applying the ALs and extended areas for assessment.

How nurses interpreted the ALs in the adapted model can be seen in the guidelines offered in the form of brief key guidance words representing the five influencing factors for each AL and additional areas for assessment. (Table 1.2).

Table 1.2 Adapted elements of nursing assessment and guidance key

PHYSICAL PROFILE:

1. PHYSICAL NATURE OF SELF: Physical Soundness or Frailty of Individual. Abnormalities due to Genetic/Inherited or Environmental causes, vital signs and normal range, Epilepsy & its frequency, Allergies Infections/Anaemia etc. Appearance of the skin, complexion

2. GENERAL HEALTH/APPEARANCE: Day to day health, whether good or prone to recurrent colds, Infections/Anaemia etc. Appearance of the skin, complexion

3. MAINTAINING A SAFE ENVIRONMENT: Physical factors to include the five senses, Dizziness, Psychological Factors — Knowledge & attitudes to safety in the home, work & play, Road Safety, Awareness of common dangers. Smoking, Alcohol, Spread of Infection, Personality & Temperament. Social Factors — Housing, Type of residential setting

4. ELIMINATION: Continent or Incontinent, what routine have they? Dietary intake — Constipation/Diarrhoea. Toilet Facilities — Habits regarding handwashing after elimination. Degree of independence relative to age/Mental health. Need for special Equipment/Aids. Urine Input/Output — Fluid balance

5. VISION: Extent of Visual Field/Wears Glasses/Eye Defects, response & sensitivity to bright lights

6. HEARING: Extent of Hearing — Screening & Testing. Response to noise levels/Sensitivity. Aids & Tolerance

7. MOBILITY: Physical Development, Mobilising habits at home/Work & Play. Range of movement. Aids needed for independence. Whether over or under active, factors limiting independence. Extent of disability, Knowledge & attitudes to exercise & physical disability

8. DEXTERITY: Gross motor skills — walking, running, swimming. Laying tables — work & play. Fine — motor skills — drawing, writing — Fine movements associated with work and play

9. DRESSING: Level of competence — what they can/cannot do. Clothing relative to age — Appropriateness. Modification to dress due to disability, Care of clothes. Suitability of footwear, preference — Time needed to dress & undress. Mobility problems

10. PERSONAL HYGIENE: Bathing/Shower/Frequency. Appearance of skin, hands & nails, hair, mouth & teeth, teeth. Pattern of self — care, dependency. Standard of cleanliness relative to clothing and dress. Handwashing routine/oral hygiene etc.

11. EATING & DRINKING: Proficiency in taking food & drink, religious restrictions, state of mouth & teeth, height & weight, emotions, dietary likes & dislikes. Timing & location of meals. Aids needed for independence, Appetite. Ability to shop. Food hygiene

12. SLEEP PATTERN: Sleeping Environment — size of room, own or shared. Usual sleeping behaviour — pattern i.e. going to bed & going to sleep — rising. Good or bad sleeper — mood on rising, Factors interfering with sleep i.e. mood/boredom — effects of medication — epilepsy

OCCUPATIONAL THERAPY
Attendance at Dept. — Access to an O.T. Involvement & types of activities available

SOCIAL EDUCATION CENTRE
Attendance times, name of Instructor, type of work & programme

EMPLOYMENT
Potential/Actual Interests

SCHOOL
Name of School/Teacher — Level of Education & Scope of achievement/development

ADULT LITERACY/LITERARY SKILLS
Attendance/Teacher — Skills being taught — Times & Location etc.

PSYCHO/SOCIO PROFILE:

13. MENSTRUATION: Whether regular cycle or irregular/Self — care, pre — menstrual tension — affects on behaviour. Knowledge & awareness

14. ADDITIONAL INFORMATION:

15. PSYCHOLOGICAL EXPRESSION: Within familiar environment, unfamiliar environment. Happy/Sad/Indifferent general mood, content. Is aggression (normal, absent or excess). Factors interfering with general behaviour i.e. anxiety/frustration/boredom etc.

16. COMMUNICATION: Physical factors, method & stage of development — speaking, seeing, hearing, reading & writing. Psychological factors — Intelligence, extent of vocabulary, accent, dialect, eye contact, gesticulation. Sign language — makaton — bliss symbolics etc. Environmental factors e.g. Type/size of room, personal space factors, individual habit, noise, congruence of body & verbal language. Orientation time of day, day of week etc.

17. SOCIAL NETWORK: (Family contacts etc.) Relationships with family member & relatives + friends. Frequency of contact with the family, neighbourhood and other support groups e.g. The Church/Societies & Clubs etc.

18. HOLIDAYS: Frequency of Holidays — Location & means of travel. Type of vacation which suits & satisfies need. Partners on excursions

19. RECREATIONAL ACTIVITIES: Types of pursuits — General interests, opportunity for recreation & frequency

20. EXPRESSION OF SEXUALITY: With behaviour, appearance & communication. Relationships/Preference/Sexual relationships/Sexual function/Dysfunction. Effects of being in ordinary life setting

21. SPECIFIC BEHAVIOUR DISORDER: Self — mutilation — Head banging/Smashes windows/Aggression to others, biting, grabbing, etc.

22. KNOWN LIKES	KNOWN DISLIKES
	Food, Work & play, Hobbies, People, Staff, etc.

22a. CHOICES TO BE OFFERED

23. SPIRITUAL/CULTURAL NEEDS: Identification of Religious commendations & beliefs/wishes. Restrictions due to culturally determined behaviour

24. SOCIAL INTERACTIONAL SKILLS: Verbal & non — verbal behaviour relative to situations/people/objects etc. Withdrawn/Domineering/Irritable. Appropriate — inappropriate actions etc.

25. SPECIALISED ASSESSMENTS/ACTIVITIES: Use of PA.C./Star/Bereweeke/Goal planning etc.

OCCUPATIONAL & EDUCATIONAL PROFILE:
Housekeeping & personal laundry skills/Domestic skills. Routine within home e.g. Cleaning/Dusting/Polishing.

Washing own clothes & linen. Kitchen work e.g. Washing up/Drying. Ironing & putting clothes away. Laying of tables/Making beds etc.

Awareness/Knowledge of money, time, days of week etc. Use of money/Orientation relative to time, days of the week. Understanding of shopping with money — Budgeting/Pocket money etc.

Health facilitation

In a post *Valuing People* (DH 2001) era, a situation exists where a proliferation of checklist assessments are being designed to identify health needs in a health facilitation framework at both strategic and individual level.

Health facilitation is a strategy that aims to improve access to primary care and also involves individual casework by practitioners to help people access mainstream services.

The Learning Disability Network *(www.ldhealthnetwork.org.uk)* regularly has calls for further information about health check tools and health action plans. Matthews (2003) developed the 'OK' Health Checklist for guidance on how the role and functions of the health facilitator could develop. The checklist is now established as a widely used health assessment tool.

Nevertheless, nurses in learning disability need to be cautious in how they perceive and apply health facilitation in terms of whether it is an attempt to redeem a professional identity within primary health care. Health facilitation is also in danger of being perceived as purely a biomedical health check activity without significant evidence in how it is being strategically employed by learning disability nurses.

Adoption of conceptual models that require consistent evaluation into their application with people have the additional value of pursuing person-centredness and working in partnership to achieve goals that are holistic.

Health facilitation is in danger of being perceived as purely health checks as a means to an end, but instead perhaps rather seen as an opportunity to develop a conceptual framework that reflects the holistic nature of the individual self – for the nurse's unique practice.

This chapter pursues how the Elements of Nursing can be developed and adapted to provide a conceptual approach to being person-centred. It shows one such approach in defining and contributing towards what constitutes a holistic contemporary learning disability assessment for nursing practice.

As the multidisciplinary and agency nature of health care is increasingly emphasised, it is important that the nursing profession has a clear sense of what constitutes its own discipline (Tierney 1998).

Adoption of models in nursing development units (NDUs) has highlighted how they were intended to clarify thinking, create shared understanding, focus on patients and allow nurses to identify more clearly their contribution to care (Pearson 1992).

From a contemporary perspective and within an era of health facilitation, health care gains and health action planning (DH 2002) a conceptual model such as the adapted Elements of Nursing model becomes a relevant framework to apply.

Health facilitation and the development of health action plans at an individual practice level for people and learning disability nurses becomes a holistic focus.

Although there are examples of health assessments (Matthews 1996), there can be an additional focus upon GP templates and health screening checks that have a biomedical interest. As a result, these approaches may not lead to a greater

Box 1.2 Health action planning: assessments to consider

- Health issues of particular relevance to that person and perceived as important to them from their own perspective, for example mental health, behaviour, psychological issues
- Actions that reflect more vulnerable health because the person:
  –Has a current illness
  –Has epilepsy
  –Has a particular syndrome with health consequences
  –Has issues relating to self-abuse-drugs, alcohol, tobacco, solvents
  –Has issues relating to their sexuality (being lesbian, gay, bisexual, heterosexual) and/or their sexual health
  –Has profound and multiple impairments
  –Is from a minority ethnic group
  –Is an older person
  –Has a sensory impairment
  –Has issues relating to physical and sexual abuse
- Health issues, applicable to this person, that are the focus of National or Local Health initiatives (For example National Service Frameworks)
- Health issues identified as particularly relevant to people with learning disabilities, including:
  –Oral health and dental care
  –Fitness and mobility
  –Continence
  –Vision
  –Hearing
  –Nutrition
  –Emotional needs
  –Medication taken and side effects
  –Records of any screening tests

Case study: David

David is a young man of 16 years and at a point of transition in education, healthcare and potentially some future form of supported living. He lives at home during the week while he attends school. However, the increased frequency in attending a respite service at weekends and holiday times is due to David's erratic behaviour, coupled with his parents' frustration and progressive inability to manage at home. David has additional health care needs in the form of tuberous sclerosis (see Box 1.3) and epilepsy.

The Assessment in Table 1.3 has been completed in partnership with David, his parents, school and respite care staff.

Table 1.4 consists of the person-centred care plan in partnership with David, his parents school and respite care staff.

Box 1.3 Tuberous sclerosis

The diagnostic and prognostic factors and symptomatology for tuberous sclerosis that nurses, professionals, carers and family need to acknowledge for appropriate quality person-centred care approaches.

Background

Tuberous sclerosis is a genetic disorder affecting cellular differentiation and proliferation, which results in hamartoma formation in many organs, including skin, brain, eyes, kidneys and heart.

Von Recklinghausen first described tuberous sclerosis in 1862. Bourneville coined the term sclerose tubereuse from which the name has evolved. Sherlock coined the term epiloia, encompassing the clinical triad of epilepsy, learning disabilities and adenoma sebaceum.

Frequency

International frequency is 1 in 5,000–30,000.

Diagnosis

- White skin patches (82% by 5 years)
- Facial fibroangiomatous rash (50% by 5 years)
- Skin fibromatous plaques (shagreen patches)
- Whitish retinal phacomata
- Intracranial calcification
- Evidence of complications
- Most children are diagnosed between 2–6 years

Prognosis

- Epilepsy 80–90%
- Learning disabilities 60–70%
- Variable lifespan that depends on the severity of the learning disability
- Severely affected infants are thought to die before age 10 years and 75% die before age 25 years
- The prognosis for the individual diagnosed late in life with few cutaneous signs depends on the associated internal tumours

(Nambi 2006 www.emedicine.com/derm/topic438.htm)

understanding of a broader or more holistic conceptualisation of what health represents as they impact upon a person's everyday living experiences.

Action For Health (DH 2002) issues guidance on how to develop health action planning and states in particular what assessments should consider, see Box 1.2 David's case study contains a variety of elements identified in Box 1.2 that reflect dimensions of health vulnerability for David, who is at a point of transition.

Table 1.3 David's person-centred assessment

PHYSICAL PROFILE

1. PHYSICAL NATURE OF SELF

David is of sturdy build for his 16 years. He has Tuberous Sclerosis which is developing rapidly, i.e. appearance of butterfly rash, adenoma sebaceum and epilepsy which is becoming more frequent. Anticonvulsant therapy is sodium valproate 600mgs tds., phenytoin sodium 50mgs tds and phenobarbitone 30 mgs b.d. Review of medication is at present six monthly

2. NORMAL HEALTH/APPEARANCE

David's daily health is usually good. However, his appearance and health varies of late, sometimes he is alert and aloof, and some days he is very lethargic and incoherent. His complexion is pale, and his hair becomes quite greasy and also has dandruff. His personal appearance regarding clothing depends on his mothers supply and choice

3. MAINTAINING A SAFE ENVIRONMENT

David is aware of and uses his five senses. He wears a "fit" helmet due to his epilepsy, and has been justified on some occasions. He is aware of all common dangers and is aware of safety factors when crossing the road. His main drawback is that he will tend to be impulsive when over excited and therefore ignore danger signals. He can be overly rough with other smaller children

4. ELIMINATION

Is fully continent (except when having a seizure). David uses the toilet on rising and usually after meals or when he has drank a lot. However, when urinating he will be messy i.e. over the seat and floor. He at times becomes constipated. Takes charcoal biscuits for flatulence He will sometimes wash his hands afterwards, but needs verbal prompting

5. VISION

David has previously been known to stumble and not see objects in front of him or at the side. He has now got spectacles, but needs prompts to wear them. Extent of visual field uncertain?

6. HEARING

Will sometimes not hear what is said to him as if elsewhere in thought. He will also carry out an action totally oblivious to anyone around him. Extent of hearing uncertain?

7. MOBILITY

Is physically mature for his age, and when he is alert and at his best he is very active. He enjoys physical exercise like walking and kicking a ball around. At school he recently went for a weeks holiday and enjoyed swimming and walking. At home and at the respite care unit he enjoys dancing to cd:uk & MTV on Sky. When not at his best he is content to sit quiet, look at magazines, watch t.v. and jigsaws

8. DEXTERITY

Gross motor skills are good-although again is dependent on David's health. Fine motor skills are also dependent on his health. He can paint, draw, some writing skills, but at times his movements can be clumsy and jerky

9. DRESSING (MOTOR SKILLS)

Clothing is supplied by his mother in which David has a choice and selection (is age-appropriate). Mother also cleans/irons clothing at home. Can manage all his clothing, but has difficulty with his buttons and can't yet tie shoe laces. He needs plenty of time to dress in the morning, and can easily be distracted-appears to have no concept of time, especially in the morning

10. PERSONAL HYGIENE

Although David dislikes having a wash in the morning he enjoys having a bath which he has nightly. (His use of shampoo can be excessive though). Finger and toe nails need careful manicure. He can brush his own teeth. He sometimes will put on clothing which is dirty and in the laundry basket

11. EATING AND DRINKING

David has a good appetite and will often have second helpings (nb. weight). His table etiquette is eratic. Seems to like all food, teeth and gums tend to bleed (nb. side effects of phenytoin). Has his meals with other children and sits at the table with Andrew and Susan. Enjoys having an evening snack at 7pm with care staff in the kitchen

12. SLEEP PATTERN

David will stay up as long as the t.v. is on and sometimes needs prompting especially if it is during weekdays. However, he will ask to go to bed around 8:30 if not already prompted. Needs to be given a call at 7am to allow him enough time to get ready. If he has a seizure during the night it will influence greatly his sleep pattern. Sometimes his seizures have necessitated a late arrival to school

13. MENSTRUATION   N/A

14. ADDITIONAL INFORMATION

Table 1.3 continued

PSYCHO/SOCIO PROFILE

15. PSYCHOLOGICAL EXPRESSION David is generally a happy child, but will have period of quietness and tiredness coupled with incongruous behaviour relative to his periods of epileptic activity. He is always willing to please and be involved in wanting to do things. He enjoys involvement with others communicating/talking/having a joke	20. EXPRESSION OF SEXUALITY David will play with himself, and occasionally will indiscriminately display his genitals. Has been on occasion found to be interfering with younger girls on the pretence of taking them to the toilet. He represents his male sexuality by dressing quite sporty and models his style of dress on how David Beckham looks in his sports gear
16. COMMUNICATION David can articulate well in a broad Midlands accent. He will gesticulate using his arms and hands to describe what he means. He has a good memory for names and enjoys repeating them to the named person. He tends to invade a person's personal space talking as if he wants to kiss you. He will attempt to kiss both female and male staff. At times his speech is slurred — indicative of possible epileptic activity. David will also shout loudly and generally act 'silly' which will potentially progressively lead to out-of-hand behaviour	21. SPECIFIC BEHAVIOUR WHICH CHALLENGES An excess use of physical aggression towards the smaller children. Has been known to pick up a smaller child and just drop them. His strong and loud verbal abuse can also become quite distressing to both staff and children and offensive in nature
17. SOCIAL NETWORKING When in the respite unit David knows the majority of children and his special friends are Andrew and Susan. He also has a friend at another unit called John who he will enjoy playing with when they meet up. His family parental bond is quite strong, and his parents take an active interest in his development and care plan when David is in the unit for prolonged periods	22. LIKES (KNOWN) DISLIKES (KNOWN) Sweets, crisps, c.d.'s, music, 'disco' & dancing, picture pop-up books. Washing, getting out of bed Talking and wearing sports clothes. Football, Manchester United and Real Madrid David Beckham 22a. CHOICES YET TO BE OFFERED
18. HOLIDAYS Previous holidays have been with his parents, but is reliant upon the school and the unit for future support in this area as his parents find him demanding not only because of his epilepsy but of his increasing challenging behaviour	23. SPIRITUAL/CULTURAL NEEDS Enjoys going to church with his parents and singing in particular, but appears to be indiscriminate to denomination. Has an innate quality of due regard for people most of the time. Enjoys being with people
19. RECREATIONAL ACTIVITIES David enjoys walking, running, playing cd's, looking through magazines and picture pop-up books, playing with toy cars and rides out in the car or MPV. Kicking a football, and watching football	24. SOCIAL INTERACTIONAL SKILLS David's verbal and non-verbal behaviour can at times be completely appropriate. However, he can be quite demonstrative and impulsive totally giving up all social graces. This in turn can lead to frustration and aggression to people and objects 25. SPECIALISED ASSESSMENTS/ACTIVITIES

OCCUPATIONAL & EDUCATIONAL PROFILE

Occupational Therapy N/A Social Education Centre N/A Employment N/A	School Attends _____ School and is progressing well according to his teacher Adult Literacy/Literary Skills N/A	House Keeping and Personal Laundry Will attempt to make his bed in a fashion Will collect what he believes to be dirty clothing, but some would be perfectly clean Will collect any dirty plates when dining room is clear, and will wipe down the tables. Will help to collect clean linen Awareness/Knowledge of Money, Time, Days of Week Is aware of the days and months but is learning both numerical and literary skills at school

Signature   Date

Table 1.4 Person-centred care plan for David

NAME: David Wright **PERSON-CENTRED CARE PLAN** Thanks to: Catherine Doherty (Specialist Epilepsy Nurse Practitioner) with South Birmingham Primary Care Trust for her assistance with the development and advise on the Care Plan

INDIVIDUAL NEED	OBJECTIVES	HOW CAN THIS BE MET?	KEY INDIVIDUALS	EVIDENCE TO KNOW IF THIS WORKS
To enhance David's quality of life & health status through Health Action Planning	To actively promote David in developing his individual life-plan — utilising tools to improve and encourage health gain	1. Offer David the opportunity of a Health Action Plan. A key stage in life as he is in Transition 2. Offer David a hand-held Health Action Plan for personal use to be accessed by the multi-disciplinary team, and those involved in his care/life	All involved in David's life	David possesses a hand-held Health Action Plan. Multi-disciplinary team to utilise Health Action Plan and identify that care is consistent
To provide David with appropriate professional support through Transition	To ensure David has all his needs assessed, and tasks allocated accordingly to meet his needs as he moves from childrens' towards adolescent/adult services	1. Allocation of a Community learning disability nurse from either transition or adult team 2. Need for a referral and allocation of a Social Worker	Parents, Community learning disability nurse, Social Worker, Educational staff & Medical Practitioners	Community learning disability nurse allocated with appropriate referral agencies notified Dates set for meetings
VISION — NEED to wear spectacles	Improve vision —? reduce need to wear spectacles as David does not always wear them	CT/MRI Scan of brain to ascertain if tubers developing & affecting visual field	Medical staff	Results of MRI Scan could be a candidate for surgery to remove tubers & improve visual field
Hearing	To ascertain the problems relating to David's hearing	1. Is it a hearing deficit or is it seizure related. Review epileptic activity 2. Check for ear wax 3. Auditory test	Parents Care staff Medical staff Practice nurse	Hearing loss could be seizure related — seizures more effectively managed Physical problem dealt with & hearing, concentration improved
Promote healthy lifestyle	Lose weight	Encourage physical activities which David enjoys. Swimming, walking, dancing. Need to undertake a personal safety plan relating to epilepsy & activities	School staff, Respite care staff, Parents, David	Reduction in weight David has a personal healthier outlook
	Healthy eating	Encourage David to become involved in cooking, shopping for food. Active discussion on healthy options of food	School staff, Respite care staff, Parents, David	David involves himself in meal planning, shopping, cooking & eating healthier foods
To alleviate Constipation	Constipation to be eradicated from David's life	Physical exercise Encourage healthy option foods Encourage increase in fluids Engage David in selecting & preparing healthy meals	David, School staff, Respite care staff, parents	David is less constipated, Non-reliant upon medication to 'open' bowels
David to have greater independence	For David to develop self-help skills in all areas of his life Focuses upon the advantages of being able to accomplish tasks	Encourage positive attitude towards self-help skills i.e. — washing, bathing, toileting, oral hygiene, dressing & undressing, personal laundry skills	David, School staff, Respite care staff, parents	Establishment of a relationship with David where a partnership in teaching new skills increases David's ability to integrate
College/Day Care placement upon leaving school	To review and make arrangements for appropriate placement post school	Assess David's needs Establish from David what he would like to do upon leaving school Discuss with David & his parents; To Review possibilities, college, employment & alternative options	School staff, David, Parents, Community Nurse, Social Worker, Employment & Co-Operative Agencies	Establish services which David may wish to access Secure name on waiting list if required & secure funding
Appropriate Short break post 18 years of age	To identify an appropriate short break service to support David	Assess David's needs holistically. Establish short break services & requirements, example day/overnight & weekend. David to visit potential services. Ensure service can support David's needs	David, Community Nurse & Social Worker	Establish appropriate service that will meet David's needs Secure funding Place name on waiting list Audit & review of service identified. CSCI Report
Physical & Verbal aggression	To modify inappropriate behaviour	Engage with David on a 1:1 session. Assess behaviour is not related to seizures pre/post ictal state. Engage in humanistic person — centred & behavioural strategies to assist in reducing negative behaviour. If necessary refer to Psychology Development of positive approaches in education to reduce negative behaviour Proactive strategies for all to follow	David, Parents, School staff, Community nurse, Respite care staff, psychology, Medical	Refer to Medical staff if a correlation between seizure activity & behaviour is identified David's behaviour both physical & verbal will be more positive

Table 1.4 continued

INDIVIDUAL NEED	OBJECTIVES	HOW CAN THIS BE MET?	KEY INDIVIDUALS	EVIDENCE TO KNOW IF THIS WORKS
Appropriate displays of sexuality	For David to understand how to show affection in an appropriate manner, including sexual activity	Engage David in Personal Relationships education which includes expression of sexuality. Ascertain that behaviour is not related to post — ictal behaviour. Assess seizure activity in relation to behaviour	David, Community learning disability nurse, Health promotion specialists & Sexuality therapists	Review with medical staff if correlation is identified
Issues with Speech	To improve David's Speech	Ascertain link between seizure activity and loss/poor speech. Review anti-epileptic medication. Could contribute to slurred speech. Slurring could indicate (pre-seizure activity). Reduce seizure activity by administering prophylactic medication	Community Nurse, Care staff, Parents, Medical Staff	Speech could be improved
Epilepsy — Increase in Seizure Activity	Reduce seizure frequency & possibly the severity of seizures. All of which could have pre & post ictal effects on David's life	Undertake the following tests as deemed appropriate — EEG/Ambulatory EEG — MRI Scan — CT Scan	Medical Staff	EEG Results could record pre & post ictal activity & could be linked to David's behaviour patterns. Scans could advise of an increase mass of tubers on the brain — giving rise to increase in seizure activity
	To record seizure activity — to ascertain triggers to seizures	Record seizure activity utilising a seizure diary, including time awake/asleep, type of seizure & activity being undertaken	School staff, Parents & Care staff	Surgery may be considered Records of seizure activity Information recorded could hold the key to seizure activity which could lead to significant lifestyle changes
Epilepsy — Reduction in seizures to improve quality of life	Improve dexterity skills, gross & fine motor movements	Changes to lifestyle dependent on outcome of seizure recordings Triggers may be established, changes to medication & times in which medication is administered	School staff, Respite care staff, Parents, Medical staff	Improved gross & fine motor skills Ability to physically function better
Epilepsy medication	Review medication — as older drugs. Discontinue older aed	Review all medication; discontinue Phenytoin; discontinue Phenobarbitone Review more frequently process will take several months	G.P./Epileptogist or Neurologist, Parents, Care staff	Reduce medication slowly 1 aed at a time. May invoke increase in seizures if sudden introduction newer aed e.g. Lamotrigene or Keppra Vigabatrin effective for seizures in T.S. pts. (Hopkins et al, 1995), but not advised due to visual field defects
	Reduce side effects linked to aed e.g. weight gain	Discontinue Sodium Valproate. Introduce a newer aed if weight is a problem	As above	Reduction in body weight. Reduction in food intake
	Reduce side effects linked to aed e.g. bleeding of gums, mental slowing sedation	Discontinue Phenytoin, introduce a newer aed A slow process over several months	As above	Reduction in bleeding of gums. Reduction in gum hypertrophy, alertness, greater levels of concentration
	Reduce side effects linked to aed e.g. mental slowness, hyperactivity Discontinue the need for blood level monitoring	Discontinue Introduce newer aed; will be a slow process over several months Discontinue older aed's and introduce newer aed's that do not require regular serum level monitoring	As above	Reduction in hyperactivity episodes Should be more alert, ability to concentrate better Reduction in AED's until discontinued. Reduces likelihood of toxicity
	Reduce seizure frequency & severity	Introduce newer aed's. Consider Vagal Nerve Stimulator (VNS) Therapy	Medical staff	Research (Parais et al 2001) has indicated good prognosis of VNS therapy in this population

DISCUSSED AND AGREED WITH INDIVIDUAL/ADVOCATE	Y	N	SIGNATURE	DATE
DISCUSSED AND AGREED WITH RELATIVES/CARERS	Y	N	SIGNATURE	DATE

SIGNATURE   DESIGNATION   DATE

Conclusion

This chapter has embraced one of the most popular and yet misunderstood and often disregarded models of nursing in the family of nursing in the UK. The inclusion of the Elements of Nursing in its original and adapted conceptualisation in the field of learning disability nursing practice has been pursued, and as Tierney (1998) has observed in practice, the model appears to be extant and not extinct.

From an academic and professional learning disability practice dimension, there is little doubt that this model has a great deal to offer, and as the academic and practice literature evidenced, it has been applied across a number of specialist fields, albeit with various and ambiguous interpretations as to its application, and in some cases, overly simplistic and naïve interpretations and applications from nurses themselves.

In the introduction to this chapter, person-centred planning was identified in its aims to consider the:

> *'Aspirations and capacities expressed by the service user or those speaking on their behalf, rather than needs and deficiencies'*

> (Mansell & Beadle-Brown 2004, p1)

For people with complex needs, the aim for learning disability nurses is to ensure a partnership where a holistic assessment and comprehensive person-centred care plan reflects individual felt and expressed needs. When achieved as accurately as possible, this process enables and promotes high quality engagement and supporting for the person – particularly with complex health needs – to maximise their independence. Advantages of adopting a nursing model for practice have been discussed. These include:

- Assisting nurses to be more coherent and organised with regard to their thinking about nursing (Clark 1982)
- Giving direction to quality practice (Pearson & Vaughan 1986)
- Enhancing autonomy and promoting empowerment for nursing (Ingram 1991), while simultaneously promoting empowerment in the person themselves

Shaping the Future: A Vision for Learning Disability Nursing (United Kingdom Learning Disability Consultant Nurse Network (UKLDCNN) 2006) identifies and quotes that a view of disability that argues that:

> *'People with impairments are disabled by a range of physical, social, economic, psychological and attitudinal barriers that prevent or limit their full participation in Society'* (Prime Minister's Strategy Unit 2005)

These barriers may be identified through the adoption of a conceptual model such as with the Elements of Nursing on an individual practice relationship level. As *Shaping the Future* goes on to state:

> *'The primary focus of nursing interventions in the social model of disability is therefore on reducing or eliminating barriers to good health and thereby increasing social inclusion'*

and – as Kitson (1999) postulates – provide what can be described as the Essence of Nursing.

References

Aldridge J (1987) Initiating the use of a nursing model: The importance of systematic care planning – a ward clinician's perspective. In: Barber P (ed): *Using Nursing Models Series. Mental Handicap. Facilitating Holistic Care.* Sevenoaks, Hodder & Stoughton, Chapter 3, pp 25–47

Aldridge J (2003) The Ecology of Health Model. In: Jukes M, Bollard M (eds) *Contemporary Learning Disability Practice.* Salisbury, Quay Books, Chapter 8, pp93–123

Barber P (1987) *Using Nursing Models Series. Mental Handicap, Facilitating Holistic Care.* Sevenoaks, Hodder & Stoughton

Barker P (2004) *Assessment in Psychiatric and Mental Health Nursing – In Search of the Whole Person* (2nd edn). Cheltenham, Nelson Thornes

Barr O (2006) The evolving role of community nurses for people with learning disabilities: changes over an 11-year period. *Journal of Clinical Nursing* **15**, 1, 72–82

Beech I (2002) Book review on Forster S (ed) (2001) *The Role of the Mental Health Nurse Journal of Psychiatric and Mental Health Nursing* **9**, 119–125

Department of Health (1990) *The NHS and Community Care Act.* London, HMSO

Department of Health (2000) *The NHS Plan.* London, The Stationery Office

Department of Health (2001) *Valuing People: A New Strategy for Learning Disability for the 21st Century.* London, The Stationery Office

Department of Health (2002) *Action for Health – Health Action Plans and Health Facilitation. Detailed Good Practice Guidance on Implementation for Learning Disability Partnership Boards.* London, The Stationery Office

Chamberlain P (1986) The STEP skill teaching system: staff training to meet the needs of people in residential units. *Mental Handicap* **14**, June, 80–82

Cutliffe JR, Goward P (2000) Mental Health Nurses and Qualitative Research Methods: A Mutual Attraction? *Journal of Advanced Nursing* **31**, 3, 590–598

Elliot-Cannon C (1990) Mental handicap and nursing models. In: Salvage J, Kershaw B (eds) *Models for Nursing 2.* Harrow, Scutari Press, Chapter 9, pp77–88

English National Board and Welsh National Board (1988) *Syllabus of Training. Professional Register–Part 5 Registered Nurse for the Mentally Handicapped 1982* Didcot, Bocardo Press

Clark J (1982) A model for health visiting. In: Newton C (ed) The Roper-Logan-Tierney model in action. London, Macmillan.

Clarke J, Gates B (2006) Care planning and delivery for people with profound intellectual disabilities and complex needs. In: Gates B (ed) *Care Planning and Delivery in Intellectual Disability Nursing.* Oxford, Blackwell Publishing, Chapter 13, pp277–301

Green C (1988) The Development of a Conceptual Framework for Mental Handicap Nursing Practice in the UK. *Nurse Education Today* **8**, 9–17

Henderson V (1969) *The Basic Principles of Nursing Care.* Geneva, ICN

Hodges B (1989) The Health Career Model. In: Hinchcliffe SM (ed) *Nursing Practice and Health Care* (1st edn only). London, Edward Arnold

Holland AJ (2000) Ageing and Learning Disability. *British Journal of Psychiatry* **176**, 26–31

Ingram I (1991) Why does nursing need theory? *Journal of Advanced Nursing* **16**, 350–353

Jeffree D, Cheseldine S (1982) *Pathways to Independence. Checklists of self-help and social skills.* Sevenoaks, Hodder & Stoughton

Jukes M (1987) Assessing the whole person. *Senior Nurse* **6**, 3, 14–16

Jukes M (1988a) Breaking the mould. *Senior Nurse* **7**, 4, 45–46

Jukes M (1988b) Model of nursing or psychological assessment. *Senior Nurse* **8**, 11, 8–10

Kitson A (1999) The Essence of Nursing. *Nursing Standard* **13**, 23, 42–46

Mansell J, Beadle-Brown J (2004) Person-centred planning or person-centred action? Policy and practice in intellectual disability services. *Journal of Applied Research in Intellectual Disabilities* **17**, 1–9

Marriner Tomey A, Alligood MR (1998) *Nurse Theorists and their Work* (4th edn) St Louis, Mosby

Matthews D (1996) *The 'OK' Health Check for assessing and planning the health care needs of people with learning disabilities.* Preston, Fairfield Publications

Matthews D (2003) Action for Health. *Learning Disability Practice* **6**, 5, 16–19

McAllister M (2007) *Solution-focused Nursing: Rethinking Practice.* Basingstoke, Palgrave Macmillan

McAllister M, Walsh K (2003) CARE: A Framework for Mental Health Practice. *Journal of Psychiatric and Mental Health Nursing* **10**, 39–48

McCann E (2003) Exploring sexual and relationship possibilities for people with psychosis – a review of the literature. *Journal of Psychiatric and Mental Health Nursing* **10**, 640–649

McNally S (2006) Person-centred planning. In: Gates B (ed) *Care Planning and Delivery in Intellectual Disability Nursing.* Oxford, Blackwell Publishing. Chapter 4, pp68–84

Minshull J, Rose K, Turner J (1986) The Human Needs Model of nursing. *Journal of Advanced Nursing* **11**, 643–649

Moss S, Turner S (1995) *The Health of People with Learning Disability.* Manchester, Hester Adrian Research Centre

Murphy K, Cooney A, Casey D, Connor M, O'Connor J, Dineen B (2000) The Roper, Logan & Tierney (1996) Model: perceptions and operationalisation of the model in psychiatric nursing in a health board in Ireland. *Journal of Advanced Nursing* **31**, 6, 1333–1341

Musker M (2007) Learning disabilities and solution-focused nursing. In: McAllister M (ed) *Solution-Focused Nursing – Rethinking Practice.* Basingstoke, Palgrave Macmillan

National Patient Safety Agency (NPSA) (2004) *Safeguarding people with learning disabilities in the NHS: An Agenda for the National Patient Safety Agency.* London, NPSA

Neuman B, Fawcett J (2002) *The Neuman System Model* (4th edn). Upper Saddle River, New Jersey, Prentice Hall

Newton C (1992) The Roper–Logan–Tierney Model in Action. Basingstoke, Macmillan

Northway R, Jenkins R (2003) Quality of life as a concept for developing learning disability nursing practice? *Journal of Clinical Nursing* **12**, 57–66

Orem D (1980) *Nursing: Concepts of Practice* (2nd edn). New York, McGraw Hill

Orlando ID (1961) *The Dynamic Nurse–Patient Relationship: Function, Process and Principles of Professional Nursing Practice.* New York, GP Putnam's Sons

Parker D (1997) Nursing art and science: literature and debate. In: Marks-Moran D, Rose P (eds) *Reconstructing Nursing: Beyond Art and Science.* London, Baillière Tindall, pp3–24

Parley FF (2001) Person-centred outcomes: are outcomes improved where a person-centred care model is used? *Journal of Learning Disabilities* **5**, 4, 299–308

Pearson A (1992) *Nursing at Burford: A Story of Change.* Harrow, Scutari Press

Pearson A, Vaughan B, Fitzgerald M (1986) *Nursing Models for Practice* (2nd edn). Oxford, Butterworth–Heinemann

Peplau HE (1952) *Interpersonal Relations in Nursing.* New York, GP Putnam's Sons (English edn). Reissued as a Paperback in 1988 by Macmillan Education Ltd, London)

Prime Minister's Strategy Unit (2005) *Improving the Life Chances of Disabled People.* London, The Stationery Office

Reed J, Robbins I (1991) Models of nursing: their relevance to the care of elderly people. *Journal of Advanced Nursing* **16**, 1350–1357

Reilly D (1975) Why a Conceptual Framework? *Nursing Outlook* 23, 566–569

Roper N (1979) Nursing based on a model of living. In: College M, Jones D (eds) *Readings in Nursing.* Edinburgh, Churchill Livingstone

Roper N, Logan W, Tierney A (1981) *Learning to Use the Process of Nursing.* Edinburgh, Churchill Livingstone

Roper N, Logan W, Tierney A (1986) Nursing models: a process of construction and refinement. In: Salvage J, Kershaw B (eds) *Models for Nursing.* Chichester, John Wiley, pp25–38

Roper N, Logan W, Tierney A (1990) *The Elements of Nursing: A Model for Nursing based on a Model for Living* (3rd edn). Edinburgh, Churchill Livingstone

Roper N, Logan W, Tierney A (1996) *The Elements of Nursing: A Model for Nursing based on a Model for Living* (4th edn). Edinburgh, Churchill Livingstone.

Roy C (1976) An Introduction to Nursing: An Adaptation Model. Cited by Galbreath JG (1990) Sister Callister Roy. In: George JB (ed) (1990) *Nursing Theories: The Base for Professional Nursing Practice. New Jersey,* Prentice Hall

Roy C (1980) The Roy Adaptation Model. In: Riehl JP, Roy C (eds) *Conceptual Models for Nursing Practice* (2nd edn). New York, Appleton–Century–Crofts, pp179–188

Sanderson H, Jones E Brown K (2002) Active support and person-centred planning: strange bedfellows or ideal partners? *Tizard Learning Disability Review* 7, 1, 31–38

Sheppard C, McAllister M (2003) CARE: a framework for responding therapeutically to the client who self-harms. *Journal of Psychiatric and Mental Health Nursing* **10**, 442–447

Subscriber Network (2006) Individual and Person-Centred Planning. Canterbury, Tizard Centre. (*www.kent.ac.uk/tizard/SubscriberNet/index.htm*)

Taggart L, McConkey R (2001) Working Practices employed in and across hospital and community service provision for adults with an intellectual disability and additional needs. *Journal of Learning Disabilities* **5**, 2, 175–190

Tierney A (1998) Nursing models: extant or extinct? *Journal of Advanced Nursing* **28**, 1, 77–85

Travelbee J (1971) *Interpersonal Aspects of Nursing* (2nd edn). Philadelphia, FA Davis

United Kingdom Learning Disability Consultant Nurse Network (2006) *Shaping The Future: A Vision for Learning Disability Nursing.*

Walsh M (1989) Model example. *Nursing Standard* **3**, 23–25

Wimpenny P (2002) The meaning of models of nursing to practising nurses. *Journal of Advanced Nursing* **40**, 3, 346–354

Website

www.ldhealthnetwork.org.uk

CHAPTER 2

Models for practice
Neuman's Systems Model

Mark Jukes and Penny Spencer

Introduction

Valuing People (DH 2001) places the person with a learning disability at the centre of assessment and planning for meeting their needs and aspirations by way of person-centred plans; and improving health care through health action plans. This strategy paper also suggests that learning disability nurses might be well placed to fulfil the role of health facilitator.

To assess the health needs of people with a learning disability, nurses will need a suitable model for assessment to identify health priorities and the cause of such health needs.

Neuman's Systems Model

Neuman's Systems Model is a holistic approach that encourages an interdisciplinary focus to health promotion, maintenance of wellness, prevention and management of stressors that are perceived as determinates for ill health. Neuman (2002, p3) describes optimal wellness, which represents the greatest possible degree of system stability at a given point in time.

Neuman's Systems Model was developed as an educational tool to help graduate nursing students to build their practice on a synthesis of knowledge gained from their education, life experience, nurse training and clinical experience. At a time when health care was becoming increasingly fragmented and specialised, this model encouraged practitioners to view the person as a whole and integrated being. Betty Neuman and her original co-author Rae Jeanne Young Memmott were both brought up in rural communities and felt this shaped their view of the world and the model. Neuman stated:

> *'My view of the world was shaped by the simple events of farm life and the hardiness of my parents in responding to them. There was reverence, dignity, and respect for all life...I was aware at an early age of the importance of God in my life and my having my needs met holistically'* (Carson & Arnold 1996, p92)

The Neuman Systems Model presents a nursing systems-based framework for viewing individuals, families or communities that is based on general systems theory. The person is viewed as an open system that interacts with its internal and external environments to maintain a balance between disrupting factors, described by Neuman as 'stressors'. Stressors can either act positively or negatively on the body, depending on the person's ability to cope with them at a given time.

The Neuman Systems model draws from and is related to Gestalt, Stress, and dynamically organised systems theories from such theorists as de Chardin, Cornu, Edelson, Lazarus and Selye (Neuman (2002, p12). Neuman acknowledges her early work in developing a teaching tool for graduate students in psychiatric and gerontological nursing and adopted the general systems theory of Ludwig von Bertalanffy (1968) and Hans Selye's (1950) work on stress and defences against stress.

Von Bertalanffy (1968) identified an image of the person in society as an unlimited entity with an active personality system, whose evolution follows principles, symbolism and systemic organisations, while not always able to see the potential of the entity or the ramifications of its actions.

Neuman identifies with levels of prevention, which are factors examined at an intra-, inter- and extrapersonal level to achieve optimal wellness and maintenance of the organism's basic structure. Neuman describes the support that nurses offer as 'intervention'. People require nursing intervention when they cannot cope with environmental stressors. The aim of any intervention is to reduce the negative stressors affecting the person and to promote an optimum level of functioning, wellness and stability.

Why Neuman and learning disability?

The Neuman Systems Model has been applied across a wide spectrum of nursing specialties including:
- Multiple sclerosis (Knight 1990)
- Family nursing (Reed 1993; Ross & Helmer 1988)
- Mental health nursing of older adults (Moore & Munroe 1990)
- Nursing women who have been abused (Bullock 1993)

It has also been used in a wide range of acute adult and child settings.

Learning disability nursing has always been concerned with the 'whole' person, and if aligned to Neuman's model, is concerned with how the person with a learning disability is in a continuous interplay and relationship with environmental stress factors, which represent physiological, psychological, sociocultural, developmental and spiritual variables. These variables directly affect a person's response to stress. Primarily, the learning disability nurse facilitates, intervenes and acts to reduce encounters with stressors, or helps to militate against the effects of stressors.

A learning disability nurse practitioner is actively involved in health promotion and education, teaching life skills and acting as an empowerment and advocacy agent (Bollard & Jukes 1999). Conceptualisation of health is where a person's health is a state of wellness or illness that is determined by the five variables identified above, and which are seen as being in a constant dynamic state of interaction. From an environmental conceptualisation there are external and internal environments. The external environment is all that is external to the person – the internal environment is the person's internal state in terms of influences from physiological, psychological, sociocultural, developmental and spiritual variables.

Owen (1995) identified with Neuman's 'total person' approach in her casework as a community learning disability nurse, with a young lady with Down's syndrome living at home with her elderly mother as carer and sister (who also has a mild disability).

As a framework and conceptual model for practice, Neuman's model was identified as particularly relevant to people with learning disabilities, because they experience variable demands and frustrations in diverse life situations. These may fluctuate and be inconsistent, depending where the person lives – and with whom.

Self-concept and self-awareness are based on how others see a person with a learning disability, along with establishment of sound personal relationships to achieve an inclusive, and positive sense of being a valued person in our society. Figure 2.1 shows Neuman's model with the major features identified, including the nursing roles.

There follows a brief summary of the description found in the original publication (Neuman & Young 1972). The client system is represented by a series of solid and broken circles. The central circle is the basic structure or energy source, which includes basic survival factors common to the species such as genetic response patterns, strengths or weaknesses of body organs and normal temperature range. The basic structure also consists of characteristics that are unique to the person, such as innate musical talent or artistic ability.

The outer – most solid – circle is referred to as the normal line of defence and represents a person's normal state of wellness or the usual state of adaptation that they have maintained over time. The broken line outside the normal line of defence is the flexible line of defence. Ideally it will prevent stressors from invading the client system by blocking or defusing stressors before they can attack the normal line of defence. The flexible line of defence is accordion-like in its function. When it expands, greater protection is provided. When it narrows and is closer to the normal line of defence, its ability to protect is diminished. Regular exercise, adequate sleep and good nutrition are practices that will expand the flexible line of defence.

The broken circles surrounding the basic structure are the lines of resistance, which are defined as the reactions that occur in the client system when a stressor succeeds in penetrating the normal line of defence. Their function is to restore equilibrium and protect the basic structure – for example, the body's increased production of white blood cells in response to the presence of disease-producing bacteria.

Figure 2.1 Neuman's Systems Model: a total approach to client needs

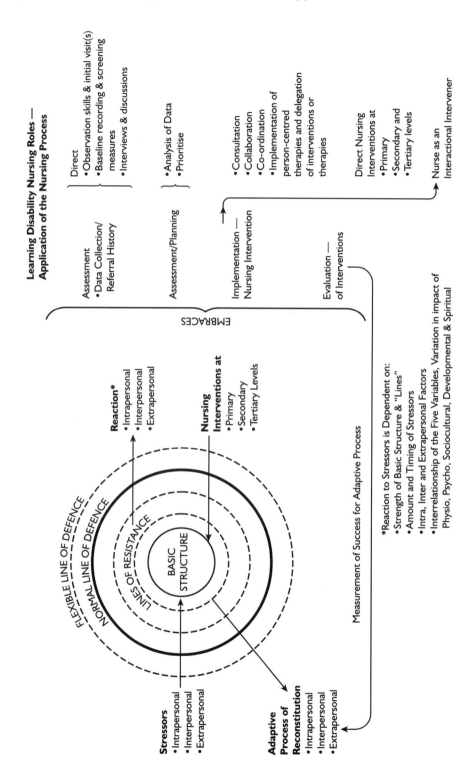

The five components

Five variables are seen to overlap and interact with, and influence all functions of the client system. Neuman (1989) stated:

> 'In all lines of defence and resistance are found elements similar, but specific functionally, related to five client variables'

All responses of the client systems should be viewed in the context of five variables that are believed to be present and interactive in all client systems:

- Physiological
- Psychological
- Sociocultural
- Spiritual
- Developmental

There are three types of stressor:

Intrapersonal: forces that occur in the individual and are often conditioned responses

Interpersonal: forces that occur between people, for example, mother–child interaction

Extrapersonal: forces that occur as a direct result of the wider environment or culture in which the person lives, for example, the impact of the benefit system on a person living in supported living.

Any stressor or reaction to a stressor will fall under one of the five variables, and often the variables overlap. For example, a mother's distress over her child's failure at school may be viewed as sociocultural if it disrupts her relationship with the child, or psychological if the mother experiences a sense of loss of self-as a 'good mother'. Box 2.1 identifies the major assumptions of Neuman's Model.

Valuing People (DH 2001) emphasises the importance of collaborative working alliances with the person as central to the relationships with professionals and others. Neuman's System Model includes the influence of Caplan's (1964) conceptual model for levels of prevention at the primary, secondary and tertiary levels, and have been adopted and adapted by Bollard and Jukes (1999) when developing a model for primary health care practice (Table 2.1).These conceptual levels of prevention are of particular importance to nurses supporting and empowering people with learning disability. Interventions can occur at different levels:

Primary: to strengthen the flexible line of defence

Secondary: to help restore the client system to equilibrium by treating symptoms that occur after penetration of the line of defence by a stressor

Tertiary: to prevent further damage and maintain stability after reconstitution has occurred.

The Neuman Systems Model fits well with the holistic concept of optimising a dynamic yet stable inter-relationship of spirit, mind and body of the person in a constantly changing environment and society (Neuman & Young 1972). The World Health Organization (1985) mandate for the year 2000 states:

> '...wellness of spirit, mind, body and environment'

in its definition of health. The systems approach permits a reorientation to a scientific approach to studying people.

Box 2.1 Major assumptions underlying Neuman's Model

- Although each person is unique, he or she is also a composite of common knowns or characteristics in a normal, given range of response in a basic structure.

- The person as a system is in a constant dynamic energy exchange with the environment.

- There are many known stressors. Each is different in its potential to disturb a person's equilibrium or normal line of defence. The particular inter-relationships of the person's variables – physiological, psychological, sociocultural, spiritual and developmental – at any point in time can affect the degree to which an individual is protected and able to use his/her flexible line of defence against possible reaction to a single stressor or a combination of stressors.

- Each person over time has evolved a normal range of responses to the environment that is referred to as a normal line of defence. It represents change over time through coping with diverse stress encounters. Is used as a standard from which to measure health deviation.

- When the cushioning, accordion-like effect of the flexible line of defence is no longer capable of protecting the person against an environmental stressor, the stressor breaks through the normal line of defence. The inter-relationship of variables – physiological, psychological, sociocultural, developmental and spiritual – determines the nature and degree of the person's reaction to the stressor.

- Each person has an internal set of resistance factors (lines of resistance), which attempt to stabilise and return him or her to the normal line of defence or potentially to a higher level of stability should a stressor break through it.

- People in a state of wellness or illness are a dynamic composite of the inter-relationship of the five variables that are always present.

- Primary prevention relates to general knowledge that is applied to individual client assessment and intervention in an attempt to identify and allay the possible risk factors associated with stressors. The goal of health promotion is included in primary prevention.

- Secondary prevention relates to symptomatology, appropriate ranking of intervention priorities and treatment to reduce their debilitating effects.

- Tertiary prevention relates to the adaptive process as reconstitution begins and maintenance factors move the person back in a circular manner towards primary prevention.

Neuman (2002, p14)

Table 2.1 Prevention-as-intervention adapted for learning disability nursing

Needs assessment		
Primary	*Secondary*	*Tertiary*
Conduct initial assessment of needs that threaten client system	Plan and conduct short intervention programmes	Review and evaluate interventions
Involve clients in assessments and provide information	Promote advocacy and empowerment	Educate, re-educate or reorient as required
Consult carers and carer participation groups	Motivate, educate and involve clients in health care goals	Co-ordinate with other disciplines
Support positive coping skills	Facilitate purposeful manipulation of stressors and reaction to stressors	Be client advocate in health education and social care
		Give client/carer feedback to commissioners of services through surveys or forums

Risk identification		
Primary	*Secondary*	*Tertiary*
Identify clients who seriously challenge within the home or other services	Set up measures to prevent situation escalating	Co-ordinate any follow-up care to support and monitor situation
Initiate a safety plan for client/carer	Ensure that programmes are in place	Educate staff and clients about safety planning
	Facilitate and share policy details among relevant people	

Disease prevention		
Primary	*Secondary*	*Tertiary*
Co-ordinate and integrate interdisciplinary theories and epidemiological profiles	Plan and facilitate services around identified needs highlighted in epidemiological profiles	Provide interventions to monitor and measure any health gain

Health promotion		
Primary	*Secondary*	*Tertiary*
Collaborate and share health promotion with clients and carers, and on an interdisciplinary level within primary care, social services and educational forums	Hold specific health promotion groups, e.g epilepsy	Provide primary or secondary prevention if required
	Carry out screening programmes within primary health care team	Refer on or apply appropriate intervention to highlight need
	Collaborate with GP, practice nurses and interdisciplinary teams	

Bollard & Jukes, 2003

Nursing models in learning disability

There is a paucity of research-based evidence to show that learning disability nurses are applying nursing models successfully in practice. However, learning disability nurses are developing adaptations from existing theory in their practice (Jukes 1987; Owen 1995; Spencer 2002; Parkes 2003; Horan et al 2004a, b). Others have developed their own theory and frameworks, such as Aldridge (2003) Turner & Coles (1997) and Hodges (1989). Parker (1990) argues that in periods of significant social and professional change, nursing models and theory can provide a degree of stability and guidance:

> '...an anchor in the sea of issues and problems'

Duff (1997) reported that a literature search found little proof of the efficacy of nursing models in learning disabilities nursing and that more nursing research was needed in this area of practice. During a prolific era of nursing model development in the UK, Jukes (1988) questioned whether there was:

> '...a professional malaise among learning disabilities nurses in using nursing models?'

and if there was a preference instead for the application of psychological functional assessment tools, which could inhibit the development of knowledge and practice in learning disability nursing.

Neuman (1989, p10) claims that in the Neuman System Model:

> 'Wholism is both a philosophical and a biological concept implying relationships and processes arising from wellness, dynamic freedom and creativity in adjusting to stress in the internal and external environment'

Neuman (1989, p8) also states that wholism is not a difficult idea to grasp, she suggests that:

> 'A clear conception of systems organisation requires skill in viewing client situations abstractly. That is, client system boundaries and related variables may lose some clarity because they are dynamic and constantly changing, presenting different appearances according to time, place and the significance of events'

Different people will also perceive things differently, so it is important to address the perceived need from the client's, carer's and the nurse's perspective. If the person cannot communicate their needs, the carer should be asked to do so, but the carer's perspective may be different to the client's. When using Neuman's assessment process, conflicting views can be identified, which require further understanding contextually as well as personally.

If a person has severe and profound multiple learning disabilities and minimal verbal communication, other forms of communication can be used in the assessment process, including:

- Maketon
- Interpretation of body language

- Art as a medium for expression of thoughts and feelings
- Pictures and symbols
- Life-story work

A person-centred approach involves gaining a person's perspective of their needs, and those of the carer or significant other before the nurse's, so that the client can feel in control of the process rather than the passive recipient. McClure (1995) acknowledges the conflict of interest between carers' needs and dependants' needs when observing community nurses and carers as co-workers. Learning disabilities nurses frequently work with the carer to support the client, often visiting the carer alone to offer support and advice to enable them to continue supporting the client. There can be conflict if this disempowers the client or the carer.

> 'Empowerment is too often viewed as a zero sum – empowering one person is thought to remove power from another. Disempowering parents is unlikely to be a helpful strategy in increasing the empowerment of people with learning disabilities. Recognising the skills and understanding which parents bring to the development of their sons or daughters should form the basis of a three-way partnership in those cases where professionals have substantial involvement in people's lives'   (Barnes 1997, p85)

Neuman's client assessment and nursing process comprises of five major stages:

1. Initial nursing diagnosis – a database determined by identifying and evaluating potential stressors

2. Stressors perceived by the client (or if the client is incapacitated, data from family or other areas (Box 2.2)

3. Stressors perceived by the caregiver (Box 2.3) asks the same questions from the caregiver's perspective (it is important to note any discrepancies or distortions between the client's perception and that of the caregiver)

4. Personal factors:

- Intrapersonal factors (Box 2.4)
- Interpersonal factors, for example resources and relationship of family, friends, or caregivers that either influence or could influence
- Extrapersonal factors, for example, resources and relationship of community facilities, finances, employment or other areas

5. Comprehensive nursing diagnosis (Box 2.5)

Neuman's five components offer a:

> '...generic guide for assessment and intervention, and is appropriate for adoption in any designated client system – an individual, a family, a community, or a social issue'   (Neuman 2002, p347)

In terms of the person who has a learning disability the client is seen as being a composite of variables (physiological, psychological, sociocultural, developmental and spiritual), each of which is a subpart of all parts, and which forms the

Box 2.2 Identifying stressors: client's perspective

(If client is incapacitated, secure data from family or other resources)

Question to ask	What is identified?
1. What do you consider to be your three major stress areas, or areas of health concern?	Three main areas of stress
2. How do your present circumstances differ from your usual pattern of living?	Lifestyle pattern
3. Have you ever experienced a similar problem? If so, what was that problem and how did you handle it? Were you successful?	Past coping patterns
4. What do you anticipate for yourself in the future as a consequence of your present situation?	Perceptual factors Reality versus distortion Expectations
5. What are you doing and what can you do to help yourself?	Present coping patterns Possible future coping patterns
6. What do you expect your caregivers, family, friends or others to do for you?	

Box 2.3 Identifying stressors: caregiver's perspective

Question to ask	What is identified?
1. What do you consider to be the three major stress areas, or areas of health concern for the person you care for?	Three main areas of stress
2. How do their present circumstances differ from their usual pattern of living?	Lifestyle pattern
3. Have they ever experienced a similar problem? If so, what was that problem and how did they and you handle it? Were you and they successful?	Past coping patterns
4. What do you anticipate for the person you care for in the future as a consequence of their present situation?	Perceptual factors Reality versus distortion Expectations
5. What are they doing and what can they do to help themselves?	Present coping patterns Possible future coping patterns
6. What do they expect their caregivers, family, friends or others to do for them?	*(Neuman 2002)*

Box 2.4 Intrapersonal factors

Physiological
- Nature and causation of disability
- Degree of mobility
- Physical health – range of body functions
- Elimination
- Medication
- Psychological state
- Sexual orientation and level of activity.
- Abuse past and present.
- Self-care and levels of support

Psychosociocultural
- Relationships
- Attitudes
- Values
- Expectations
- Lifestyle
- Behaviour pattern
- Coping patterns
- Housing

Spiritual beliefs
- Hope
- Sustainment
- Resilience

Developmental
- Daily activities – past and present
- Degree of normalcy.
- Use of local facilities
- Communication
- Respite
- Future needs

(Neuman 2002)

whole of the client. The client is seen as an open system in total interface with the environment. These headings are a useful way of indicating areas in which interventions could be formulated.

Neuman describes stressors as environmental factors that have potential for disrupting the system stability. A stressor may be any phenomenon that might penetrate both the flexible and normal lines of defence, resulting in positive or negative outcomes.

Interprofessional working

Community learning disability nurses are rarely the line manager for the staff supporting a client – their role is largely one of facilitation and liaison. This can lengthen the decision making process when finding alternative daytime activities or support to meet direct care needs as a client may have behavioural input by staff from health, activities funded by social services where the providers are

Box 2.5 Formulation of a comprehensive nursing diagnosis

This is accomplished by identifying and ranking the priority of needs based on total data obtained from the client's perception, the caregiver's perception, or other resources such as medication reviews, lab reports and results, or other significant people and agencies.

A priority for nursing action in each of the areas of prevention as intervention is to determine the nature of stressors and their threat to the client system. Nursing goals are prioritised in terms of:

- Primary prevention (prevention or treatment)
- Secondary prevention (treatment)
- Tertiary prevention (follow-up after treatment)

Primary prevention	Secondary prevention	Tertiary prevention
Date:	Date:	Date
Goal 1:	Goal 1:	Goal 1:
Goal 2:	Goal 2:	Goal 2:
Goal 3:	Goal 3:	Goal 3:
Intervention:	Intervention:	Intervention:
Outcome:	Outcome:	Outcome:
Comments:	Comments:	Comments:

independent, small, private organisations or individuals. Where there is a lengthy dialogue between the agencies, Neuman's model can be used to document the differing perceived needs, and priorities established to co-ordinate meeting the clients assessed needs through multi agency working.

The government consultation paper *Partnerships in Action* (DH 1998a) includes proposals to encourage health authorities and social services to work together by removing constraints in the systems and introduce incentives and collaborative arrangements. It is proposed to introduce a bill to allow health, social services and education to move budgets in response to each other's commissioning arrangements to integrate service provisions. It is designed to meet the needs of the most vulnerable people in society where it is often difficult to separate what is a health care need and what is social care.

The green paper *Independence, Wellbeing and Choice* (DH 2005) sets out to examine whether Person-centred planning can be linked to a single assessment process and the care programme approach to provide a comprehensive assessment for complex cases, and to reduce the number of professionals assessing and reassessing clients.

Neuman's Systems Model:

- Provides a framework for interagency working,
- Places the client at the centre
- Encourages sustained and careful listening to the person (as with person-centred planning)
- Puts people in the context of their families and communities, their systems, and their support networks

Julian's case study (below) pursues the ethos and application of Neuman's model, and shows the process in which a community learning disability nurse has internalised and applied the model as a means for intervention.

Case study: Julian

Julian is 13 years old. He has what can be classified as having moderate to mild learning disabilities, attention deficit hyperactive disorder and epilepsy.

He lives at home with his mother, who has recently separated from Julian's father, and his 18-year-old sister, who has just gone away to university.

Recently, Julian's mother has been concerned that there has been an increase in the number of seizures Julian is having. His levels of aggression and inappropriate behaviours towards others are also becoming unmanageable.

Julian's school is telling his mother they can no longer meet his needs and are also concerned about his now more frequent challenging behaviours.

In desperation, Julian's mum seeks help from her GP, who refers Julian to the community learning disability team, and he is allocated to the community learning disability nurse.

The community nurse makes a number of assessment and intervention visits with Julian, his mother and sister (when at home from university), the schoolteachers and significant other people and resources. The community nurse has adopted Neuman's model as an appropriate means for identifying and planning intervention strategies.

Figure 2.2 shows how the five variables are applied to the case study.

Julian's care is defined through how the five variables have influenced him before referral and the family separation, with the maintenance of his normal line of defence.

As a core family unit his father, mother and sister have all been involved in how his physiological, psychological, sociocultural, developmental and spiritual variables through their interaction with each other have been maintained both in the internal and external influences in the environment.

Figure 2.2 Neuman Systems Model adapted for learning disability nursing: how the five variables can be applied to the case study

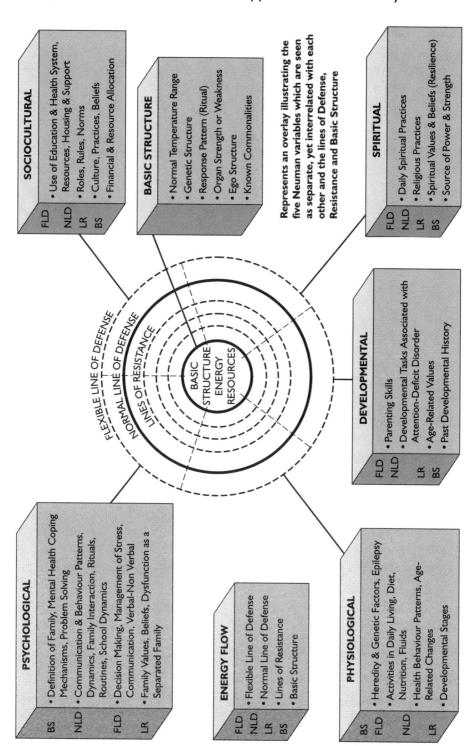

Case study: Julian (continued)

Julian's basic energy/core structure consisting of the five client system variables, must be protected by the lines of defence and resistance to keep Julian safe and dynamic. The normal line of defence defines Julian's current health status.

Before his father left, and his sister went to University, the triad of his mother, father and sister had helped in achieving Julian's sense of self and integrity in the home and outside at school while interacting/integrating in the immediate community.

The flexible line of defence protects Julian from immediate or short-term environmental stressors that potentially or actually destabilise his normal line of defence, that is, his usual health/wellness status. It is important to assess the strength and nature of each interacting variable in the flexible line of defence to determine how well it functions as a protective shield or as a composite. Examples in Julian's case would be

- Sleep pattern
- Perception and experience of recent events
- Nature of perceived/lack of social support
- Behavioural responses through an altered pattern of support systems
- Engagement/interactional changes

The normal line of defence is penetrated by one or several stressors that come from intra-, inter- or extrapersonal sources, shown in Box 2.7. To achieve stability in the normal line of defence, the CNLD adopts the use of the three prevention-as-intervention modalities in Box 2.8 to facilitate an optimal client system health/wellness condition.

Using Neuman's System Model allowed Julian's needs to be identified and addressed in his care plan. It shows the need for ongoing dialogue between all parties to achieve the desired outcomes for the client.

The client's care programme shows the need for partnership between the client and his paid and unpaid carers, between the client and the agencies funding his care, between health and social services to meet the client's needs.

Pitkeathley (1999) defines partnership as:

'...participating in ways that meet the needs of all the people involved and enables all the people in the partnership to participate in a way that is suitable for them...this needs understanding of where all the parties are coming from, what there needs are and what they bring to the partnership'

She also acknowledges that it is easy to pay lip service to carer partnerships, but difficult to carry through in practice.

Conclusion

A definitive definition of what learning disabilities nurses do has been sought for a number of years in relation to the unique contribution made by learning disabilities specialist community nurses in facilitating and empowering the person

Box 2.7 Julian's identified stressors

Intrapersonal

- Increased epilepsy activity
- Altered neurological functioning
- Sleep pattern altered – long periods of wakefulness, deprivation
- Little insight or expression into altered behaviour pattern
- Role alterations in and outside the family
- Nutrition inadequate at home and inconsistent at school – weight loss.

Interpersonal

- Roles altered and relationship with mother through absent members of family, mother is more authoritative and exerts restrictions on Julian
- Little knowledge and insight from mother about Julian experiencing loss
- Julian has little insight into the altered family structure and changed dynamics
- No communication with father or sister
- Personal distress exhibited through altered relationship with mother
- Schoolteacher and classroom assistant relationship with Julian is stressful when attempting to manage in the classroom

Extrapersonal

- Geographic isolation and distancing from father and sister
- Limited transport (mother cannot drive)
- Financial loss due to separation and sister at university
- Family not known to social services

with a learning disability. *Continuing the Commitment* (DH 1995b) and *Learning Disability Nursing in a Contract Culture* (RCN 1994) emphasised the contribution of learning disabilities nurses in a variety of settings in ensuring that people with a learning disability have access to mainstream health and social care to lead as normal a life as possible.

Signposts for Success (DH 1998b) recommended multidisciplinary approaches and partnerships in care as a way of meeting the specialist needs of people with learning disabilities while acknowledging their individuality. The Healthcare Commission's *Draft three-year strategic plan for assessing and encouraging improvement in health and health care of adults with learning disabilities 2006– 2009* again highlights the inequalities of access to mainstream services and the increased prevalence of ill heath among people with learning disabilities.

Community specialist learning disability nurses need to be more visible in a variety of client/carer forums (Manthorpe et al 2002), and proactive in collaboration with other professionals to empower people who need to access mainstream and specialist services. For numerous clients there is no neat line between what constitutes health care and what constitutes social care. Using the Neuman Systems Model to assess and plan Julian's care allows for the process of working with stressors from a variety of sources to allow Julian to identify and to be assisted to return to a more

Box 2.8 Prevention-as-interventions modalities

Primary prevention

Interventions intended to reduce the possibility of the client's encounter with stressors, and strengthen the client system's flexible line of defence and raise awareness of the issues of family dynamics.

- Provide information about support for families of people with learning disabilities in GP practices, social services, education and leisure centres
- Provide education programmes, advice and help centres, drop-in centres
- Target information at GP practices, schools, community centres, supermarkets and pharmacy information boards.
- Deliver presentations in schools and primary health care centres.

Secondary prevention

Nursing actions that help to protect the basic core structures of the client's and family's systems once the normal line of defence has been invaded by stressors.

- Initiate and develop a short-term safety plan in collaboration with Julian, his mother and school staff for those occurrences of aggression and violence
- Consult with dietician on how to stimulate interest with a variety of food
- Assess epilepsy activity, and have existing anticonvulsant serum levels monitored – advice on further management of seizures may be required
- Assess existing medication and identify principal doctor/consultant to co-ordinate and be responsible for continuing to monitor epilepsy.
- Assess sleep pattern
- Obtain baselines over a series of visits for behaviour and give practical advice on behaviour management at school and in the home
- Work with Julian one-to-one, to allow him to express himself in terms of his overt distress – commence a life book
- Work with mother on her coping skills and develop a coping strategy for relating and communicating with Julian
- Teach anger management principles with mother
- Liaise with educational and systemic psychologist/counsellor

Tertiary prevention

Nursing interventions designed to maintain wellness once a client system has achieved stability through secondary prevention interventions.

- Continue parent group support system
- Continue individual and interdisciplinary alliances and networking and monitoring measures

homeostatic balance in his life. It also emphasises the need for co-ordinating various agencies to work together to meet Julian's needs, and showed that Julian's social world is dynamic and constantly changing, and the importance of appreciating that people's perception of events changes with time, place and interactions with others. Using Neuman's Systems Model as a framework for interaction enabled realistic goals to be set and achieved with interagency working.

References

(websites accessed 7 June 2007)

Aldridge J (2003) The Ecology of Health Model. In: Jukes M, Bollard M (eds) *Contemporary Learning Disability Practice.* Salisbury, Quay Books. Chapter 8, pp93–123

Barnes M (1997) Families and empowerment. In: Ramcharan P, Roberts G, Grant G, Borland J (eds) *Empowerment in Everyday Life.* London, Jessica Kingsley

von Bertalanffy, L (1968) *General Systems Theory.* New York, Braziller

Bollard M, Jukes M (1999) Specialist practitioner in community learning disability nursing and the primary health care team. *Journal of Learning Disabilities, Health and Social Care* **3**, 1, 11–19

Bollard M, Jukes M (2003) Developing a model for primary care in learning disabilities. In: Jukes M, Bollard M (eds) *Contemporary Learning Disability Practice.* Salisbury, Quay Books. Chapter 7 pp79–89

Bullock LFC (1993) Nursing interventions for abused women on obstetrical units. Association of Women's Health, Obstetric and Neonatal Nurses (AWHONN) *Clinical Issues in Perinatal and Women's Health Nursing* **4**, 3, 371–377

Carson VB, Arnold EN (1996) *Mental Health Nursing: The Nurse-Patient Journey.* Philadelphia, WB Saunders Company

Caplan G (1964) *Principles of Preventive Psychiatry.* New York, Basic Books

Department of Health (1995a) *The Health of the Nation – A Strategy for People with Learning Disabilities. London,* DH

Department of Health (1995b) *Continuing the Commitment.* London, HMSO

Department of Health (1998a) *Partnerships in Action.* London, The Stationery Office

Department of Health (1998b) *Signposts for Success.* London, The Stationery Office

Department of Health (2005) *Independence, Wellbeing and Choice.* London, The Stationery Office

Duff G (1997) Using models in learning disability nursing. *Professional Nurse* **12**, 10, 702–704

Healthcare Commission (2005) *Draft three-year strategic plan for assessing and encouraging improvement in the health and healthcare of adults with learning disabilities 2006–2009.* London, Healthcare Commission *(www.healthcarecommission.org.uk/_db/_documents/04021628.pdf)*

Henderson V (1969) *Basic Principles of Nursing Care* (revised edn). New York, S Karger

Hodges B (1989) The health career model: In: Hinchcliffe SM (ed) *Nursing Practice and Health Care* (1st edn only). London, Edward Arnold

Horan P, Doran A, Timmins F (2004a) Exploring Orem's self-care deficit nursing theory in learning disability nursing: Philosophical parity paper: Part 1. *Learning Disability Practice* **7**, 4, 28–33

Horan P, Doran A, Timmins F (2004b) Exploring Orem's self-care model in learning disability nursing: Practical application paper: Part 2. *Learning Disability Practice* **7**, 4, 33–37

Jukes M (1987) Assessing the whole person. *Senior Nurse* **16**, 6, 14–16

Jukes M (1988) Nursing model or psychological assessment? *Senior Nurse* **8**, 11, 8–10

Knight JB (1990) The Betty Neuman System Model applied to practice: a client with multiple sclerosis. *Journal of Advanced Nursing* **15**, 447–455

Manthorpe J, Alasewski A, Gates B, Ayer S. Motherby E (2003) Learning disability nursing: user and carer perceptions. *Journal of Learning Disabilities.* **7**, 2, 119–135

McClure L (1995) Community nursing and carers: what price support and partnership? In: Cain P, Hyde V, Howkins E (eds) *Community Nursing: Dimensions and Dilemmas.* London, Arnold

Moore SL, Munroe MF (1990) The Neuman Systems Model applied to mental health nursing of older adults. *Journal of Advanced Nursing* **15**, 293–299

Neuman B (1982) *The Neuman Systems Model.* Connecticut, Appleton-Lange

Neuman B (1989) *The Neuman Systems Model* (2nd edn). Connecticut, Appleton-Lange

Neuman B (1995) *The Neuman Systems Model* (3rd edn). Connecticut, Appleton-Lange

Neuman B, Fawcett J (2002) *The Neuman Systems Model* (4th edn). Upper Saddle River, New Jersey, Prentice Hall

Neuman B, Young RJ (1972) A model for teaching total person approach to patient problems. *Nursing Research* **21**, 264–269

Owen M (1995) Care of a woman with Down's syndrome using the Neuman Systems Model. *British Journal of Nursing* **4**, 13, 752–758

Parker ME (1990) Developing perspectives on nursing theory in practice. In Parker ME (ed) *Nursing Theories in Practice.* New York, National League for Nursing

Parkes N (2003) Abuse and vulnerability. In: Jukes M, Bollard M (eds) *Contemporary Learning Disability Practice.* Salisbury, Quay Books, Chapter 11, pp151–164

Peplau H (1952) *Interpersonal Relationships in Nursing.* New York, G.P. Putnam & Sons

Pitkeathley J (1999) How to use Government policies to make partnerships really work. *Nursing Management* **6**, 1, 32–37.

Royal College of Nursing (1994) *Learning Disability Nursing in a Contract Culture.* Leeds, Nuffield Institute for Health

Reed KS, (1993) Adapting the Neuman Systems Model for family nursing. *Nursing Science Quarterly* **6**, 2, 93–97

Ross MM, Helmer H (1988) A comparative analysis of Neuman's Model using the individual and family as the units of care. *Public Health Nursing* **5**, 30–36

Selye H (1950) *The Physiology and Pathology of Exposure to Stress* Montreal, ACTA

Spencer P (2002) Support system. *Learning Disability Practice* **5**, 7, 17–20

Turner M, Coles J (1997) Meeting the needs of people with learning disabilities: developing an interactive model of care. *Journal of Learning Disabilities* **1**, 4, 162–170

World Health Organization (1985) *Targets for Health for All.* Geneva, World Health Organization

CHAPTER 3

Models for practice
Roy's Adaptation Model

Neville Parkes

Introduction

In this chapter, Roy's model of nursing will be discussed in respect of its eminent suitability for use in 21st century services for people with a learning disability. We propose that if the model is used correctly, it lends itself to a person-centred approach.

Although Roy's model is a model of 'nursing', we argue that the basic assumptions of the model should find some commonality among both health and social care professionals in services for people with a learning disability. The model views health from a holistic (bio- social- physiological and spiritual) perspective. The reader should not wrongly assume the term 'model of nursing' means that this model promotes only a biomedical-focused or a disease-based approach to care.

This chapter will identify that some concepts and terminology in Roy's model are likely to be counterproductive if used by a worker in current services for people with a learning disability. The author has proposed some changes in the terminology used and a more flexible way to view 'adaptation' to ensure the model is more suitable for contemporary learning disability services.

Activities throughout the chapter are aimed to generate reflection and discussion for the reader and colleagues. There will be a reflection on a case study of clinical work undertaken from personal practice as a community nurse for people with a learning disability, to demonstrate the utility of the model. The case study uses work undertaken in a community peripatetic role. This does not exclude the use of the model elsewhere, for example in compulsory treatment placements or in community-based residential services.

Models of nursing

At its simplest, a model of nursing explicitly defines what nursing 'is' by seeking to describe and inform theoretically what is nursing practice. A nursing model develops a coherent theory of specific concepts related to nursing practice – nursing, health, the human and the environment. The intricacies of the theory and constructs of a model of nursing go much beyond the parameters of this chapter – for more information, see Fawcett (1989) and George (1980).

Roy's model

Roy's model views the human as a bio-psycho-social adaptive system in a constant state of interaction with the environment (Villareal 2003). The environment, according to Roy, includes factors such as the person's physiological and psychological processes and external factors such as the person's home, places they work and attend recreation, as depicted in Figure 3.1. Andrews and Roy (1986, p18) define the person (in focus) as an intrinsic part of their group or society and that they are involved in a social system.

Figure 3.1 The human response to internal and external environment

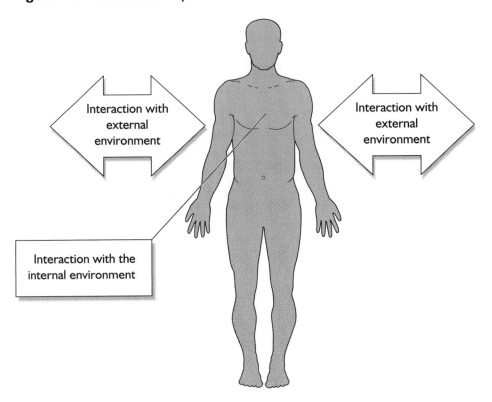

The reaction to stimuli, referred to as outputs (internal or external) is suggested by Roy to be either adaptive or ineffective. Roy suggests that adaptation is met when the integrity of the person is maintained. Adaptation is defined as when:

'The person is able to meet most goals of survival and growth'

(Galbreath 1990; Logan 1990)

Ineffective reactions/outputs are when the person is unable to meet these goals. Roy's view of the role of nursing is to promote adaptation through manipulation of stimuli the person receives.

The four adaptive modes

Roy suggests that adaptation is processed through four adaptive modes which interact constantly in the internal and external environment

- Physiological
- Role function
- Self-concept
- Interdependence

Figure 3.2 is my interpretation of how Roy views the adaptive modes.

Figure 3.2 Four adaptive modes

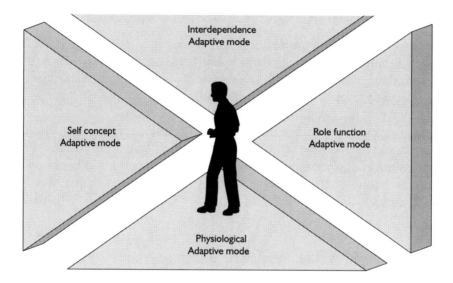

Physiological adaptive mode

Roy describes this adaptive mode as one that relates to the physiological somatic functions that pertain to physical and chemical aspects related to the individual (Villareal 2003, p378). The five needs outlined by Roy and Andrews (1999) are:

- Oxygenation
- Nutrition
- Elimination
- Activity
- Protection

Roy suggests that homeostasis is maintained when these elements of the physiological mode are in balance.

Self-concept adaptive mode

Roy uses this adaptive mode to describe how the person interacts and functions in society (Andrews & Roy 1996, p123–124). It is the composite of beliefs and feelings that the person holds, and relates to the personal insights including the physical self (via body sensations and body image) and spiritual self. This is pertinent for many people with a learning disability, as their viewpoints of their selves relate directly to their functioning, e.g. if a man with a learning disability refers to himself as a 'naughty boy' it is probably indicative of his own belief about himself as a child, which most likely indicates the social system he is in. This is also pertinent when dealing with sexuality issues (Parkes & Hodges 2006).

Role concept adaptive mode

The role concept adaptive mode focuses on how a person functions in society. It is linked to developmental steps – for example, what is appropriate for a five-year-old child is not for an 80-year-old person. Roy requires the nurse to consider how a person functions within their primary role (their main day-to-day roles, e.g. a family member) and their secondary roles (which are not permanent).

Independence adaptive mode

This adaptive mode relates to the relationship between individuals, the quality of support and the client needs that the nurse must consider. It helps the nurse to identify a person's level of ability and independence and the level of support that they require in physical, psychological and emotional domains

Assessing a person with a learning disability in the interdependence adaptive mode can enable the nurse to identify strengths and gifts that the person with a learning disability has, for example a person who can support his or her carers in some daily living tasks. It may enable some insights into the function of social support networks.

Stimuli

Roy asserts (Figure 3.3) that each individual, through their adaptive modes, receives:
- Focal stimuli – personal experiences
- Contextual stimuli – from the external environment
- Residual stimuli – views, beliefs and experiences

This can be demonstrated by the example of a person having a headache. The focal stimulus is the person having a headache, the contextual stimulus is a room with fluorescent lighting which may have contributed to the cause of the headache; the residual stimulus is that the person believes (through experience) that they require analgesia and time in a less well-lit environment.

Roy views that humans have two subsystems:
- Regulator – the physiological processes that are not in the direct influence of conscious thinking, such as the impulse from the brain stem to regulate the heartbeat
- Cognator – the processes that are affected via conscious thought.

The nursing process using Roy's model has two assessment levels (Andrews & Roy 1986, pp4–8). These include an identification of the client behaviours and the stimuli that impinge on the individual. The second level assessment is characterised by identification of problems, goal setting intervention and evaluation. The nurse

Figure 3.3 Focal, contextual and residual stimuli

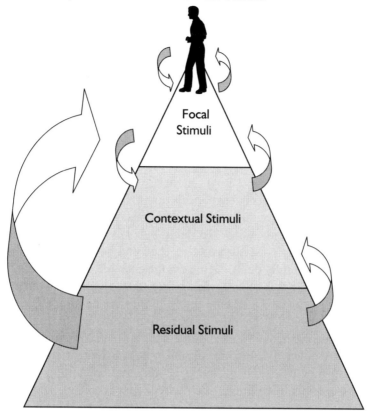

selects areas of concern to the client or their carer or family.

Using Roy's model in practice

Roy's model has been applied to a wide variety of needs and in a wide variety of nursing settings, for example:

- Smoking cessation (Villareal 2003)
- Alzheimer's disease (Thornbury & King 1992)
- Psychosexual concerns (LeMone 1995)
- Psychological distress (Yeh 2003)
- Sexuality and multiple sclerosis (Gagliardi 2003)
- Accident and emergency nursing (Ingram 1995)
- Community health nursing (Dixon 1999)

There are few examples in the literature of nursing models used in learning disability nursing, even though people with learning disabilities have a full spectrum of health care needs. Duquette (1997) describes how Roy's model was used successfully with children with special needs in the school setting. Parkes (2003) discusses Roy's model of nursing applied to a man with a learning disability who is a survivor of sexual abuse. Horan (2004) discusses the use of Orem's model applied to people with a learning disability; Aldridge (2003) proposes a specific model tailored for people with a learning disability.

The concept of adaptation as outlined by Roy is likely to be unhelpful in contemporary services for people with learning disabilities. A person with a learning disability could be seen as being at 'fault' (or other equivalent terms). Such approaches in most cases are antithetical to person-centredness. Defining adaptation in a way that views human responses as being positive (adaptive) or negative (ineffective) in some cases can be relatively straightforward – for example, if one is judging the efficiency of how one is breathing or taking in fluids. Some things, even when dealing with physiological issues, may be more debatable and even controversial, for example the debate about dietary intake and cholesterol (Tang et al 1998).

The assumption of health in Roy's model is congruent with how Seedhouse (1991, p29) critiques such a concept of health as an 'idealised state'. This simplistic definition of health assumes that anything that does not achieve an optimum level of human function is 'unhealthy'. To define what is an optimum level is very problematic. For example, Seedhouse (1991, p6 and p41) highlights that disease and health can be culturally defined. He cites the example of foot binding in China. It was highly valued in that culture while in Western cultures the woman would be viewed as having deformed feet; conversely, in Western culture, a selfish egotistic businesswoman would not be seen as being sick while in the past this type of behaviour has been seen as evidence of mental illness in communist countries.

Services for people with a learning disability need to be cautious about adopting this or similar view of health, as many people with a learning disability have enduring physiological conditions such as epilepsy, cerebral palsy or thyroxin deficiency. In this approach they can never achieve an *(sic)* 'idealised state'. The problems of judging adaptability have been discussed by Dixon (1999, p294) in the community health field.

It is also difficult to apply Roy's role function and self-concept adaptive modes to real situations in learning disability services. For example, the health or social care worker may need to decide whether the person with a learning disability is 'adaptive' if they attend a large day centre undertaking age inappropriate activities that they enjoy. The viewpoints on this situation are likely to be numerous, for example:

- The person *is* adaptive because they are empowered by doing what they like and enjoy
- The person *is not* adaptive because they are attending a segregated service undertaking activities that will 'devalue' them
- The person is as adaptive *as they can be* in a 'devaluing' system.

All these viewpoints are based on ideological standpoints. In many other examples in the field of learning disability, such judgments are far from simple.

Learning disability nurses need to be cautious about promoting a notion of 'adaptability' based on notions of optimum health (however defined) This is likely to set goals for people with learning disability that expect them to lead a peculiarly sanitised and virtuous existence, which may be perversely stigmatising.

Case study: Jason

Jason's case study – drawn from personal professional experience – shows how Roy's model can be applied. His name has been changed, and the inclusion of the following has been discussed with his parents, as he does not have capacity to give permission to do so.

Profile

Jason is 17 years old with a severe learning disability. He uses short phrases and single words to convey his needs. He requires constant support and supervision. He lives with his mother and father and his non-disabled younger brother Ryan who is 14. Jason exhibits many features of autistic spectrum disorder (Attwood 1998; Wing 1976) although no formal diagnosis was available while working with him (but has been gained subsequently). He exhibited stereotypical routine behaviours, he did not respond well to change and he anxious about forthcoming events. He exhibited difficult behaviour that included verbalised anger, throwing objects, property destruction and violent behaviour towards his younger brother Ryan. This behaviour is problematic for the family. They had received ongoing support from the community learning disability team for many years before my involvement, and this continued when I stopped working with Jason.

Assessment

Tables 3.1–3.3 outline the first level assessment undertaken for three of the adaptive modes. It was difficult to assess his self-concept because of his learning disability.

Jason is generally in good health. The behaviours that are most likely to be linked to his anxiety, which is in turn linked, to the stimuli he gets from his environment.

The relationship between Jason and Ryan is extremely volatile, resulting in the two leading very many separate lives in the same house. This raised many concerns for Jason's mother and father, as it makes events such as family outings and holidays difficult. Increased stress for siblings of disabled children has been identified by Gath (1989).

Ryan's lack of understanding of Jason's learning disability and autism is congruent with Bagenholm and Gillberg (1991), who identified that many siblings could not explain their brother or sister's condition. Begun (1989) identified that adolescence was a time when times of conflict and stress are more likely to occur. Conway and O'Neill (2004) identified, in their study of siblings of children with autism, that the impact of the behaviour of their autistic brother or sister impacted on their sleep, friendships and feeling different and in some cases learned to feeling isolated.

Jason's mother identified that holidays were extremely stressful as Jason is out of his familiar environment (thus having no routine to reassure him) and in close proximity to Ryan. The difficulty this raises was characterised by the striking image of his mother describing the time the family visited Disneyland – which was a very expensive holiday. Jason had no particular interest in this except for the small sparrow-like bird he could see in the foreground – he is very interested in birds – ignoring Disneyland in the background. Although his mother recounted this with some amusement, she added it was quite soul-destroying.

Jason's mother (and probably other members of his family) used words and phrases that were highly abstract, complex and often sarcastic – reflecting many people's experience of the day-to-day banter of family life. It was clear from my observations that Jason was likely to have not understood the qualitative meanings, probably picking up on one or two key words. This, in some cases, could have led to him not being fully reassured or getting the comments that he was seeking. This in turn could have led to him becoming anxious and exhibiting difficult behaviours.

The interaction between Jason and his mother was good-natured and Jason often enjoyed the voice tone of some words. He responded well to phrases that he was familiar with.

However, it is likely Jason has a 'failed theory of mind' (Baron-Cohen et al 1985). Jason would most likely lack or be severely limited in his understanding of nuances, and intuitive understanding resulting in his understating of language being quite literal (a typical characteristic of people with autism).

Table 3.4 shows how a second level assessment was developed for Jason, using the adaptability continuum.

Evaluation

DRO and reward programmes: The differential reinforcer of other behaviours (DRO) programme and the reward programme for Ryan not to provoke Jason both had some effect in that Jason and Ryan could spend a few minutes together. This approach was used at times when conflict was likely to occur, usually when both brothers Ryan and Jason returned home from school. It was not undertaken in school holidays, as Ryan spends most of his time out of the family home with his friends and undertaking sporting activities. The DRO ran for a number of months and appeared to have some success.

Information about autism: Ryan commented that he found the information about autism helpful – but it is not easy to judge the effect of this.

Sequential planning diary: This was felt to have some success in reducing Jason's repetitive questioning. A behavioural team from whom Jason subsequently received service developed the diary further.

Family visits: Regular visits to discuss progress with the family provided some time to reflect on the use of phrases and words used to communicate with Jason. It is difficult to qualify how this was interpreted. Jason's mother commented that she felt that she was using less abstract phrases for Jason, but acknowledged it was an ongoing issue.

The family took a holiday without Jason. Respite care and some care from a relative were provided for Jason with support from the community nursing ream to ensure Jason was coping. This was a clear success as Jason was very settled and commented he enjoyed being there The family had a good holiday. Jason's mother said that they missed Jason and felt quite guilty for not taking him.

Table 3.1 Physiological adaptive mode: Jason

First level assessment	Focal stimuli	Contextual stimuli	Residual stimuli
	Jason becomes anxious, movement and his voice levels raise	Change in the environment, his mother is unable to give him exclusive attention	Difficult to assert what Jason believes but likely to want to understand and know sequencing of events. He finds change distressing because of this. Likely to find his routine behaviour a coping strategy
Jason has difficulty sleeping due to nightmares	Jason has intermittent sleep and is awake early most mornings	He sleeps in his bedroom	It is considered by his community nurse that this may be an adverse effect of his medication
Jason exhibits dramatic changes in behaviour related to the above	Jason receives mood-stabilising medication (carbamazepine) and a beta blocker prescribed by his consultant psychiatrist	Given to him by his parents and monitored by his community nurse/ GP	
Jason is generally otherwise healthy	No obvious health difficulties		

Table 3.2 Role concept adaptive mode: Jason

First level assessment	Focal stimuli	Contextual stimuli	Residual stimuli
Jason is a son	He becomes anxious if his mother is unable or unwilling to give him exclusive attention. He directs this towards himself or objects or to his younger brother	This occurs if there is an unexpected change or if a future change is mentioned to him that does not occur in the very near future for example someone says, 'in two days we will go to town'. Or there is a lack of routine or structure, particularly when he is at home in holidays and weekends	Jason, it is surmised, believes that he should have exclusive access and attention to his mother. The family understands Jason's need for routine but find it difficult to ensure their lives 'revolve' around Jason by accommodating his needs all the time
Jason is a brother	Ryan is present. Ryan will sometimes precipitate Jason's anxiety by making comments or gestures and/ or react to his aggression with his aggression	Jason becomes distressed and angry when his brother Ryan is present with his mother	Ryan has no awareness of autism. Jason is likely to view Ryan as someone who takes his attention from his mother and with resulting anxiety
Jason is a student at a special school	He is very quiet, and has no particular friends, but enjoys many activities undertaken at the school, such as swimming and cookery	He will accept more changes at school. He appears to feel relaxed in a routine environment	His parents find his apparent flexibility in this environment quite frustrating as he would not do similar things at home
Jason attends a respite care facility every two weeks	He appears to feel relaxed in a routine environment	Similar to above, it is believed he finds the routine supportive	

Table 3.3 Interdependence adaptive mode: Jason

First level assessment	Focal stimuli	Contextual stimuli	Residual stimuli
	Jason is dependent for support and supervision from his parents/ carers/ school staff	He is supported and supervised continually	It is believed that Jason will need this level of supervision and support for all his life
			Family find it difficult and stressful especially holidays when Jason is in a different environment without his routine and familiar surroundings
	Jason has some daily living skills		It is felt Jason could develop some skills, e.g. learning to wash his own hair
	Jason needs prompts and reassurance about the sequence of events	His mother will use phrases that have double meanings or even sarcasm that are congruent with typical family life, which Jason can find amusing but often reacts by displaying difficult behaviours or repeating the same question numerous times	His mother is unaware of the way her interaction may precipitate his difficult behaviours. She uses this type of response as 'stress release'

Table 3.4 Second level assessment for Jason, using the adaptability continuum

Highly adaptive zone	OK zone	Debatable zone	Ineffective zone	Strategies to promote adaptation
Jason is in good health	Jason is able to feel relaxed in environments with structured routines such as his respite care placement and his school	The family attempt to accommodate Jason's routine – this includes attempting to go on holidays as a family.	Jason does not receive any prompts from his family for sequential planning and is likely to be made more anxious by this Jason finds being in his brother's company anxiety-provoking Jason's brother does not have any awareness of autism	Some sequential planning using a pictorial diary/planner with some proviso for inadvertent changes A differential reinforcer of other (DRO) behaviours program to lessen aggressive behaviours when Jason's brother is present Jason's mother will instigate a reward programme for Ryan for not provoking Jason Provide some reading materials and discuss with Ryan about his brother's needs Jason to stay in respite care and his relatives while the family go on a holiday

I propose that the way to move forward is to expand the concept of adaptation, as described by Roy, enabling a more pragmatic approach in determining when to develop interventions.

Figure 3.4 places behaviours into zones on a continuum. The 'highly adaptive' and the 'ineffective' zones represent the established position of Roy's model. The 'OK' zone and the 'debatable' zone represent a flexible way to decide, discuss and assess individual issues. To make a judgement, the nurse must consider a number of factors (Box 3.1).

Figure 3.4 The adaptability continuum

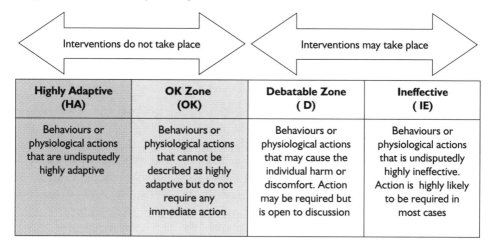

Highly Adaptive (HA)	OK Zone (OK)	Debatable Zone (D)	Ineffective (IE)
Behaviours or physiological actions that are undisputedly highly adaptive	Behaviours or physiological actions that cannot be described as highly adaptive but do not require any immediate action	Behaviours or physiological actions that may cause the individual harm or discomfort. Action may be required but is open to discussion	Behaviours or physiological actions that is undisputedly highly ineffective. Action is highly likely to be required in most cases

Box 3.1 Considerations when defining adaptability

(many of these overlap)

- Current health/illness-based evidence
- Ethical considerations (see Seedhouse 1998) for a detailed discussion on how health care workers should work ethically
- Social mores/norms – what most would see as socially acceptable behaviour in that person's culture?
- Competence – to what level can the individual understand and make a valid choice in relation to the issue?
- Relevant laws
- Risk management (for a useful guide to risk management in services for people with a learning disability see Titterton (2005), Saunders (1999) and Chapter 15
- Human rights – is the personhood of the individual respected?
- Service issues – relating to the resources and implications for the service

To show how the zones should operate, Box 3.2 discusses the issues raised by a woman with a moderate learning disability who smokes 20 cigarettes a day. She lives in a group home where she is 'allowed' to smoke in a designated smoking area. She can afford the cigarettes and has received some health education about the long-term health risks. In Box 3.2 the issues are outlined to enable a complex consideration.

Box 3.2 Defining adaptability for a client who smokes

Current health/illness-based evidence: In this case the evidence of health risks relating to smoking are overwhelming

Ethical considerations: She can make a choice, she smokes in a designated room, she can afford the cigarettes she is most likely to understand the risks. Therefore this individual's behaviour is ethical

Social mores/norms: Although many may object to smoking, it is only in some circumstances that it deemed to be unacceptable

Competency: The service user has demonstrated she has the capacity to understand and make an informed decision

Relevant laws: The Health Act 2006 will apply to smoking in this environment

Risk management: There is some risk of fire, ashtrays needed to be available and the room must be checked regularly. The room should have adequate smoke alarms. Non-smoking service users should be encouraged not to be present when she smokes to avoid risk of passive smoke. The room is well ventilated after the service user has finished smoking. Otherwise the risk is manageable.

Human rights: She has right to smoke in certain parameters i.e. in the smoking area of the residential home.

Service issues: The service provides the individual with somewhere to smoke that does not infringe on others' rights. The service may be subject to changes in rules in future, which may make this less tenable.

Considering this contentious example of a person who smokes brings into focus a number of difficult and challenging issues for health and social care services, which exemplifies the issues of definition outlined previously. Undoubtedly the behaviour, in this case smoking, is ineffective to the physiological system. However the person-centred approach (in this case) identifies that this person is making a valid decision.

An ethical approach for learning disability support services may, in this type of situation, justify continuing to educate (not browbeat) the person about the risks associated with smoking. This could be combined with ongoing monitoring for consequences of the smoking such as hypertension, bronchitis and cancer. Sometimes nurses need to be courageous in enabling a person with learning disability to make problematic or unattractive choices.

Reflection exercise

Here are some examples to help you reflect, discuss and debate issues with your colleagues. The aim is to enable a reflective approach, which goes beyond defining behaviours as 'adaptive' or 'ineffective'. When discussing any of the examples with colleagues it is not important to reach a consensus, as would be case with a real client issue. There are deliberately no answers in this chapter – as this may stifle reflection or discussion.

Which is the most appropriate zone for each of these cases, and why?

- A woman in the autistic spectrum with a mild learning disability will, at set times in the day, drink a daily total of six cups of tea (approximately 1200 ml) with no deviation.
- A woman with a mild learning disability often has sex with men she meets while socialising in various public houses. She does not practise safer sex.
- A gay man with learning disability kisses his partner in a public place and is physically assaulted by a member of the public.
- A man with a moderate learning disability who receives direct payments to enable him and his informal carers to organise his services makes racist comments towards his black workers and does not want them to help him access community facilities.
- A woman with a borderline learning disability has lived in a community-based group home for 15 years. She states at her planning/review meeting that she wants to return to live at the large learning disability hospital from which she was discharged.
- A woman with severe learning disabilities swears at her parents when she wants them to leave her alone. The parents are extremely upset and want her to stop swearing at them.
- A man with cerebral palsy does not want to wear the specialist built-up shoes he has been prescribed.

Manipulating stimuli

Avoid using the term *manipulating stimuli* that Roy and Andrews (1999) use when referring to nursing interventions. It is a rather dated and impractical, clumsy term and does not lend itself to partnership working as it assumes that 'stimuli' are under the direct control and influence of the nurse. In many settings, for example clients living with their families, the stimuli are not under the nurse's direct control. Patton (2004) comments that the term 'manipulation' may lead nurses to assume a paternalistic approach in that they may consider it is a legitimate approach to decide what care a person should receive.

The nurse can usually encourage and educate clients and their families rather than 'manipulating' which has negative, underhand connotations and is far from person-centred. This chapter proposes a collaborative, multidisciplinary approach in accordance with the *Code of Professional Conduct* (Nursing and Midwifery Council 2004, Clauses 4.1–4.7 and the *NHS Improvement Plan* (DH 2004).

Summary

The approaches described show the holistic nature of Roy's model. It enabled a complex understanding of the social world Jason was in – working with the key players in that world enabled some positive movement along the adaptability continuum.

The approach was successful in identifying that the nurse can work legitimately with key players in the person's social world with the goal of enabling some positive movement. In this case study, this included working with Ryan to reward him for not provoking Jason, providing him with information and working with Jason's mother on her interaction style with Jason. If the nurse used an over-focused approach – only focusing on Jason – then it is likely that the nurse would not have given due consideration to his family's needs. However, the nurse suggested that the family might take their holiday without him (which was a positive outcome for them and Jason). To reach this action involved the nurse taking a considered view of the family situation and Jason's position in it.

Using an over-focused approach may have the veneer of a person-centred approach (de facto the person is in the centre) but workers in learning disability services need to acknowledge, understand and work with the people who provide support that service user receives. If an overfocused approach had been undertaken with Jason and his family, the work would have been basically tinkering with the symptoms while not considering the real underlying causes.

Roy's model as a person-centred approach

Using this adapted version of Roy's model it is proposed that it is a way to develop a person-centred approach, as Roy's intrinsically requires the nurse to appreciate the world the person is in. Roy's model could be used work in concert with other processes, such as person-centred planning, community care assessments and discussions in multidisciplinary teams.

Valuing People (DH 2001) and the *NHS Improvement Plan* (DH 2004) emphasise that agencies and stakeholders are required to work together in partnership. Roy's model can allow the nurse to assess the client's existing support. If the nurse considers the client's issues from a holistic perspective, they can offer judgments that are accurate and they can authoritatively comment on the influences that go beyond a level of superficiality, for example, having the potential both to identify who exists in the client's life and demonstrate the carer's beliefs and subsequent care practices that impinge on the client.

In adopting Roy's model the nurse needs to be able to reflect on the concept of adaptability beyond simplistic notions. They should not be grasping at ideology or apply overfocused and simplistic approaches that may appear to be 'good' for the person but fall short of a person-centred approach (as in the smoker example given earlier). This may raise many issues for services for people with a learning disability, which may be challenging and may be difficult to respond to – but this is the nature of developing a truly person-centred approach.

Another major challenge for the nurse is defining the system the client is in. If, for example, a worker was working with a man with learning disabilities who lives on a large housing estate and is harassed by his neighbours. Then it is legitimate that the worker should take steps to facilitate a response from the appropriate agencies. Any worker taking a blinkered approach and ignoring this is likely to be in breach of their formal and moral duties.

Defining the limits of the level of intervention the nurse should seek to influence in relation to the client's social system can raise a number of issues. For example, people with a learning disability, it is well recognised, are a devalued group through many micro- and macro-societal forces. It is unlikely to be considered a legitimate role for a health or social care worker to write a care or intervention plan that includes development of a pressure or campaign group. However, helping people access campaigns for wider social issues that have direct or indirect relation to people with a learning disability may be – in some cases – legitimate.

Roy's model by nature is an individualist model that is congruent with Western views of autonomy. Naidoo (1986, p20) highlights critiques of individualism in health care that view health as a matter of free choice while ignoring the social structures, for example quality of housing, that impinge and influence on health. A balance needs to be achieved between a person's choice, consequences of that choice and their responsibility and their competence – which may be far from easy.

Roy's model allows the nurse to consider others in the network by assessing the interdependence adaptive mode and the contextual stimuli – for example, in the case of a person who likes to play loud music – to the chagrin of other people he lives with. This has the potential to circumvent an overfocused approach. Individual interests could be sought and a way established to enable a level of harmony (for example, he agrees to play his music when other people are out of the house and he uses headphones at other times).

Exceptions to this approach should be when people are obviously highly incompatible. There is a challenge – to what extent does the nurse take the others in the social system into account to meet the individual's needs? Adopting this approach does not mean that people with a learning disability should have to accept the status quo that exists in their social networks. Use of the model can be more emancipatory – it can signpost the client's best interest in a myriad of issues, identify needs that may be quite complex and may help to identify poor or abusive practices.

Service user priority-led service

The nurse must have the client's needs paramount in their interventions and be able to justify their work on this basis. It may be legitimate to move away from describing learning disability services only as 'person-centred' as it may fall short of describing the real ethos that services should develop and may not fully acknowledge the role of key players in the service user's life. I propose the term 'service user priority-led service' (SUPLs) This enables a more accurate description of a concept that is congruent with the ethos of *Valuing People* (DH 2001), which identifies working in collaboration with informal and formal caregivers. Otherwise

Table 3.9 Suggested alternatives to Roy's terminology

Roy's model terminology	Suggested alternative(s)
Stimuli	Influence
Adaptation	Development
	Improvement
	Progress
Focal	First hand experience (s)
Contextual stimuli	Environmental*
Residual	Beliefs
	Viewpoints
	Experiences
Internal environment	Physiological
	Psychological
Manipulation of stimuli	Seek to influence
	Work collaboratively with…
Adaptive mode	Area of life
Ineffective outputs	The client has needs
	The client requires support

Note: avoid using 'the environment' to mean internal physiological and psychological processes

we are in danger of not seeing the wood for the trees when it comes to working effectively with service users and their supporters and carers.

Roy's model has the potential to enable workers in services for people with learning disabilities to identify appropriately the complexities of physiological and social influences on the individual in focus (Parkes 2003). It enables an appreciation of the individual in the social world that they are in. Parkes (2003) comments that if a wider picture is not taken then there could be risk of pathologising the person with a learning disability rather than appreciating that the issue is a manifestation of the influence and power exerted by the social system the person is in.

Roy's model offers a way to assess what is happening in a person's life and its likely impact on them and the social system they are in. It has the potential to enable a holistic overview of the client's life and enable (in partnership with them) to prioritise the timing and level of interventions and support. To illustrate, by reflecting on the example of a man with learning disability who is clinically obese, if an overfocused view was used by assuming that the cause of his obesity was made *only* by his lifestyle choices. This could prevent a more accurate assessment of his informal carer's practices by the amount and type of food prepared for him and the level of physical activity he could undertake. Although this may be a highly simple example, it highlights a possible problem; if an overfocused approach is adopted and one attempts to change behaviours on an individual level with the client, such as healthy eating sessions, giving symbolised leaflets, exercise sessions in day services without taking into account the power and influence of the social system that they are in. Many readers of this chapter may have their own experience of overfocused approaches used with people with and without learning disabilities.

It is a paradox that to achieve a person-centred service, services for people with a learning disability should need to consider the wider social system that the person with a learning disability is in.

Nurses who adopt this approach will need to be cautious in using the terminology devised by Roy because other nurses and workers, service users and carers may not be familiar with the terms. The terms need either to be explained to others in the multidisciplinary team, service users and carers needs to be given or – more advantageously – translated into everyday language. Table 3.9 suggests some everyday terms to communicate the basic tenets of Roy's model.

I thank Jason and Ryan's family for their permission for me to include details of my work with them. I have the utmost admiration for them and enjoyed the work I undertook with Jason and his family.

References

Aldridge J (2004) Learning disability nursing: a model for practice. In: Turnbull J (ed) (2004) *Learning Disability Nursing*. Oxford, Blackwell Publishing

Andrews H, Roy C (1986) *Essentials of the Roy Adaptation Model*. Norwalk, Appleton–Century–Crofts

Attwood T (1998) *Asperger's Syndrome: A Guide for Parents and Professionals*. London, Jessica Kingsley.

Bagenholm A, Gillberg C (1991) Psychological effects on siblings of children with autism and mental retardation: a population-based study. *Journal of Mental Deficiency Research* **35**, 4, 291–307

Baron-Cohen S, Leslie AM, Frith U (1985) Does the autistic child have a 'theory of mind?' *Cognition* **21**, 37–46

Begun AL (1989) Siblings' relationships involving developmentally disabled people *American Journal of Mental Retardation* **93**, 5, 566–574

Conway S, O'Neill K (2004) Home and Away. *Learning Disability Practice* **7**, 7, 34–38

Department of Health (2001) *Valuing People: a new strategy for learning disabilities for the 21st century*. London, The Stationery Office

Department of Health (2004) *The NHS Improvement Plan: putting people at the heart of public services*. London, The Stationery Office

Dixon EL (1999) Community health nursing and the Roy Adaptation Model. *Public Health Nursing* **16**, 4, 290–300

Duquette A (1997) Adaptation: a concept analysis. *Journal of School Nursing* **13**, 5, 30–33

Fawcett J (1989) *Analysis and Evaluation of Conceptual Models of Nursing*. Philadelphia, FA Davis

Gagliardi B (2003) The experience of sexuality for individuals living with multiple sclerosis. *Journal of Clinical Nursing* **12**, 571–576

Galbreath JG (1990) Sister Callista Roy. In: George JB (ed) *Nursing Theories: The Base for Professional Nursing Practice*. New Jersey, Prentice Hall

Gath A (1989) Living with a mentally handicapped brother or sister. *Archives of Disease in Childhood* **64**, 4, 513–516

George JB (1980)(ed) *Nursing Theories: The Base for Professional Nursing Practice*. New Jersey, Prentice Hall

Horan P (2004) Exploring Orem's self-care deficit nursing theory in learning disability nursing. *Learning Disability Practice* **7**, 4, 28–37

Ingram L (1995) Roy's adaptation model and accident and emergency nursing. *Accident and Emergency Nursing* **3**, 3 150–153

LeMone P (1995) Assessing psychosexual concerns in adults with diabetes: pilot project using Roy's modes of adaptation. *Issues in Mental Health Nursing* **16**, 1, 67–78

Logan M (1990) The Roy adaptation model: are nursing diagnoses amenable to independent nurse functions? *Journal of Advanced Nursing* **15**, 468–470

Naidoo J (1986) Limits to individualism. In: Rodmell S, Watt A (eds) *The Politics of Health Education: Raising the Issues*. London, Routledge & Kegan Paul

Nursing and Midwifery Council (2004) *Code of Professional Conduct: Standards for Conduct and Ethics*. London, Nursing and Midwifery Council

Parkes N (2003) Abuse and vulnerability. In: Jukes M, Bollard M (eds) *Contemporary Leading Disability Practice*. Salisbury, Quay Books

Parkes N, Hodges N (2006) Working with and supporting men with a learning disability who are gay, bisexual or attracted to the same sex. In: Jukes M, Aldridge J (eds) *Person-Centred Practices: A Therapeutic Perspective*. London, Quay Books, MA Healthcare

Patton D (2004) An analysis of Roy's adaptation model of nursing as used in acute psychiatric nursing. *Journal of Psychiatric and Mental Heath Nursing* **11**, 221–228

Roy C, Andrews H (1999) *The Roy Adaptation Model* (2nd edn). Stamford, Appleton & Lange

Saunders M (1999) *Managing Risk in Services for People with a Learning Disability*. Nottingham, Association of Practitioners in Learning Disability

Seedhouse D (1991) *Health: The Foundations for Achievement*. Chichester, John Wiley

Seedhouse D (1998) Ethics: The Heart of Health Care. New York, John Wiley

Tang JL, Armitage JM Lancaster T, Silagy CA, Fowler GH, Neil HAW (1998) Systematic review of dietary intervention trials to lower blood total cholesterol in free-living subjects. *British Medical Journal* **316**, 1213–1220

Thornbury JM, King LD (1992). The Roy adaptation model and care of persons with Alzheimer's disease. *Nursing Science Quarterly* **5**, 3, 129–133

Titterton M (2005) *Risk and Risk Taking in Health and Social Welfare*. London, Jessica Kingsley

Villareal E (2003) Using Roy's adaptation model when caring for a group of young women contemplating quitting smoking. *Public Health Nursing* **20**, 5, 377–384

Wing L (ed)(1976) *Early Childhood Autism* (2nd edn). Oxford, Pergamon Press

Yeh CH (2003) Psychological distress: testing hypotheses based on Roy's adaptation model. *Nursing Science Quarterly* **16**, 3, 255–263

Websites

(accessed 8 June 2007)
Roy's model of nursing
www.bc.edu/bc_org/avp/son/theorist/nurse-theorist.html
www.bc.edu/schools/son/faculty/theorist.html

Other nursing models and theory
healthsci.clayton.edu/eichelberger/nursing.htm
www.enursescribe.com/nurse_theorists.htm
library.stritch.edu/nursingtheroies/nursingtheories.htm

CHAPTER 4

The Interactive Model

Maureen Turner

Introduction

This chapter aims to explore the benefits of care delivery to people with learning disabilities based on a model of care that has been specifically designed and developed to meet the complex health and social care needs of this client group. It also explores the influence that changing attitudes from society, medicine, professions allied to medicine and government reports have had on the use of a wide and changing range of frameworks and philosophies of care. These frameworks of care have been used to underpin practice but they have not always met the complex needs of the individual. Evaluation and exploration of these various care philosophies and models of care help to identify omissions in care delivery, and justify the need for a model of care developed from within the profession of learning disability nursing.

A model of care developed within the field of learning disability nursing enables care interventions to be based on appropriate research and sound evidence. Learning disability nurses have the knowledge and skills to access and use a wide range of evidence – the preregistration nursing curriculum includes knowledge of biology, psychology, sociology and nursing.

Various models of care have been used as frameworks on which to provide care for this client group but they were often models adapted from the field of adult nursing, which predominantly provides care to those who are sick or dying. This made them inappropriate as a basis for care delivery to people with learning disabilities as, generally speaking, people with learning disabilities are not sick.

Consequently these models had to be changed and adapted to such an extent that they became fragmented, and the nursing philosophy of the model was lost. It must be argued that people who are sick or dying can often still make an informed choice and may not desire the interventions that are considered most suitable for their condition according to the appropriate research and literature. Learning disability nurses must be able to justify their care practice, as people with learning disabilities may be limited in the choices that they can make. Other disciplines, including medicine and psychology, have also influenced care practices, and changing government agendas have dictated changes in service provision and ultimately care practices.

Although it is central to contemporary practice to empower people with learning disabilities to make choices, people with learning disabilities can only make choices within their ability and limitations to do so. Care interventions must be based on appropriate evidence that can be scrutinised and the intervention justified when the person with a learning disability has been unable to make an informed choice.

To appreciate the importance of developing a model of care specifically for people with learning disabilities we need to understand how previous care approaches have not appropriately met the needs of this client group.

History and background

Throughout history, politicians, professionals from the fields of medicine, psychology, nursing and social work, as well as the general public through various pressure groups, have debated the ways in which people with learning disabilities should be cared for. These opinions have influenced both service provision and care delivery.

Changing care philosophies in more recent years have focused on empowering people with learning disabilities to self-advocate, but the willingness to listen to this client group has tended to be with a view to planning appropriate services, rather than taking account of how individuals themselves would like to be cared for.

The reason for this is that service providers have a vested interest in care delivery being organisation-driven, rather than providing services to entirely meet the needs of the individual.

For many years, people with learning disabilities were cared for in residential services that were the result of varying government reports. These reports have developed as a consequence of changing public attitudes towards people with learning disabilities, rather than the desires of this client group being acknowledged.

Historically, society's attitudes towards people with learning disabilities demanded their exclusion from living ordinary lives and the government responded by the passing of various acts of parliament including the Mental Deficiency Act (1913) and two Mental Health Acts – the Mental Health Act (1959) which was superseded by the Mental Health Act (1983). The recommendations outlined in these acts impacted on the way that people with learning disabilities were to be cared for. However, government acts – while intended to protect and meet the needs of individuals – over time actually become disadvantageous. It was the result of public opinion and legislation that led to the rise of institutions to care and protect people with learning disabilities.

Many people with learning disabilities have been subjected to many years of residential care in establishments that incarcerated them from society and would now be considered as institutions that offered little in the way of care or individuality. This new model of care intends to address many of the problems created for the individual by institutional living. An interactive model of care requires the practitioner to consider the impact of the individual's past life on their current health state and – through effective care planning – address the physical and emotional difficulties created by such environments.

Care in the institution was not based on sound evidence and research but on organisation- driven institutional regimes. The intention in this new model of care is that all interventions in place to address the complex needs of the individual will be based on sound evidence. To address the possible emotional and behavioural issues created by the institution, it is important for the practitioner to understand the concept of institutionalisation, and the effect this may have on the health and well-being of the individual.

Goffman (1961) states that the characteristics of the total institution include lines of command and chains of responsibility that become the care model and there is a social gap between those who control and those who are controlled. There is a staff culture and an inmate culture of varying degrees of sophistication. The institution will have a meaning and purpose, not only in its own frame of reference but also for the community outside.

Hospitals for people with learning disabilities provided large overcrowded wards with poor staffing levels that barely managed to meet the basic physical needs of the individual.

Morris (1965) described nurses providing basic care that consisted of people being washed and dressed en masse. Collective sleeping arrangements were provided that gave no privacy.

It was custom and practice for residents who were considered more able, to care for those with profound disabilities by providing the hands-on care. Meals were taken in a communal dining room, with little hope of teaching self-help skills in feeding, or finding out the likes and dislikes of the individual.

Consequently, people with a learning disability living in this environment became dependent on others for their basic care needs. Many adults with learning disabilities currently living in either the community or small group homes have previously received care in a hospital for people with learning disabilities. It is essential, therefore, that a model of care specifically developed to meet the needs of people with learning disabilities promotes independence through the development of self-help skills, advocacy, social skills and interventions to treat the emotional needs of the individual. This requires the practitioner to consider how each area of an individual's life has interacted to produce the uniqueness of the person, and to meet their needs using the most appropriate knowledge and research.

This principle does not only apply to people with learning disabilities who received care in hospital but to any individual who has a learning disability, as they too will have had a range of life experiences and major life events that impact on their health and well-being.

A person with learning disabilities may express their emotional needs and difficulties by displaying inappropriate behaviour that in part may have been learnt from dysfunctional environments. According to Emerson (1992), high levels of challenging behaviour were seen in institutions but this behaviour was the product of care practices in the institution due to the number of clients in relation to the number of staff. It is understandable how individuals used inappropriate behaviour to get their needs met. Although the literature acknowledges the negative impact of the institution, family dynamics and community living may not always be conducive to achieving maximum health and well-being.

Emerson (1992) also articulates that:

> 'Those individuals in a setting who show the most serious challenging behaviours are likely to receive the greatest amount of staff attention; therefore, if antisocial behaviour is the result of faulty learning, learning theory could be used to change behaviour'

By altering the reinforcement that a given set of behaviours receive, people with learning disabilities could be taught that the same needs may be met by behaving in a more desirable way and this led to a care framework based on behavioural psychology. There is no doubt that the introduction of behavioural intervention therapies saw improvement in both the behaviour and self-help skills of individuals. However, basing care delivery using a behaviourist approach does not meet all the needs of an individual.

This interactive model of care may guide the practitioner to encompass therapeutic interventions based on behavioural research in a care plan but not at the exclusion of other interventions designed to meet the complex needs of the individual. The other aspects of a person's life that need to be considered are their physical emotional and social needs. The intention of this model is that all internal and external factors impacting on the life and health status of the individual – regardless of where they have been cared for – need to be addressed through appropriate care planning and care delivery.

Interventions implemented to address these needs may include building self-esteem through care tasks that enable a person to feel good about themselves. This could be achieved by promoting the internalisation of a positive self-image or creating the opportunity for them to address their emotional needs and unresolved emotional conflicts through a variety of evidence- based therapeutic interventions. Teaching and developing a wide range of self-help and social skills can improve the self-worth of the individual; and any care task that promotes maximum physical health, improved work and leisure activities and communication skills will result in health gains.

The change towards housing people with learning disabilities in much smaller groups – whether they live in the community or in a residential health care setting – has provided the time for more appropriate care interventions to be delivered. For this reason, along with changing attitudes, it is felt that this new model of care is timely and appropriate for current service provision.

It is not only the field of psychology that has influenced how care is delivered to people with learning disabilities. Changes in service provision and care practices have equally been dictated by changing government agendas. *Better Services for the Mentally Handicapped* (DHSS 1971) heralded the development of community care and the notion of living an ordinary life.

Several reports were published following *Better Services* that continued to acknowledge that people with learning disabilities can live a valuable life in the community. Although these reports altered service provision they did not directly deal with the negative experiences of the individual or ultimately change the value base and attitudes of staff. Consequently, change in values, beliefs and philosophy underpinning the care of people with learning disabilities evolved simultaneously with the development of the new services.

The aim of this new model of care is to promote the notion of an ordinary life by facilitating the opportunity for people with learning disabilities to achieve maximum health and well-being, which will enable them to move towards greater independent living that is in keeping with the recommendations of the report *Valuing People* (DH 2001).

Changing attitudes and care philosophies

Wolfensberger (1972), a psychologist, articulated an ideology that to some extent apposed the notion of behaviourism and gave greater credence to the value of the individual. His theories of normalisation articulated the need for people with learning disabilities to live as normal a life as possible and his later theories of social role 'valorisation' described the importance of the person with a learning disability being and feeling valued. Wolfensberger's theories of normalisation were published simultaneously with the changing government agenda and supported the recommendations for small group and community living.

Wolfensberger explained the value for people with learning disabilities of:

- Being given choice over their life decisions
- Being meaningfully occupied
- Being dressed age-appropriately
- Living a productive life as any other member of society

These theories were meant to underpin care practice but in some instances were misinterpreted and seen as a model of care. On the basis of these theories people with learning disabilities were often put into the position of making choices that they were incapable of making – again the result of misinterpretation.

The new interactive model of care embraces these theories as part of the model philosophy to underpin care practice but also recognises the limitations of the individual and suggests that people with learning disabilities should be encouraged to make choices that are informed.

The care planning process considers how an individual may be supported to make appropriate choices. The justification for this is that it is stressful and detrimental to health if choices have to be made which one is incapable of making and often results in the choice being ill-informed. The philosophy of giving choice to people with learning disabilities may seem to portray the ideal –according to Hood and Leddy (1997):

> *'A philosophy is the beliefs and values of individuals or a group*
> *which may because of intellectual enquiry appear reliable'*

However, it must also be considered that philosophies, regardless of their intended ideal, may place the person under stress that is detrimental to their health and well-being. The balance between offering choice and putting people under unnecessary pressure has to be achieved through planning appropriate care.

The impact of Wolfensberger's theories was another philosophical shift that meant care staff became more focused on meeting the social care needs of people with learning disability rather than that of changing their behaviour, but according to Gates (1998) many of their complex health care needs were being overlooked. This again provided the justification as to why a specific model for people with learning disabilities was required. The new model of care enables the practitioner to use knowledge and research from a wide range of sources to develop appropriate care plans that meet the individual's health and social care needs.

Underpinning care practice with theory

Community care has been hailed as the definitive care principle and the philosophy of living an ordinary life has significantly improved the quality of life for people with learning disabilities. However, as Henley (2001) states:

> 'There is the need for caution that, in pursuing care in the community concepts and seeking "rights" that are beneficial for ordinary citizens and for some people with learning disabilities, we do not ultimately deprive many other people with learning disabilities of basic "rights" that are of infinitely greater value to them'

Those basic rights may include the opportunity to express unresolved emotions and conflicts that may impact on the health and well being of the individual. The notion that previous experiences can lead to unresolved conflict that in turn affects the mental well-being of the individual is central to analysing the relationship between a person's history and mental well- being at the assessment stage of this new model and providing appropriate care interventions at the planning stage.

According to Thompson and Mathias (1998) people with learning disabilities suffer from the full range of mental disorder with the highest reported illnesses being affective disorders such as anxiety and depression, which may be related to the lack of opportunity for self-expression. The new model of care considers that one care intervention might be to encourage self-expression with the aim of achieving one ultimate care goal, that may be to treat mental ill health or reduce challenging behaviour. Alternatively, practitioners should consider a wide range of interventions available to treat mental ill health by exploring the interactions of all aspects of a person's life.

Central to this interactive model of care is the belief that all aspects of an individual's life need to be considered at the assessment stage and that all of a person's needs must be considered in the context of their life and not just as one or a list of problems. This stems from the belief that what makes the 'Self' is the unique relationship between all aspects of an individual's life (Figure 4.1).

The Nursing and Midwifery Council Code of Practice states that care practice should be based on sound evidence. Behavioural intervention therapy is based on research and sound evidence from the field of behavioural psychology and is

Figure 4.1 The components of self

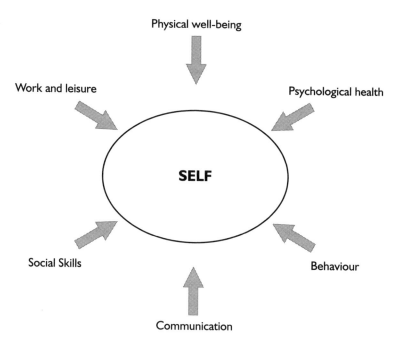

therefore justification for practice. However, Hood & Leddy (2003) suggest that theory is the study of both a class of phenomena and associated uniformities and the relationship between defined concepts. Behavioural psychology may not consider the relationship of concepts necessary for the basis of caring for and meeting the complex health and social care needs of people with learning disabilities. The theory of behavioural psychology concentrates on the uniformities of changing behaviour. Also, it could be argued that behavioural psychology was initially derived from experiments with animals and later applied to human behaviour – the relationship between concepts to meet complex individual need may be missed. Equally, this principle can be applied to the theories of normalisation and social role valorisation that may not guide practitioners to consider the complex physical health care needs of people with learning disabilities.

In the interactive model of care, the role of the nurse is to use a wide range of knowledge, research and theories to provide the most appropriate range of care interventions to address all aspects of a person's life that makes them unique, and to minimise the risk of omissions in both the health and social care needs of the individual.

Nursing models

Hood and Leddy (2003) categorise models into two types – conceptual models or growth models of change. Conceptual models consist of concepts and the relationship between those concepts, for example the individual and their environment. A conceptual model is a systems framework that facilitates the understanding of a range of influences on the whole person.

The interactive model considers the relationship between all factors – internal and external – that function in the life of the person with a learning disability and influence their current health state. The role of the practitioner is to use their knowledge and skills to analyse and synthesise the information collected at the assessment stage to plan appropriate care to meet the complex needs of the individual. (Figure 4.2).

The analysis and synthesis of information during the assessment summary enables the practitioner to plan interventions that are inter-related rather than using a reductionalist approach to care (Figure 4.3).

According to Hood and Leddy (2003) the emphasis placed on each concept varies between models. It is the emphasis of the concept that may make the model an unsuitable framework of care for people with learning disabilities. For example, King's (1989) systems interaction model focuses on:

> '...individuals whose interactions in groups in social systems
> influence behaviour in systems'

While it is important to assess the interpersonal systems of a person with learning disabilities, the implementation of such a model may mean that other factors impacting on the life of a client are missed. According to King (1998), as

Figure 4.2 The components of care

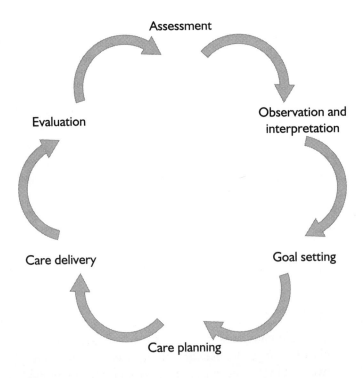

Figure 4.3 The components of optimum health and well-being

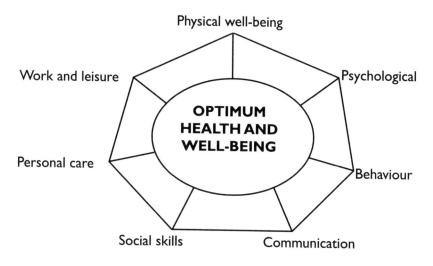

the person interacts with the environment they adjust to deal with the stress. The fact that a person with a learning disability has cognitive impairment may mean their ability to adjust is limited and a different philosophy and focus are required to achieve maximum health and well-being.

The intention of the interactive model is that the nurse is able to intervene in any area of the clients' life that they are unable to manage for themselves and assist them to adjust to deal with their life stresses.

Growth models of change, according to Hood and Leddy (2003):

> 'focus on helping the person's growth to realise or attain full human potential'

Orem's (1980) self-care model is described by Hood and Leddy as a growth model of change, although other theorists have described it as a conceptual model. The underpinning philosophy of caring for people with learning disabilities has been to promote independence and consequently Orem's model has been widely used in caring for people with learning disabilities. However, the model has become fragmented through its adaptation, changing its main philosophy of the model.

The interactive model acknowledges the need for people with learning disabilities to receive education and training to reach their potential for maximum independence – but continues to value the individual in areas where it is impossible for them to succeed. An example of this may be acknowledging that a person with additional physical disabilities may never be continent of urine. This requires learning disability nurses to use their knowledge of biology and continence management. Alternatively, it may be possible to teach an individual new skills and this requires the learning disability nurse to use their knowledge of behavioural psychology to facilitate the teaching of self-help and social skills. The model philosophy acknowledges that the person with a learning disability has the right to receive help in any area of their life they cannot manage for themselves.

The central theory to Orem's model is that of self-care deficit – the absence of the ability to maintain continuous self-care or to maintain health. It could be argued that many people with learning disabilities are unable to maintain self-care or maximum health without intervention. It must also be argued that people with learning disabilities are likely to need long-term intervention to maintain self-care and maximum health and well-being and that the loss of independence in self-care is not a short-term problem. This necessitated a model that can accommodate long-term life changes and accepts the limitations of the individual.

Orem also discusses health deviation in relation to self-care which may require the individual or nurse to seek medical treatment or treatment from other professionals In Orem's self-care model, the need for treatment may be the individual's recognition of need for treatment or the health deviation is an emergency that requires immediate treatment.

The need for the person with a learning disability to seek treatment for a problem with their physical or mental health may be directly related to the aetiology of their learning disability, which they cannot recognise. It is from the analysis of the data collected during the assessment process that particular health issues previously unrecognised by either the client or the carer can be treated.

Equally it must be argued that theories and models developed by nurses from other countries and professional backgrounds may not be suitable for specific client groups. As McKenna (1997) asks:

'Would a theorist whose background was surgical nursing be credible
as an originator of a mental health nursing theory?'

Applying this principle to the care of people with learning disabilities it appeared essential to have a model developed from the knowledge and experience of learning disability nursing. The learning disability nursing curriculum equip nurses with the knowledge and skills that make them credible to develop a model of care specific to their client group.

The Interactive Model

The theory on which nursing models are based can also be entrenched in academic terminology that is difficult for unqualified staff to understand. It is important to recognise this as an issue as a great deal of the hands-on care is carried out by a range of carers and a framework that could be used by all staff is required.

The evidence for the development of a model of care specifically designed and developed for people with learning disabilities arose from a small research study that examined whether learning disability nurses considered a wide range of motivations for a person with learning disabilities and challenging behaviour. This study showed that staff perceived attention-seeking to be the most likely reason why an individual challenged their carers and the service. This is despite the fact that registered learning disability nurses gain knowledge of biology, psychology, sociology and nursing.

The conclusions that were drawn from this study alluded to the influence of behavioural psychology and the move towards a social care model influenced by Wolfensberger's theories of normalisation, both of which had changed the nursing curricula and changed the knowledge base of staff – which led to omissions in meeting the complex health and social care needs of the individual.

In addition, a wide range of nursing models and frameworks for practice were being used on which to plan care but this was not always evident in care delivery. This may have been partly due to the fact that other nursing models taken from the field of adult nursing were being used, but had been altered and fragmented to fit the requirements of people with learning disabilities so the philosophy of the model was often lost. In this model – specifically developed for people with learning disabilities – the model philosophy should be evident in both the care plan and the care tasks that are delivered.

The model philosophy states that:

> 'People with learning disabilities have a right to expect to receive care that meets all of their needs: physical, psychological emotional, social, environmental, education and training. They should also expect to receive care based on sound knowledge delivered by competent practitioners that facilitates their right to receive help in any area of their life that they cannot manage independently'

> (Turner & Coles 1997)

This philosophy statement acknowledges those areas of a person's life that promote health and well-being that are not directly associated with illness. For example, promoting the independence of an individual through teaching self-help skills will result in increased self-esteem and self-value, which are conducive to positive health and well-being.

Because it has been specifically designed for people with learning disabilities rather than implementing adaptations of existing models, the interactive model of care recognises the individual's abilities and limitations in a way that is not devaluing.

Consequently, this model acknowledges the impact that the aetiology of the person's learning disability has on his/her life (if singular). To some extent, this apposes the social models of care suggesting that it is the harmonious relationship between all aspects of a person's life that promotes optimum health and well-being. The model philosophy embraces contemporary practice and ideology and promotes the principles of normalisation and social role valorisation but in clients' ability to benefit positively, rather than identifying these issues in care plans as token gestures to appeal in some way to contemporary thinking. People with learning disabilities can – through tasks that they are able to achieve – demonstrate their value in the community in which they live and make informed choices that are within their ability to make. The model has also been developed to accommodate the consistently changing needs of the person with learning disabilities receiving long-term care – if the health or social care needs of the person change, the appropriate components of the care plan can be adapted to meet these changing needs.

The components of the interactive model are:

- Physical health
- Psychological health
- Behaviour
- Personal care
- Communication
- Social adjustment
- Work and leisure

Social adjustment includes such issues as sexual and spiritual needs, as well as the person's current ability to advocate for themselves.

Assessment checklist

The first stage of the process is the assessment stage, which requires the nurse or carer to collect all the information available on a person. This includes:

- Age
- Gender
- Physical health
- Psychological health
- Behaviour
- Lifestyle, including:
  –Communication
  –Community skills
  –Sexuality
  –Spirituality
  –Work and leisure
- Past history and experiences
- The aetiology of the learning disability

The art of care planning and care delivery using the interactive model is to then consider the aetiology in relation to all other aspects of the person's life which would include their behaviour, environment, history, emotional state, ability and competence in all skills of daily living and work.

The assessment checklist gives examples under each heading to enable the carer to complete the assessment accurately and identify current care interventions. It should **not** be seen or used purely as a checklist but as the first step in finding out as much information as possible about the person.

No rating scale or score chart is used as part of the assessment process, as these can appear demoralising to both the client and carer, particularly if the individual has additional disabilities which may make it impossible to move towards a specific goal in one area of their lives. This acceptance of the person and their limitations values the individual without judgment or conditions. For example, a person with cerebral palsy may not progress to the point of being successful in the area of mobility, so having a measure for this is demoralising.

Assessment summary

The next stage is the assessment summary, which requires the registered nurse to use their knowledge and skills to observe and interpret the interactive relationship between all areas of an individual's life. For example, if the assessment shows that appetite is altered, sleep pattern is disturbed, there is a lack of motivation for self-help skills and other activities, behaviour has become more challenging and the person grew up in an institution it may be reasonable to explore with other professionals the possibility of clinical depression. To arrive at this possibility the registered nurse is required to analyse and synthesise the information collected during the assessment processes. The same analytical process is then used to plan appropriate care interventions to address the identified issues.

The assessment summary requires practitioners to use their knowledge and skills to interpret and analyse the information taken from the assessment checklist and consider the interactions that function internally and externally to maintain the current health state of the individual. This will lead the practitioner to the main care goal and identify the tasks of nursing that need to be delivered to improve the person's health status.

The goal of nursing, therefore, is to achieve one ultimate goal through as many components as are necessary to address the specific needs of the individual – rather than a reductionist approach that identifies several problems but does not consider the inter-relationship of a wide range of aspects impacting on a person's

---

Interactive Model of Care: Assessment toolkit

To put the interactive model of care into your practice, you might find it helpful to use the suite of assessment tools published by the School of Nursing and Midwifery at De Montfort University (1998).

The toolkit contains nine assessment sheets and summary sheets to bring together the information in sheets 1–9 and help you draw up and develop a nursing care plan.

1 Name, address, carer details, details of disability

2 Life history, likes, dislikes, professionals involved in care

3 Physical health problems and medical treatments

4 Psychological health problems and medical treatment

5 Maladaptive behaviours and possible reasons for those behaviours

6 Personal care activities and how much the person can do for themselves

7 Communication skills and problems of poor communication

8 Social skills and problems of poor social skills

9 Work and play activities that the person takes part in

The assessment toolkit is available from: Maureen Turner, School of Nursing & Midwifery, Faculty of Life Sciences, De Montfort University, Leicester, LE1 9BH, England

life. For example, the goal may be to treat depression in a person with learning disabilities. Although medication may be considered as the answer to treatment, it is important to consider care interventions that are equally justified as a means of treating depression, using all components of the model.

The assessment process would clearly identify any physical factors that may be contributing to the individual's needs, such as pain or another health problem. Using the example above it is the responsibility of the registered nurse to consider any health issues that are linked to depression.

The nurse should also consider any psychological factor that may influence the person's behaviour or illness – such as altered memory, altered cognitive ability or any other emotional problem. The relationship between these and other aspects of a person's life also need to be considered, for example that these may be exasperated due to the person's inability to communicate coupled with a lack of activity or meaningful relationships. The past experiences of the individual also need to be taken into account – it may be that they have lived in residential care since childhood and are therefore devoid of meaningful relationships on a day-to-day basis. While the institution did not promote individuality and self-esteem, many relationships were formed in residential care that staff were not always aware of, and with the move to community care these were often lost.

Care planning

Once the assessment summary has been completed, care is planned to address the issues identified. At this stage, it is important to acknowledge what the person can do for themself to address their own needs and for the registered nurse to justify the care intervention based on sound evidence where the individual cannot identify and address their own needs. This may be achieved by care tasks that address the negative effects of institutionalisation and a training plan that teaches self-help skills with a view to promoting independence by improving communication. This will empower the individual to make their needs known and express their feelings. If the person cannot communicate verbally, referral to a speech and language therapist may help them access alternative forms of communication.

The use of art and drawing may also be considered to enable expression. This promotes even greater independence and may prevent the frustrations that have the potential to lead to mental ill health, challenging behaviour and low self-esteem.

Encouraging interest and pride in their appearance through the use of make-up and mirrors helps the person to feel good. By encouraging them to look in the mirror and feel pleased with their appearance they can internalise feeling good and develop self-worth.

Increasing their daily activities encourages and develops motivation this could include involving them in the preparation of food, which may help with appetite loss and create a sense of belonging. By participating in the chores of the home and additional activities, the person can develop meaningful friendships and relationships. The Interactive Model does not address these issues separately, but analyses the interaction of each area of a person's life and develops care plans that

Case study

This is a hypothetical case example

Past history and significant life events

The data collected at the assessment stage identified a 40-year old woman diagnosed with autism who has lived in a hospital for people with learning disabilities since the age of 10. She had lived in a number of different hospital wards, but always those that were labelled for people with challenging behaviour.

Both parents, although elderly, visited regularly.

Her attendance at school had been poor due to her behaviour, particularly biting other children.

Physical health

- There was evidence of premenstrual tension and heavy periods
- She had a history of occasional epileptic seizures
- She was fully continent
- She had a good appetite
- Her weight was in keeping with her height
- She was constantly trying to obtain fluid to drink

Psychological health

- Her moods could change rapidly particularly in response to requests to leave the unit
- She also showed signs of anxiety and agitation
- She occasionally became distressed and tearful
- At other times she laughed and looked cheerful

Behaviour

- She did not mix with the other residents and repeatedly drank water out of the toilet bowl. She permanently carried a large bag full of rubbish that drew attention to her when she was outside the unit.
- Outside activities required three members of staff to accompany her due to the presentation of high levels of challenging behaviour Her challenging behaviours included biting, scratching, hair pulling and screaming, which increased before menstruation. Her behaviour prevented any attendance at daycare activities.
- She would not eat with the other residents and often took food from the plates of others
- Although her family visited regularly she would often ignore their presence and her behaviour precluded them from taking her home.

Personal care

- She was competent in all self-help skills but disliked cleaning her teeth, so the back ones had been neglected
- She liked perfume and make up
- She enjoyed having her hair brushed

Case study (continued)

Communication
- She could communicate with single words
- She could make her needs known through gesture
- She had good comprehension of the spoken word
- She could communicate her likes and dislikes

Social adjustment
- She had no meaningful relationships with her peers
- She could wait her turn or share
- At times she would interact with care staff
- It was difficult to establish her sexual and spiritual needs
- She could not go out into the community alone
- She had no concept of time or money

Work and leisure
- She enjoyed swimming when she was actually in the water
- She liked looking at magazines
- She liked drawing jigsaw puzzles
- She liked listening to music

The assessment summary

The assessment summary considered the possibility of her drinking water from the toilet bowl being the result of diabetes insipidus, of which there was a family history. The test for this revealed that there was no physical problem and the conclusion was that this had to be a behavioural problem.

Closer observation and assessment of her reactions when being encouraged to go out or undertake a task identified an increased level of anxiety. It was also felt that drinking from the toilet may be associated with her feelings of anxiety.

The hoarding of rubbish was felt to be related to insecurity resulting from institutional living. As she had lived in wards for people with challenging behaviour, many of her problems could be linked to feelings of insecurity and lack of self-esteem, self-worth and value. The kind of environments she had lived in meant that she would have had little opportunity to choose or develop meaningful relationships.

Care plan

Her care goal was to reduce the number of behavioural incidence and use of PRN medication.

- Her behaviour linked to her menstrual cycle was recorded and appropriate medication prescribed.
- Due to her age and problems with menstruation a well woman check needed to be undertaken when her behaviour was conducive to this being carried out without stress.
- Initially her challenging behaviour was managed by no eye contact and making her sit calmly with only her needs/desires being met for calm sitting behaviour.

- Through analysis of the assessment summary her behaviour in relation to leaving the unit appeared to be due to her anxiety that could be associated with her diagnosis of autism. The task of care delivery was to reduce her levels of anxiety and fear. She was encouraged to walk to the end of the path outside the unit but always leaving the door open so that she could go back at any point. The justification for this is that it is less anxiety provoking if the individual can freely go back to a secure place. On returning to the unit she was given a drink of tea, as this was something she did enjoy. The distance of going out gradually became further away from the unit until she would get on the unit transport but was able to get off immediately. Her parents also encouraged her to sit in their car. This progressed over a two-year period and she now goes out to all kinds of community activities and also goes home at the weekends. Her elderly relatives can manage her at home for the first time in several years.

- In collaboration with the speech and language therapist she was given photographs of various facial expressions that depicted a range of different moods. She used these to show staff how she was feeling – this enabled staff to react appropriately and allay her anxieties. By providing the opportunity for this woman to identify how she was feeling, the need for her to be challenging was diminished. After almost two years of intervention there were no behavioural incident forms completed and she had not received any PRN medication.

- Once she could communicate how she was feeling, staff could offer her the reassurance she was seeking. This provided the opportunity to implement daycare activities designed around tasks that she enjoyed but with the purpose of improving her self-help, social and communication skills. For example, she liked to draw but this activity also encourages self-expression. Games that are played as part of the daycare activities encouraged sharing and turn taking as well as teaching numerical skills.

- This woman was encouraged to become part of the community in which she lived by first of all closing the curtains in the evening for everyone. This was followed by setting the tables for meals. She was also encouraged to sit opposite to one other woman at meal times and pass a drink or the condiments to her. Staff consistently used both of their names and encouraged giving each other eye contact. The justification for this intervention being that doing tasks for others develops a sense of belonging. Interacting with one other person begins the development of relationships with others. This also provided the opportunity for staff to thank her and make her feel valued and encouraged the social appropriateness of meal times. This has also facilitated the opportunity for her to learn to share and take turns.

- In the evening she would go to her room and play music or look through a catalogue with a member of staff who consistently encouraged her to identify items of clothing that she liked. The outcome of this is that she now chooses to sit with the same woman she sat with at meal times at various times of the day looking at magazines and is clear about her likes and dislikes.

Case study (continued)

- A mirror was purchased and after she had chosen her clothes in the morning she was told that she looked nice but equally was encouraged to look in the mirror and point to herself and say 'I look nice'. Simultaneously, the task of promoting self-esteem was carried out in daycare and she followed a programme of having her nails painted which encouraged choice, promoted self-esteem and provided the opportunity for her to experience pleasurable touch. She was also prompted to use the mirror to look at the back of her mouth and watch the toothbrush cleaning her back teeth. She had to choose her own clothes and time was taken at bathtime to chose and use toiletries and perfume that acknowledged that she is a 40-year-old woman.

- The day care staff met regularly with the care team to ensure that one plan of care was being delivered with the same aims of care. Again the aim of focusing on personal appearance was to address some of the problems that appeared to have been created by years of institutional living. Both the unit and day care programme encouraged her interest in food preparation that again involved participating with others.

- Her large bag was replaced by smaller and smaller bags as she became more confident and willing to surrender her rubbish, using behavioural techniques. She currently carries a small block in her hand that appears to give her the security she needs without drawing attention to herself.

- All activities set for this woman had to be achievable for her to be consistently successful with the intention of promoting her self-value and self-worth.

- She was encouraged to make as many choices in her daily life as she could, although it was recognised that her ability to self-advocate could take years of building up on the ability to make small choices.

This care plan had twelve components to achieve the one care goal of reducing the number of behavioural incidents and reducing the amount of times PRN medication is given. Although the more complex the life of the individual the more components there would be to the care plan.

Evaluation can be obtained from this kind of quantitative data and the care plan should be live and on going. Each component of the care plan can be supported by the appropriate literature.

This woman now enjoys a full programme of activity and can go out into the community with just one member of staff. To be able to participate in a range of activities including accessing community facilities must have enhanced her quality of life. Her physical appearance has changed and she does look happy.

– through appropriate care delivery – will achieve the ultimate care goal.

Central to the Interactive Model is the belief that through appropriate nursing tasks any negative influences can be addressed and altered. The uniqueness of the individual determines how these influences interact and impact on their life.

For example, for a person with cerebral palsy the impact of having a physical disability can be addressed by setting achievable goals through care delivery that enables them to feel valued, maximises their ability to become more independent and uses their strengths, likes and dislikes. This also means identifying – in the care plan and through care delivery – what the person can do for themselves and those tasks that the carer needs to undertake while retaining the person's dignity and respect.

For a person with cerebral palsy, this may mean the carer is required to undertake many of the tasks of daily living; while for the person with learning disabilities who desires to lose weight this may mean providing the appropriate information.

Conclusion

It may be argued that many registered learning disability nurses do intervene appropriately with clients to meet their complex health and social care needs. The intervention model of care provides the framework to ensure that:

- There are no omissions
- The intervention can be justified from a wide range of evidence
- All aspects of an individual's life have been considered.

The focus of this model is on the assessment summary and care delivery. The tasks of nursing that are delivered improve quality of life for the person.

The influences on the practice of caring for people with learning disabilities has been derived from a wide range of professions, government and pressure groups in society and the development of this model was to some extent influenced by the inappropriateness of some care practices. This is mainly because previous models and frameworks for care have focused on a range of problems without those problems and needs being considered in the context of the person's life.

The intervention model of care was evaluated as part of the process of applying for practice development unit status for a unit that had implemented this model of care. The indications were that this approach to care delivery has increased activity for some people who were precluded from many activities because of their behaviour. Also care plans and medication charts indicate that there is an increase in medication being used for general health issues rather than to reduce challenging behaviour. The conclusion that may be drawn from this is that staff teams can focus on all aspects of an individual's life – not just those that present a problem to the care providers.

People who were quite socially isolated have started to form relationships with each other and have much greater access to community facilities. The use of PRN medication appears to have fallen and fewer behavioural incident forms have been completed.

This model shows that all professionals involved with a person's care can use the same model. For example if the one care goal is to improve communication the speech therapist can use the same model to achieve the same goal. The model also encourages carers to refer people to the appropriate professional rather then assuming that they can undertake tasks for which they are not qualified.

The greatest notable change appears to have been in the perception of staff towards clients. It seems that by giving staff a greater understanding of the motivation for a client's behaviour their attitude towards the client has changed.

This model of care can underpin the care delivery for any person who has a learning disability and requires intervention to improve their quality of life.

References

Department of Health and Social Security (1971) *Better Services for the Mentally Handicapped.* London, HMSO

Department of Health (2001) *Valuing People: A new strategy for learning disability for the 21st century.* London, The Stationery Office

Emerson (1992) cited in: Bromley J, Emerson E (1995) Beliefs and emotional reactions of care staff working with people with challenging behaviour. *Journal of Intellectual Disability Research* **39**, 4, 341–352

Gates B, Beacock C (eds) (1998) *Dimensions of Learning Disability.* New York, Addison–Wesley–Longman

Goffman (1961) cited in Morris P (1965) *Put Away: a sociological study of institutions for the mentally retarded.* Routledge & Kegan Paul, p21

Henley CA (2001) Good intentions – unpredictable consequences *Disability and Society* **16**, 7, 933–947

Hood LJ, Leddy SK (1997) cited in Hood LJ, Leddy SK (2003) (eds) *Conceptual Basis of Professional Nursing.* Lippincott Williams & Wilkins, pp181–194

Hood LJ, Leddy SK (2003) (eds) *Conceptual Basis of Professional Nursing.* Lippincott Williams & Wilkins, pp181–194

King (1989) cited in Hood LJ, Leddy SK (2003) *Conceptual Basis of Professional Nursing.* Lippincott Williams & Wilkins, pp181–194

McKenna H (1997) *Nursing Theories and Models (Routledge Essentials for Nurses)* p224

Mental Deficiency Act (1913) cited in Morris P (1965) *Put Away: a sociological study of institutions for the mentally retarded.* Routledge & Kegan Paul, pp12–13

Mental Health Act (1959) London, HMSO

Mental Health Act (1983) London, HMSO

Morris P (1965) *Put Away: a sociological study of institutions for the mentally retarded* Routledge & Kegan Paul 12–13 pp10, 12, 17

Nursing and Midwifery Council (2004) *Code of Practice.* London, NWC

Orem D (1980) Cited in: Hood LJ, Leddy SK (2003) *Conceptual Basis of Professional Nursing.* Lippincott Williams & Wilkins, pp193–195

Thompson A, Mathias P (1998) *Standards and Learning Disability.* Baillière Tindall

Turner M Coles (1997) Meeting the needs of people with learning disabilities: developing an interactive model of care. *Journal of Learning Disabilities for Nursing, Health and Social Care* **1**, 162–170

Wolfensberger W (1972) Cited in Mullick JA, Kedesdy JH (1988) Self-injurious behaviour: its treatment and normalisation. *Mental Retardation* **26**, 4, 234–239

CHAPTER 5

Models for practice
The Ecology of Mental Health Framework

John Aldridge and Dave Ferguson

Introduction

Although conceptually based on the Ecology of Health Framework (Aldridge 2003; 2004) this framework is not intended to assess holistic health in a general sense, but specifically as a means of understanding the dynamics of the mental health of people with learning disabilities. It is therefore a conceptual framework of mental health, rather than a nursing model in the conventional sense.

The framework has been developed in answer to the need for a nursing assessment, as opposed to a psychiatric diagnostic tool and is intended to be complementary to, rather than an alternative for, tools such as the Mini PASS-ADD Interview Pack (Moss 2002) and other aids to diagnosis. The framework therefore avoids psychiatric terminology such as 'depression' or 'schizophrenia', and instead focuses on the range of universal elements that may influence mental health and mental illness.

As a nursing assessment, it is part of the range of multidisciplinary assessments that might be used in mental health, rather than an alternative. It may be used to complement assessments, including diagnostic assessments carried out by members of the multidisciplinary team, to gain a broad picture. The Ecology of Mental Health framework will also enable the nurse to identify those issues requiring nursing action, as opposed to a narrower concept of psychiatric treatment.

Priest and Gibbs (2004) note that there is a frequent association between challenging behaviour and mental illness in people who have learning disabilities and that it is often difficult to differentiate between the two. Professionals are often faced with a referral to an individual whose behaviour is strange or challenging. A deeper analysis of such behaviour may show that is driven by a range of possible causes:

- Physical factors, such as pain
- Learning and reinforcement
- Mental illness
- Environmental and interpersonal factors.

The Ecology of Mental Health framework acknowledges these factors and aims to:

- Provide a framework for the identification and analysis of mental illness and/ or challenging behaviour in people with learning disabilities
- Enable hypothesis building by prompting the user to develop a theory of what has influenced the individual's behaviour and why the individual has become ill
- Identify issues in the role of the nurse
- Identify issues for shared working in the multidisciplinary team.

It can be seen that the framework therefore operates at both a descriptive and analytical level and is broadly designed to help the user explore the relationships between the range of factors that may influence an individual's illness or behaviour.

The conceptual basis of the framework

Mental health may be thought of as an ecological system, that is, a system in which the individual's behaviour may be influenced by the inter-relationships between a large number of factors. The ecology of the individual's mental health may be diagrammatically represented as an elongated cube, of which the front face is seen (Figure 5.1).

In this cube are a number of concentric layers that represent the range of influences on the person's mental health. We may imagine the front face as a slice across the cube, as a 'snapshot in time' that represents the Present. We can see that stretching back behind this is the Past. A further elongation of the cube (that we cannot clearly see) represents the Future (Figure 5.2).

The behavioural interface

The individual's behaviour forms the starting point for an analysis of the range of possible influencing factors (Figure 5.3) because their behaviour is usually the reason for referral and because it forms the interface between the person and their external environment. Behaviour is therefore broadly influenced by a range of factors that may be called 'internal factors' or 'external factors'. Behaviour in mental health terms falls into two main categories:

- Behaviours that are cause for concern
- Behaviours related to coping and responding

'Cause for concern' behaviours

In mental health work, it is often the individual's behaviour that alerts to the need for intervention and support. The person may complain that they are coping poorly, but very often it is aspects of the individual's behaviour that cause others to comment that they are 'not themselves' and that they are behaving oddly in some way. It is the person's behaviour, therefore, that usually leads to them being considered for mental health assessment. This behaviour needs to be uncharacteristic, to represent a marked change in the individual's usual behaviour

Figure 5.1 The Ecology of Mental Health model

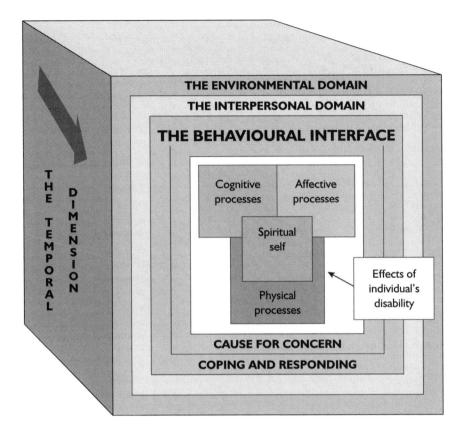

and needs to be relatively enduring to be a cause for concern. 'Cause for concern' behaviours are indicators of mental illness and fall into four broad areas that are present to a greater or lesser degree in all mental illnesses:

Distress: This is behaviour that suggests the individual is disturbed or deeply unhappy in some way. For instance, the person may spend long periods crying, be irritable, show signs of marked anxiety or fear or be tense and watchful. They may feel physically ill and be convinced that they are dying of some disease.

Dysfunction: We may notice that the person is no longer coping with aspects of their daily living:

- In domestic and personal care, they may look unkempt and dishevelled, they may no longer be keeping their home as clean and tidy as before.
- In social relationships, they may become withdrawn, disinterested in social situations, unable to relate to others.
- In work and occupation, they may no longer be able to carry out the duties of their job or to occupy themselves in a constructive way.

Figure 5.2 The past, present and future elements of the model

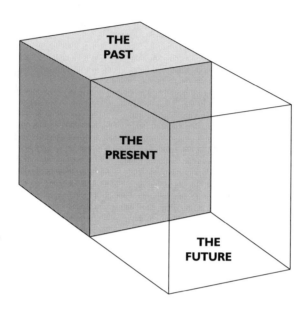

Figure 5.3 The behavioural interface

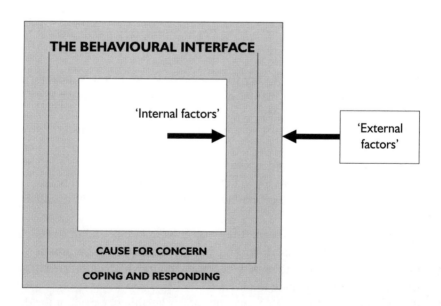

Deviance: from social, cultural and personal norms. The person may behave in markedly unusual ways that go beyond eccentricity:

- Odd and bizarre behaviour that may be very noticeable and at variance with their own society or culture
- Extremes of over or underactivity and unusual patterns of rest and activity
- Extremes of routines, habits and rituals

Risk, vulnerability and dangerousness: Morgan and Wetherell (2004) note that people who are mentally ill are often seen as posing a threat to members of society and that there are recorded instances of mentally ill people who have committed acts of violence. The implication here is that mentally ill people are dangerous and pose a threat to others. Certainly, this may be true in a small number of cases, but Barker (2003) also points out that mentally ill people are also vulnerable and that this vulnerability is often a noticeable feature of their illness. Vulnerability may be a more prevalent feature of mental illness than dangerousness. If we combine dangerousness and vulnerability under the heading of 'risk', then we might observe risky behaviours as:

- Putting self at risk
- Putting others at risk
- Putting the environment at risk

Disorientation: Some mental illnesses may cause the person to be confused and lacking appropriate awareness in a number of ways:

- Confusion as to *time* – not being aware of the true time of day, time of the year or of the year itself
- Confusion as to *place* – lacking appropriate awareness of where they are (for example, thinking they are in their parental home when they are actually in residential care)
- Confusion as to *activity* – the individual may forget what they are doing and wander around aimlessly, often with little sense of where they are
- Confusion as to *person* – talking to and relating to people as though they were someone else (e.g. their mother who died years ago).

Many of the cause for concern behaviours are often found in people with learning disabilities and are part of the phenomenon of 'diagnostic overshadowing' (Reiss et al 1982). We need to differentiate between behaviours that have been an enduring and consistent part of the individual's character and those that have appeared reasonably recently.

Coping and responding behaviours

While being aware of behaviours that cause concern, we also need to achieve a balanced view between positive and negative factors. Indeed, the Stress–Diathesis (Goldman 1992) and Stress–Vulnerability (Zubin & Spring 1977) models of mental illness emphasise that mental illness tends to be caused by the relationship between stressors and the individual's ability to cope with them. We therefore need to identify behaviours that help the individual to cope with everyday life and to respond to demands and hassles. These behaviours might be divided into two main kinds, based on the Lazarus and Folkman (1984) Transactional Model of Stress and Coping and the Knussen et al (1992) Ways of Coping (Revised) Questionnaire.

Adaptive strategies are behaviours that:
- Are helpful in the long term
- Are effective
- Enable the development of coping

They include:
- Using social, family and informal networks
- Using professional supports
- Practical coping, including learning new skills, taking action and exercising choice
- Emotional coping, including seeking emotional support, sharing feelings, stoic acceptance and use of humour
- Cognitive coping, including developing understanding, reframing, positive thinking and problem solving

Maladaptive strategies are behaviours that:
- Do not help in the long term
- May be harmful
- Are ineffective

They include:
- Avoidance, simply avoiding situations that are stressful
- Denial, refusing to accept that there is a problem
- Blaming others
- Wishful thinking
- Misuse or overuse of alcohol, drugs, smoking, comfort eating
- Using aggression
- Self-harm
- Passive acceptance and helplessness
- Withdrawal from social interaction

Figure 5.4 shows the inter-relationships between factors in the stress–coping model.

The personal domain: internal factors

The personal domain consists of those factors that in some way relate to the person themselves, that are part of their physical or psychological make-up and can be divided into: (Figure 5.5):
- The effects of the individual's disabling condition
- Physical processes – the Physical Self
- Cognitive processes – the Thinking Self
- Affective processes – the Emotional Self
- The Spiritual Self

Figure 5.4 The interplay between factors involved in mental health and mental illness

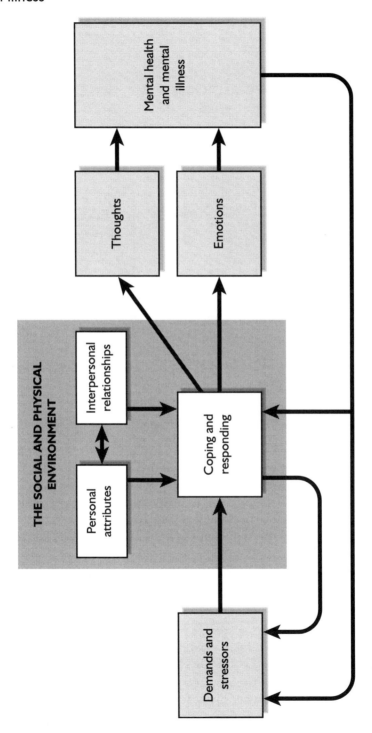

Figure 5.5 Internal factors – the personal domain

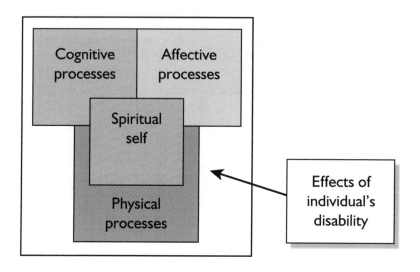

The effects of the individual's disabling condition

Certain learning disabling conditions carry risk factors for some kinds of mental illness and predispose the individual to become ill.

For instance, Down's syndrome carries risk factors for:

- Depression (Cooper & Collacott 1996)
- Alzheimer's disease (Cooper 1997)
- Hypothyroidism, which may present as 'pseudodementia' (Holland 1994; Tsouris & Patti 1997)

Other conditions may have characteristics that are close to the symptoms of mental illness and create a further example of diagnostic overshadowing. However, if they are sufficiently severe, they could constitute a mental illness. For example, characteristics in the autistic spectrum that overlap with mental illness are

- Anxious personality – the individual's 'ambient anxiety' may normally be quite high
- Obsessional traits – the individual may have a number of fixed behaviour patterns and be resistant to changes in routine
- Lack of 'interpersonal understanding' and socially dysfunctional behaviour

Individuals with Asperger's syndrome may also be at higher risk of depression and may be misdiagnosed with schizophrenia (Klin & Volkmar 1995; Eisenmajer et al. 1996; Attwood 1998).

We need to differentiate between characteristics that are part of the individual's disability and those that are suggestive of a mental illness, but we should also be alert to the increased likelihood that a person may be at higher risk. We need to guard against jumping to premature conclusions. If we are assessing a person with

Down's syndrome who is aged 50 and losing their abilities it does not necessarily mean that they are developing dementia. In any case, the role of the framework is not to reach a psychiatric diagnosis, but to identify those aspects of daily life with which individuals have difficulty and to identify why those difficulties exist.

The level of the person's learning disability will also have an effect on their cognitive functioning, their level of understanding and their communication skills. These factors in particular may make the process of assessment and therapy extremely difficult, especially if the individual's disability is severe.

The Physical Self

The relationship between mental and physical health is almost impossible to separate and a holistic view acknowledges the interdependence of the two. A full understanding of the person and their behaviour must therefore incorporate their physical self and physical health because our physical being at least partially determines who we are and how we regard ourselves. A further issue is that people with learning disabilities tend to have a higher level of health need, but a lower use of health services (Simpson 1995; DH 2001).

Physical ill health is more common in people with mental illness than in the general population (Bird 1999) and we need to be alert to the possibility of a mentally ill person additionally being physically ill. We need to screen for physical conditions and physical illness to ensure that

- The person is not physically ill as well as mentally ill
- Their symptoms are truly indicative of mental illness, rather than a physical illness
- There is not an underlying physical condition that is causing or exacerbating the person's mental illness

Although a thorough physical examination and screening are advisable, there are certain physical systems that would be of particular interest (Table 5.1).

The Thinking Self

We are thinking beings who have consciousness and awareness. We think about ourselves and our experience and our behaviour is to a certain extent governed by our thoughts. We may make a conscious decision to behave in a certain way because of what we think or believe and our understanding of the world. However, not all behaviour is consciously determined – large parts of our cognitive processes take place at a preconscious or unconscious level.

As long ago as 1985 Lovett observed that traditional behavioural approaches to working with people with learning disabilities emphasised the ability to objectively describe individuals' behaviour while ignoring the thoughts and emotions that impel that behaviour (Lovett 1985). It now seems clear that to understand why a person is behaving in a certain way we need to understand what they are thinking and how this motivates them. However, we should also acknowledge the level of the individual's intellectual impairment and the effect this has on cognitive functioning and their ability to communicate their thoughts and ideas.

Table 5.1 The relationship between physical systems and mental illness

Physical system	Some reasons for interest
Neurological	Partial complex epilepsy presenting as pseudo-hallucinations
	Epileptic seizures causing alterations in consciousness and attention
	Tumours affecting sensory and cognitive processes
Endocrine	Hypothyroid presenting as pseudo-dementia
	Hormones creating mood variation
Pain and discomfort	Causing lowered mood
	Causing sleep disturbance
	Causing loss of appetite
	Causing irritability and 'challenging behaviour'
Blood and circulation	Anaemia causing loss of energy
Gastrointestinal	Malfunction causing weight loss
	Discomfort causing loss of appetite

The Thinking Self may be subdivided into:
- Cognitive maturity
- Cognitive problem solving
- Attention and concentration span
- Memory
- Moral reasoning
- World view, world knowledge, ideas, beliefs and ideologies
- Effects of medication on cognitive processes

Cognitive maturity is of particular interest because it relates directly to the individual's learning disability or intellectual impairment. While we should not necessarily take it too literally, Piaget's (1952) theory of cognitive development may be used as a convenient basis for a framework for understanding the way in which a person's thinking develops and matures.

This by no means implies that we should think of people with learning disabilities as being childlike, or that we should treat them as children. It does, however, acknowledge that their understanding and thinking may be 'developmentally young'. This then gives us a basis for understanding both the individual's experience of the world and how we might offer therapeutic opportunities. Table 5.2 oversimplifies Piaget's theory, but may offer some insights.

To place a person in one of the stages of cognitive development, we might ask:
- How does the individual appear to experience the world?
- How do they use language?

Table 5.2 A simple overview of Piaget's developmental stages

Stage	Experience	Thought processes and behaviour	Use of language
Sensori-motor	'A here and now world'	• Pleasure/displeasure • Immediacy of needs and responses • Exploration through the senses • Development of object permanence and basic schemas	• Pre-linguistic until late in this stage. • Early use of words as labels (though over-inclusive) forms a bridge to pre-operational thought
Pre-operational	A magical world'	• Influenced by *appearance* of objects, rather than other characteristics • Pretend and symbolic use of objects • Egocentric view • Pre-logical reasoning • Problem solving by guesswork	• Internal representation through early use of language, allows the person to think about things and to apply reasoning • Basic use of language to describe experience • Thoughts externalised (running verbal commentary on thoughts)
Concrete operations	An ordered world'	• Use of inductive logic to problem-solve (development of general principles from own experience) • Ability to deal with more than one characteristic of objects • Grasp of principles of reversal of processes • A need for concrete objects to aid thought and problem solving	• Developing vocabulary and sophistication of language allows relative complexity of ideas • Use of language as a means of discovery, inc. use of reading and writing • Language more internalised
Formal operations	'A logical world'	• Development of deductive logical thought (novel answers from general principles) • Grasp of abstract concepts • Ability to carry out abstract mental problem solving	• Creative use of language to manipulate ideas at an abstract level

- What does this tell us about their likely understanding and thought processes?
- How might we interview and explore issues with them?
- How might we offer therapy?

Assessing the person's **moral reasoning** may be particularly appropriate if they have been involved in offending behaviours or seriously challenging behaviours. Moral reasoning is about the individual's understanding and beliefs regarding right and wrong. A formal and structured assessment could be based on either Piaget's moral stories (Piaget 1932) or Kohlberg's (1963) moral dilemma – a summary of both can be found in Eysenck (2004) and Gross (2005). In practice, an adaptation of Piaget's moral stories will probably be found to be more useful.

A more informal approach might be taken by talking to the person about their behaviour to see if they have an awareness of the morality of their behaviour or a regard for the rights of others.

Memory is particularly impaired in dementia, but may also be affected in mood disorders. People with learning disabilities often lack the skills to rehearse and retain information and their working memory may anyway be quite poor. General areas of investigation might include:

- Long-term memory – the individual's recall of distant events
- Short-term memory – the individual's recall for recent events
- Does the person seem consistently disoriented to time and place?

If dementia is suspected, more formal assessment tools, such as the Dementia Questionnaire for Persons with Mental Retardation (Evenhuis et al 1990) or the Dementia Scale for Down syndrome (Gedye 1995) could be used.

Assessment of the individual's **'world view'**, their knowledge and beliefs may be particularly useful if they seem to be expressing strange ideas. However, it is important to differentiate between delusory beliefs and those that result from an imperfect understanding or lack of information (see the section on cognitive–developmental maturity). We can ask:

- To what extent is the person appropriately oriented to current events, people and places, both in their own lives and in the media (in the constraints of their experience)?
- Does the person express ideas that are markedly odd, bizarre or seriously at odds with reality?
- Does the person express compulsive thoughts or ideas?

The effects of medication on cognitive processes may be particularly relevant if the individual is already taking psychotropic medication, antimuscarinics or anticonvulsants. These may affect consciousness and alertness and in some cases, side effects may even cause abnormal sensory experiences.

Generally, relatively little is known about the effects of powerful psychotropics on people with learning disabilities and it is possible that their response to these may be atypical.

The Emotional Self

Clark et al (1991) comment that staff and carers often do not pay sufficient attention to the emotional needs of people with learning disabilities, but this may be for a number of complex reasons. The most tempting explanation is that it is relatively easy to care for people at a physical level because this can be done in a mechanical and routinised way. It is more demanding to respond to peoples' emotional needs and it may be that these are simply ignored. However, Black et al (1997) report that difficulty in recognising, managing and communicating both their own and others' emotion is common among people with learning disabilities. It may be difficult for a carer to assess and respond to peoples' emotions because they express them in atypical or restricted ways.

Emotions are at least as important as thoughts in motivating peoples' behaviour and in some ways may be more important to our assessment. Although people with learning disabilities may be intellectually impaired, there is no evidence that they are emotionally impaired. Everyone experiences emotions (even young babies); even though they may not be able to identify and communicate what emotion they feel. In mental health work, mood disorders are a substantial sector of the range of mental illness and people with learning disabilities are probably at greater risk of developing mood disorders than any other kind of mental illness. In assessing the Emotional Self, we need to build up a picture of the person's emotional experience, particularly under these headings:

- Emotional maturity
- Predominant mood palette, including emotional range and predominant emotions
- Stability of mood
- Emotional response to personal stressors
- Emotional understanding ('emotional literacy')

Emotional maturity is a similar concept to cognitive maturity in that it recognises that people may differ in their capacity to understand, to deal with and express emotional issues. As before, it in no way implies that people with learning disabilities are emotionally like children or that they should be treated emotionally like children. Emotional maturity is chiefly about:

- The need for emotional support from others – as we grow older we rely less on others for our emotional security, moving from dependence to interdependence
- The degree to which we refer to others for approval – we become more self-referenced as we grow older
- Our ability to deal with frustration and emotional stress
- Our ability to understand our own and others' emotions and to express this in acceptable ways.

The predominant mood palette refers to the analogy between an artist's palette, which may contain a range of colours and mood involving a range of emotions (Figure 5.6). Each person's mood palette is individual to them and

Figure 5.6 An example mood palette for Depressed Mood

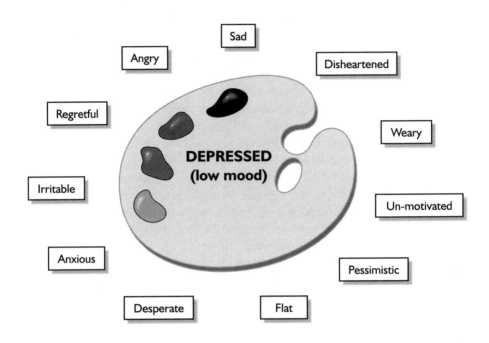

may contain a different range of emotions to that of another person experiencing the same mood. Particularly in the case of mood disorders we need to know the individual's predominant mood and the emotions associated with each mood.

The range of emotions may differ greatly from one individual to another and is not necessarily related to intelligence or cognitive maturity. Some people seem to experience a relatively small range of emotions, others experience a much greater variety. Much depends on the individual's ability to express and communicate their emotional state to others or to be able to recognise and name some of the finer shadings of emotion.

Although we may use the words 'anxious' and 'apprehensive' it may be quite difficult in clear terms to define the difference between them and each of us may perceive these emotions in an idiosyncratic way.

Stability of mood refers to the degree to which the individual's mood alters from one situation to another or from one day to another. We may also need to know what affects changes in mood. Is there a pattern to mood fluctuations and does variation occur gradually or suddenly?

In many cases, we need to know about the individual's **emotional response** to personal stressors. What kinds of situations do they find stressful and how do they respond emotionally to them? Again, what each person finds stressful is likely to be individually determined. We cannot make predictions about levels of stress merely because we believe that they *ought* to be stressful or not stressful. What non-learning disabled people find stressful does not always relate to those things that people with learning disabilities find stressful (Ramirez et al 2000).

The term **'emotional literacy'** refers to individuals' understanding of and insight into mood. Reed (1997) notes that before an individual can report on their emotional state they must be able to understand what it means to be happy, sad and so on. She further notes that this understanding is a developmental task and that there may be specific impairment in emotional understanding in people with learning disabilities. A method of testing emotional understanding is offered in Reed and Clements (1989).

The Spiritual Self

The Spiritual Self is the core of the individual and encompasses how they see themselves (in a physical sense), what they think about themselves and how they feel about themselves, as well as self-identity. As with many other psychological aspects of the framework, it may be very difficult to develop a clear picture of the individual's Self. The Spiritual Self incorporates:

- Religious, cultural and ethnic self
- Locus of control and self-confidence and self-determination
- Self-concept and self-knowledge
- Self-esteem
- Self-expression and communication

The religious, cultural and ethnic self describes the individual's sense of self-identity in relation to the society in which they live. A sense of self may be influenced by religious belief, although this is not always the case in our increasingly secular society. Religion offers explanations for such questions as 'Where do I come from? ' 'How should I live my life?' and 'What happens when we die?' and therefore may inform not only Self but also thoughts, feelings and behaviour.

Locus of control: (Rotter 1966) describes the extent to which people see themselves as being in charge of their own lives. *Internal* locus of control is when the individual believes that they influence their life through their own decision-making. *External* locus of control is where the individual believes that other people make things happen in their life.

We need to remember that for people with learning disabilities the power often does lie with others and therefore external locus of control may be an entirely accurate reflection of power relationships. Locus of control is closely related to Seligman's (1974) concept of learned helplessness and may offer a useful insight into the experience of people who spent their formative years in institutions.

Self-concept and self-knowledge relate to the degree of insight that the individual has into himself or herself as a person. It incorporates body image and beliefs (as opposed to emotions), for example 'How do I see myself?' 'What sort of person am I?' 'What things am I good at and what things am I less good at?'

Self-esteem is about the emotions that a person has in relation to himself or herself and relates closely to the relationship between self-image and self-ideal.

The individual may feel satisfied, comfortable and happy with themselves (positive self-esteem) or dissatisfied, uncomfortable and unhappy with themself (low self-esteem). One of the problems with self-esteem is that it may be wholly realistic or unrealistic or partly realistic and partly unrealistic. Low self-esteem is often involved in mood disorders and can lead to the negative assumptions and negative predictions that are often at the centre of Cognitive–Behaviour Therapy (Beck & Emery 1985).

Self-expression covers the individual's skills and abilities to express their thoughts and emotions to others by whatever means they can use. It covers not only verbal and alternative means of communication but also behaviour, facial expression and body language.

The environmental domain

The environmental domain encompasses everything that surrounds the person and includes people, places and structures. It is, in effect, the social element of a bio-psycho-social view. The domain includes:

- The cultural, ethnic and religious environment
- Neighbourhood, housing, living conditions and circumstances
- Socioeconomic status and financial circumstances
- Family membership
- Social and friendship networks
- Formal support networks

The cultural, ethnic and religious environment describes some of the background influences that might have a bearing on the individual's beliefs and outlook, their relationships with others and patterns and codes of behaviour. This environment often defines a set of norms and expectations for individuals.

'Culture' is often taken to mean a set of beliefs and values shared by religious and ethnic groups but it can be applied to any group in society. An identifiable culture may often be found in regional areas of Britain, as well as people of different social class ('class culture') and ages ('youth culture'). It could be argued that people with learning disabilities themselves might share a common culture, especially if they are well embedded in the 'learning disability system'.

Neighbourhood and housing examines where the person lives, who they live with and the nature and suitability of their accommodation. People with learning disabilities may live in their parental home, in various kinds of supported living or in their own home or accommodation. In some cases this accommodation meets their needs and is a pleasant and positive place to live, while in other cases the accommodation does not meet their needs, and is not a pleasant place to live. The positive or negative nature of the accommodation may be influenced by the kind of neighbourhood in which it is situated, its geographical location and availability of local services and the freedom or constraints it places on the individual. The physical state of repair and decoration and whether the person has their own room or has to share may strongly affect how they feel about where they live.

Socioeconomic status describes the wealth or poverty of the person. How much money do they have and how stable are their financial circumstances?

Family membership covers anyone who is regarded as being in the family (including people such as adopted 'aunties') and who may have a significant influence on the individual. We may need to differentiate between the immediate and extended family if grandparents, uncles or cousins have a significant involvement. We need to know 'who is there' and who might potentially exert an influence over the person. The dynamics and interactions between family members are covered under the interpersonal domain, below.

Social and friendship networks incorporate anyone outside the family, but who is not employed to work with them, with whom the individual has a relationship. Social networks can be thought of as a set of concentric circles, with the closest relationships at the centre and the most formal at the outside. However, McConkey (2005) points out that people with learning disabilities are often poor at differentiating between kinds of 'friendship', that they often cite staff members as friends and that social networks are often very small. The nature of such relationship networks may often be a cause of dissatisfaction in peoples' lives.

Formal support networks include people and organisations who have a professional relationship with the individual. Although we might prefer people to be as independent as possible and should not be prescriptive about who 'ought' to be involved, there needs to be a balance between over- and undersupport. It might be useful to develop a map of who is involved and what they do for the individual. As well as looking for people who are involved we might also look for those who we might expect to be involved but who are not – the holes in the person's support network.

The interpersonal domain

The interpersonal domain covers the interactions between the individual and other people and organisations in their life. It is about *how* they relate to one another and whether the interactions are helpful or harmful. The domain includes:

- Opportunities for choice, autonomy, independence and self-efficacy
- Occupational patterns, skills and preferences
- Recreational patterns, skills and preferences
- Stability and continuity in circumstances and relationships, including attachment and loss
- Family dynamics and relationships
- Effects of learning and reinforcement on the person's health and behaviour
- Cultural and family expectations
- Social handicapping
- The individual's experience of integration or segregation

Opportunities for choice, autonomy and independence is not about the person's capabilities and skills in making choices but about the extent to which their relationships and support networks *allow* them to make choices, to be autonomous and independent.

Occupational patterns, skills and preferences examines the way in which the person spends their 'working day'. This might include day centre activities or even the absence of any meaningful daytime activity. What is important here is how *fulfilling* and *satisfying* the individual finds their daytime activity. They may have aspirations toward a 'proper job' but be frustrated in their search for paid employment. Alternatively, work may be a source of stress for some individuals.

Recreational patterns, skills and preferences explore the degree to which the person's free time is spent in a meaningful and satisfying way. For most people their free time is an opportunity to spend time with friends in activities of their own choosing, that are fun and fulfilling. For some people with learning disabilities there may be an excess of 'free time' in which little happens, they do not meet their friends, do not take part in the local community and which has little satisfaction for them. However, we should note that greater opportunities for social inclusion and leisure facilities may not always be welcomed by people who have little prior experience of these activities. Carers may unwittingly promote stress and anxiety by insisting that people make use of local facilities. What we need to know is: *'How does the person spend their leisure time and how satisfying do they find it?'*

Stability and continuity in circumstances and relationships, including attachment and loss is an attempt to explore the degree to which the individual can make attachments and the degree to which those attachments can continue unbroken. The need to form at least one enduring relationship with another person is arguably an inherent human trait that implicitly leaves us potentially at risk of the experience of loss. In the case of people who have been bereaved of parents they have lived with all their lives, the pain of loss is often intense and may not be acknowledged by professional carers. People who have been placed in care from an early age may have experienced discontinuous relationships with a succession of carers and peers with whom they have lived. What we need to know here is: *'Who are the significant people in the person's life and have they been able to maintain fulfilling relationships with those people?'*

Stability and continuity also extends to a sense of personal coherency in terms of where we live and how we lead our lives. In the case of people with learning disabilities there are many opportunities for change in their living circumstances over which they may have little control.

Family dynamics and relationships is about the way that the individual interacts with members of their family. This is especially important if the individual is still living in the parental home but may still be meaningful and influential, even when the person is in supported care. Families may exert either a positive or negative influence on peoples' lives and may, indeed, be part of the picture of the individual's mental health. We may be interested in a number of factors:

- Cohesiveness and harmony – How close are the family members? Where does the family fit on the continuum shown in Table 5.3?
- Communication – the ability of family members to share information, emotions and intentions appropriately with one another. Vaughn and Leff (1976) and Leff (2001) were the first authors to suggest a relationship between expressed emotion (EE) and mental illness. EE describes the critical and negative feelings that are often expressed toward the person with mental illness, rather than being withheld or moderated (Table 5.4)

Table 5.3 Family cohesiveness and harmony

Low		High
Disengaged	**Connected**	**Enmeshed**
Too much freedom Too little support	A balance between freedom and support	Too little freedom Too much control Oversupportive

Table 5.4 Family communication

Low		High
Closed	**Open**	**Random**
Little or no communication Avoidance of showing emotions to one another Low EE	Issues discussed Emotions shared appropriately	Unselective and inappropriate discussion of topics High EE

Table 5.5 Family roles, problem solving and adaptability

Low		High
Rigid	**Flexible**	**Chaotic**
Roles and relationships rigidly defined Poor problem solving because members unable to change	Roles and relationships defined but able to adapt to changing circumstances Able to use flexibility to problem-solve	Roles and relationships hardly defined at all Poor problem solving because members unable to organise themselves

- Roles, problem solving and adaptability. The ability of family members to change the power structure, role relationships and relationship rules in response to changes in family lifecycle and circumstances (Table 5.5)

Effects of learning and reinforcement on the individual's health and behaviour recognises that any behaviour, including 'illness behaviour' may be reinforced. Very often, what we are faced with is the person's behaviour and, at first, we may have little insight into why the person is behaving in a certain way. There are four possible categories of explanation (Table 5.6).

Cultural and family expectations explores the effect that the value base and 'unwritten rules' of one's culture, religion and family have on an individual's

Table 5.6 Illness behaviour and reinforced behaviour

Illness behaviour?

		No	Yes
Reinforced behaviour?	**Yes**	Behaviour only attributable to learning and reinforcement	Illness behaviour that has been reinforced
	No	Behaviour attributable neither to illness nor reinforcement	Illness behaviour only – no effects of reinforcement

social and interpersonal behaviour. These are the 'oughts, shoulds and musts' of society that are often internalised by individuals and relate strongly to one's ego-ideal, the kind of person we feel we ought to be to live up to others' expectations. Most people can live with some degree of dissonance between how they are and how people would like them to be. However, for some individuals, this dissonance is a focus for feelings of guilt and inadequacy.

Social handicapping relates strongly to the individual's experience of stigma and the disadvantage that comes with a label of intellectual impairment. McClimens (2005) summarises the argument that, in many ways, learning disability is a socially constructed concept that has led to people being viewed differently, disadvantaged and treated differently merely because they carry that label. Such an experience may lead to low self-esteem, low self-confidence and possible emotional difficulties.

The individual's experience of integration or segregation is closely linked to the nature of service provision that the individual has used. Although many people with learning disabilities have lived all their lives in their family home their experience of 'community life' may have varied greatly. Some families' response to their child's disability and perceived stigma has been to isolate themselves and to become self-contained. Others have carried on life in a very ordinary fashion. One could argue that, until recently, the special school system and provision of daycare in relatively isolated day centres has not met peoples' need for social inclusion. The extremes of isolation were seen in many of the old institutions, where some individuals experienced abuse and exploitation. We might think that for people with learning disabilities inclusion in the mainstream of society would be welcomed with open arms but, for some individuals, life in the community with a greater range of choices is a source of anxiety because they lack the necessary coping skills.

The temporal dimension

This is a thread that runs throughout all the other assessment categories, rather than being an assessment category in itself. It represents the passage of time in the person's life and consists of three elements.

- The Present is the picture of things now, at the time of assessment. What can we see and observe?

- The Past, which relates to the individual's personal history and the history of their possible illness. We need to know whether the cause for concern behaviours have always existed, or whether this represents a recent change in behaviour. What was the person like before people became concerned about them? What has their lifestyle been like and have there been any significant changes? We may also need to know if there has been a lack of change, for instance if failure or discontinuity has been a noticeable feature of their life. However, it may sometimes be difficult to obtain a clear picture of an individual's life history, especially if they cannot tell us about it and if there has not been a consistent 'significant other' in their life.

- The Future prompts us to think about whether we can 'peer into the crystal ball' and foresee what the future holds for the individual. How do they view their future? Are there any events on the horizon, such as the death of a parent that the individual is worried about?

We would need to think, for example, about the past, present and future of an individual's anxiety, their history and development. The temporal dimension is strongly grounded in the theories of Life Story Work (Hewitt 2006; Hussain & Racza 1997).

Using the framework as an assessment tool

The Ecology for Mental Health framework is very large and complex and would take considerable time to assess fully. It is important to remember that the framework is an attempt to provide a structure for assessing the mental health of all individuals, regardless of the nature of their illness, the level of their disabilities and the nature of their living circumstances. It follows that only some of the assessment elements apply to some of the people some of the time. It is extremely unlikely that all the elements will apply in every case. What is needed is a selective approach, where the practitioner assesses only those elements that are relevant to a particular individual. However, there are some general rules for using the framework:

- Always assess all the 'cause for concern' behaviours.
- Try to gain as complete a picture as possible of the individual's coping and responding behaviours.
- Use the personal domain, the environmental domain and the interpersonal domain as a 'shopping list' of issues and only assess those that you think may be relevant.
- Always try to apply the temporal dimension to all of the other assessment categories. Think about the past, present and future of everything.

The need for a triangulated approach to assessment

In conventional mental health practice it is usual to use a patient interview as the primary method of assessment. However, in learning disability practice this may be difficult due to communication and intellectual impairment. It makes sense, therefore, to use a 'triangulated' approach to assessment whereby we attempt to gain our information from a number of sources and then to examine the degree to which these sources agree with one another. These strategies are likely to be helpful:

- Interview the individual, if necessary using visual aids, photographs and alternative communication. Again, a life story work approach would be helpful as a means of exploring the individual's ideas and feelings about their life and relationships.
- Interview other significant people who have known the individual for a reasonable length of time. These might be parents, carers, friends and neighbours. You may need to search out people who the individual knew some time ago but with whom they do not currently have contact.
- It may be useful to examine records and notes on the individual. However, we should be cautious here because the records that were often kept in long-stay hospitals were often sparse and do not necessarily contain the information we are looking for.
- Use your own observations, spend time getting to know the person and developing a therapeutic relationship with them. It is unlikely that people with learning disabilities will want to share intimate thoughts and feelings with a stranger.
- It may be useful to attempt to use rating scales and specific symptom scales, such as the Zung Anxiety Rating Scale, although few of these have been developed and validated for use with people who have learning disabilities.
- Be prepared for the assessment framework to pose more questions than answers to begin with. The task of mental health assessment is always difficult and may be doubly so when working with people with learning disabilities. The framework should help you to develop hypotheses about why the person seems to be mentally ill and what factors influence their behaviour.
- By testing out the hypotheses you will be able to 'peel away the layers' and eventually be able to arrive at an explanation that works and that provides a sound base for a therapeutic approach. None of this is easy and it may take considerable time before you arrive at a sound and workable decision.

There now follows a discussion by Dave Ferguson of a case example from his own practice, showing how the framework has been used to explore an individual's mental health.

Case study: Mike

Mike lives in a residential/hostel project in an inner city area of Southampton provided by a Housing Association. The residence is for people with mental health problems.

Mike is labelled as having a mild to moderate learning disability and has a diagnosis of schizophrenia. However he is under the care of a consultant psychiatrist in mainstream mental health services as his last psychometric test (1998) showed full IQ score of 77, which disputes his learning disability diagnosis. This is a contentious issue and there have been disputes between professionals as to the accuracy of this.

Mike has attended a special purpose employment workshop and received support from an outreach employment agency for approximately four years; however, at the time this referral was made this had stopped, as Mike's mental health had deteriorated.

Initially a meeting was held between the social work manager, care manager and myself at Social Services offices. This meeting was designed to discuss the referral that was made, to understand why the learning disability team felt he did not meet their referral criteria and to gain some insight into Mike's needs from social services perspectives and to make plans to undertake the assessment with Mike.

The assessment with Mike was undertaken over four sessions. Staff from the hostel were occasionally asked questions to inform the assessment process.

Assessment using the Ecology of Mental Health Framework

The behavioural interface – 'cause for concern' behaviours

Deviance from social, cultural and personal norms
Mike's care manager has expressed concern that Mike has had thoughts of harming himself and harming others. Mike has been said to be preoccupied with knives and has talked about how it might feel to cut his eyes out as well as how much harm he could do to others.

In the assessment interview sessions, Mike has expressed interest in what might happen if he cut out his lungs, he will then follow this questioning with a wry smile (observed on three occasions) and then claim this to be a 'silly question'.

Mike has also mentioned that he wonders what it would be like to swap his brain with someone else's and the same with someone's body – he will then state that he thinks this is funny.

During the assessment period, Mike has questioned what it would be like to harm others. There is always the probability, given his history, that this would need to be carefully observed, as he has previously physically assaulted a member of staff.

One issue that arose during the initial assessment interview with Mike, his care manager and his key worker was that he stated that one evening (not specific) he had woken up in the car park at the end of his road with only his boxer shorts on. He claimed a female member of the public had alerted him. Mike did not appear to be particularly concerned about this or the risks to him (physical health, physical harm) nor of the impression this may have given to the woman who alerted him, but naturally there was concern expressed by staff. I believe that his key worker and care manager have discussed this matter with Mike. This episode appears to carry some truth as a member of the night staff opened the front door to Mike standing in his boxer shorts. The member of the public did not make any report to the police as this was checked with the local police station. The incident was not written in Mike's file by the night staff, so detailed information is limited but it is understood that this episode did happen.

Case study: Mike (continued)

Mike does not appear to have any constructive coping strategies, however the fact that he arises at midday could be perceived as a way in which Mike deals with his day-to-day life.

Vulnerability
Mike has indicated that he experiences some harassment from other residents. He has identified this as financial exploitation, being scapegoated and reports from care manager indicate that possible sexual harassment has also been experienced. Mike is very reluctant to talk about these issues.

Issues for further investigation
- Risk assess potential harm to self-and to others
- When Mike asks questions about cutting out eyes and lungs, is he really curious or is this symptomatic of his diagnosis?
- Assessment to support Mike regarding harassment issues

Care planning issues
- Educate to protect Mike regarding personal safety
- Protect others from possible risks

The personal domain

The Physical Self

General physical health, wellness, fitness and energy
Reports from carers and care manager would suggest that Mike is usually healthy and there is no recent occurrence of illness. There are no known allergies

Personal mobility
Mike is freely mobile and experiences no difficulty in this area

The care manager reports that Mike functions in the mild to moderate range of learning disability. However, a report from the consultant psychiatrist has cited that psychometric testing in 1998 to determine Mike's level of intellectual disability gave a full score of 77. This score does not meet the eligibility criteria for learning disability services and some professionals have disputed this score. Mike has, however, been educated throughout the special schools system both locally and as an out of area boarder and I do think it would be helpful for another psychometric test to be requested from a clinical psychologist in the learning disability service to determine level of current cognitive functioning, which may help to determine appropriate future service provision.

Mike has been diagnosed with schizophrenia. He is seen by the consultant psychiatrist in mainstream mental health services and although at the time the referral was made, Mike was in an active phase of his illness and this requires constant monitoring at this stage.

Mike is prescribed:
- zuclopenthixol 300 mg IM weekly (administered by practice nurse)
- olanzapine 10 mg at night
- procyclidine 5 mg twice daily

During the assessment process Mike has had thoughts of harming himself and harming others. He has been said to be preoccupied with knives and has talked about how it might feel to cut his eyes out as well as how much harm he could do to others.

In the assessment interview sessions Mike has also expressed interest in what may happen if he cut out his lungs, he will then follow this questioning with a wry smile (observed on three occasions) and then claim this to be a 'silly question.'

Mike has also mentioned that he wonders what it would be like to swap his brain with someone else's and the same with someone's body – he will then state that he thinks this is funny.

Mike has also shared details of his auditory hallucinations. He does not associate any of the above with hearing voices. In contrast to this Mike's care manager has said that Mike's voices are set characters that give him ideas of self-harming and also to some of the issues mentioned above.

It has been difficult to ascertain from Mike what this phenomenon may mean to/for him and I believe that difficulties in understanding and processing this information have highlighted:

- His difficulties in understanding what may appear to be abstract and complex questions (is this indicative of his level of learning disability?)
- Whether these are command hallucinations

Issues for further investigation
- Efforts need to be made to obtain an accurate estimation of the frequency and pattern of 'schizophrenia related behaviours'
- Risk assess potential harm to self-and others
- Request psychometric test from clinical psychologist in learning disability services

Care planning issues
- Monitor medication

The Thinking Self

Cognitive–developmental maturity
Mike's psychotic illness appears to have begun in childhood. Reports indicate that from the age of three he received special school education. At the age of six he was reported to have withdrawn into psychotic states – poor temper control and aggressive outbursts.

There does not appear to be great difficulty in reading and writing skills and previous reports indicate that Mike can do basic arithmetic.

Memory
Mike appears to have good long-term memory but his short-term memory is not so good. He can talk about events that happened in childhood although the accuracy of these memories has not been tested. He repeats the same information without significant variation.

Case study: Mike (continued)

Moral reasoning

Mike appears to have basic understanding of right and wrong although his actual level of understanding has not been formally tested.

World view/world knowledge

Mike does not at times appear to be orientated in time and place – this has been mentioned in relation to the car park incident. Mike does have some difficulties in remembering dates, etc. – again this has not been formally tested. There are, at this stage, no recognisable patterns of ideas or beliefs but he expresses bizarre ideas concerning self-harm and harm to others and these require further investigation.

Issues for further investigation

Determine any recognisable patterns of ideas and beliefs

The emotional self

Mike has at times appeared preoccupied and tense but not agitated. This is particularly obvious in his difficulty in sitting still. This has been mostly observed in the assessment interview sessions – Mike constantly moving position, playing with hair, getting up and sitting down.

In relation to the above, on a number of occasions Mike has been asked if he has found the sessions particularly difficult – he has always responded that this is not the case.

At the time of the assessment Mike did appear to have a lot of opportunity for individual autonomy but did not demonstrate this. Currently, Mike appears quite passive and will follow whatever he is asked to do.

I have observed some symptoms of anxiety in Mike but have not been able to ascertain if this has been an issue of discussion with Mike in the past. I have observed throughout the interview process that Mike finds it difficult to sit still, plays with his hair etc. Mike has had some difficulties in answering or discussing issues with me. However I think any observed symptoms of anxiety are more likely to be symptomatic of Mike's schizophrenia but there may be issues too regarding his level of learning disability and understanding of complex and abstract questions – as mentioned earlier.

Issues for further investigation

- Undertake a modified coping strategies questionnaire
- Consider undertaking anxiety rating scale

Care planning issues

- Work with Mike on increasing appropriate coping skills.

The spiritual self

Self-esteem, self-regard and self-knowledge

I have undertaken some focused assessment work to concentrate Mike on self-esteem, self-regard and self-knowledge. Mike has some insight into self – for example, he has a degree of insight into his mental health needs but does not appear to fully understand the implications and consequences of this on his life and those around him. Mike will state that he knows he 'gets on people's nerves' but cannot seem to fully appreciate the impact this has on others or indeed their view/perception of him. I believe that this does make him vulnerable from others and Mike would benefit from further work to facilitate a greater degree of insight, as this could be indicative of lack of emotional understanding/intelligence. This work, however, would need to be undertaken *after* psychometric testing had taken place to determine the appropriate level to pitch the assessment.

Self-expression and communication

Mike communicates verbally and does not appear to have any difficulty in this regard. In the assessment interviews he would normally speak fluently and clearly.

Occasionally, Mike has found understanding some questions put to him in the assessment process confusing, and he will ask for clarification. At times he has appeared to become slightly tense but not particularly distressed or uncomfortable during this process, and indeed has appeared to 'enjoy' telling his story.

Issues for further investigation

Assess degree of insight

The care manager and key worker (initial discussion in session one of this assessment process) have both expressed concern about the kind of support that Mike requires in relation to his level of learning disability. Psychometric testing would determine his level of cognitive functioning and this assessment would help to guide and signpost Mike to the most appropriate service(s) to meet his current and future needs.

Mike has been noticed to have deteriorated in daily living skills and to some degree in self-care skills. For example, he requires constant verbal prompting (and at times physical support) to take care of personal hygiene; he no longer makes himself snacks or drinks, and rarely leaves the house alone. This may be due to his mental health status but as no record appears to be available to suggest Mike's 'best' level of functioning. A daily living skills assessment has been given to staff to undertake with Mike to establish a baseline. From this exercise there will be data from which changes in Mike's skill level can be better monitored and actions taken to respond and support this area.

Issues for further investigation

- Assessment to determine level of cognitive impairment
- Assessment of daily living skills to be completed by residential staff

Care planning issues

- Monitor activities of daily living and self-help skills
- Respond appropriately to any deterioration or improvement (i.e. maintenance) in these areas

Case study: Mike (continued)

The environmental domain

Neighbourhood and housing, living conditions and circumstances

Mike has expressed concern regarding his perception of living in his neighbourhood. In this area there are a number of socially disadvantaged individuals, including others with mental health needs, accommodation for those who are homeless, a large mental health inpatient provision and 'red light area.' He perceives himself to be vulnerable, but appears to have little understanding of how to protect himself.

Mike's living accommodation is primarily geared to people with mental illness, so whatever his level of cognitive impairment may be, he is vulnerable if these particular needs are not overtly responded to.

Social and friendship networks

Mike would appear to get on well with most of the other residents and staff in the hostel. Mike has said he gets on particularly well with Sue and Martha (residents) but that he has no friends outside the home environment.

Mike does not appear to venture out of the home much and appears to lack any motivation to do so. He spends most of his time in his room, watching T.V.

Mike states that he likes living in the area although he claims it is 'a bit rough' – citing prostitutes in particular, and expressing concern that they might rape him and he could catch AIDS.

Formal support networks, involvement of professionals

Mike's support comes mainly from statutory services (social services, mental health services, and primary care services) and accommodation from the housing association. The specialist employment workshop has been involved to assist in employment/occupation.

When well, he visits his mother (who has schizophrenia) every eight weeks. His parents divorced when he was a child and his father has remarried. He has a brother with whom he has no contact and a younger stepbrother and stepsister with whom he has limited contact. His father is in contact with Mike but generally by 'phone although he has attended some previous care programme approach (CPA) meetings.

Issues for further investigation

There is probably some merit in further visiting the hostel to undertake an observational assessment to develop a clearer picture of Mike's lifestyle - particularly what he does and who he shares his life with

Care planning issues

*   Increase Mike's personal and daily living skills.

The interpersonal domain

Opportunities for autonomy, independence and power

Mike's current living arrangements would appear to have some flexibility, so Mike does have some degree of autonomy. However, this arrangement can also mean that Mike can 'choose' to not participate in house activities or indeed in planning meaningful daily occupation – this again can lead him to having some degree of vulnerability and also where I think his ability to plan (based on independent thought and from informed choice) can be compromised.

Given Mike's psychiatric diagnosis his skill level in this area will fluctuate.

Occupational patterns, skills and preferences

At the start of this assessment Mike was not attending any daytime activities. However, Mike has since returned to gardening one day a week and has stated that he is enjoying this occupation.

Mike could be described as 'unmotivated' in terms of activity. He appears to do very little and spends a lot of his time in his room. He also has a tendency to stay in bed and usually arises at about midday. This would seem to imply some motivational difficulties. It is possible that this could be due to his mental health status and/or side effects of medication but I also wonder if it may also indicate that there is very little that is structured for him to get out of bed for.

Stability and continuity in relationships, attachment and loss

There would appear to be a succession of staff changes in Mike's current living accommodation. Mike particularly liked and got on well with his key worker, who has since left. Mike does appear to need to develop a trusting relationship with staff and also requires a coherent and consistent approach in his care.

Staff changes are unavoidable – however, given Mike's vulnerability, changes certainly impact on his personal development and growth.

Mike states he gets on well with family and has also acknowledged one or two people he lives with as being close to. Alongside this, however, Mike's vulnerability is also exposed in that he is at risk of being too trusting and open to exploitation from others.

Care planning issues

- Work with Mike to assist in planning for meaningful daily and recreational occupation
- Baseline assessment required of personal and daily living skills

Conclusion

Mike is a 30-year-old man with a diagnosis of schizophrenia. He presents with a level of cognitive impairment that requires further assessment and has been educated under the special school system.

Mike has a number of needs that will either require further investigation or which can be actioned immediately through the house care planning process. Both of these areas have been highlighted at the relevant stages in this assessment and I have also listed them below to aid further discussion and debate.

Mike requires support that will need to be multiagency and professional in nature. He currently receives support from social services (learning disability care management) and mainstream support from mental health services (outpatient appointments with consultant psychiatrist) and primary care health services (administration of depot injection from the practice nurse and any additional health needs which can be treated by GP).

I am not confident that Mike's current living arrangements wholly meet his needs. His mental illness does to some degree meet the criteria of the hostel but his illness vulnerability is compounded with the (questioned) level of his learning disability.

I believe that at this stage in Mike's life he will require increased support from professionals who understand the nature of his intellectual impairment and his mental illness. Co-ordinated shared working (through CPA process) would provide a more coherent response to addressing and meeting Mike's unique needs.

There is obviously a 'danger' in suggesting that Mike does require this increased level of support at this stage in his life – the mainstream services he currently uses may question whether they are the appropriate service to meet his needs – but I would argue that as no question has been raised to date this should not be an issue. These mainstream services *are* appropriate and meet Mike's needs well. I do not envisage any need to change this – merely to add to and complement them.

Mike's assessment shows how complex and at times how confusing the clinical picture can be when a person with a degree of learning disability also has a mental illness. This has been further complicated by the difficulty often experienced in obtaining detailed information regarding the individual.

Recommendations

Issues for further investigation

- Risk assess potential harm to self, to others and from others
- Further assess that when Mike asks questions about cutting out eyes and lungs, is he really curious or is this symptomatic of his diagnosis?
- Baseline required of personal and daily living skills – staff given 'pathways to independence' assessment to complete
- Efforts need to be made to obtain an accurate estimation of the frequency and pattern of 'schizophrenia related behaviours'. Consultant psychiatrist has been written to for details
- Assessment to determine level of cognitive impairment
- Undertake a modified coping strategies questionnaire
- Possibly undertake anxiety rating scale
- Assess degree of insight
- There is probably some merit in further visiting the hostel to develop a clearer picture of Mike's lifestyle, particularly what he does and who he shares his life with

Care planning issues

- Educate to protect Mike regarding personal safety

- Protect others from possible risks
- Protect Mike from possible risks
- Increase Mike's personal and daily living skills
- Monitor medication
- Monitor activities of daily living and self-help skills
- Respond appropriately to any deterioration or improvement (i.e. maintenance) in these areas
- Work with Mike on increasing appropriate coping skills
- Work with Mike to assist in planning for meaningful daily and recreational occupation

Conclusion

The mental health of people who have learning disabilities is a complex issue. Often the professional receives a referral to a person who presents with behaviour that is odd and a cause for concern to those who support them. Diagnostic overshadowing 'muddies the water' that is often already murky and full of uncertainty. Professionals often need to decide if the individual's behaviour can be explained by a mental illness, or whether it is part of their learning disability.

Even when diagnosis has been confirmed, we are still faced with the problem of what to do about the person's difficulties. To treat illness effectively – do more than treat the symptoms – we need to understand what has caused the illness and what maintains it.

The Ecology of Mental Health Framework provides a structure in which to explore the various factors that might influence a person's mental health. As we can see from the example of Mike, there are no quick and easy answers and often the framework poses a number of further questions. Assessment of mental health using the framework is a little like peeling away layers of varnish on an old painting. It is only by careful and patient work that we uncover the true picture underneath and begin to really understand what is going on.

The framework is not a 'tick-box' assessment, but helps us to build hypotheses about the dynamics of a person's mental illness and how we might help to promote their mental health.

References

(Websites accessed 7 June 2007)

Aldridge J (2003) The Ecology of Health Model. In: Jukes M, Bollard M (eds) *Contemporary Learning Disability Practice.* Salisbury, Quay Books

Aldridge J (2004) Learning disability nursing: a model for practice. In Turnbull J (ed) *Learning Disability Nursing.* Oxford, Blackwell

Attwood T (1998) *Asperger's Syndrome: a guide for parents and professionals.* London, Jessica Kingsley

Barker P (2003) Person-centred care: the need for diversity. In Barker P (ed) *Psychiatric and Mental Health Nursing.* London, Arnold

Beck AT, Emery G (1985) *Anxiety Disorders and Phobias: A Cognitive Perspective*. New York, Basic Books

Bird L (1999) *The Fundamental Facts: all the latest facts and figures on mental illness*. London, Mental Health Foundation

Black L, Cullen C, Novaco RW (1997) Anger assessment for people with mild learning disabilities in secure settings. In: Stenfert Kroese B, Dagna D & Loumidis K (eds) *Cognitive Behaviour Therapy for People with Learning Disabilities*. London, Routledge

Clark AK, Reed J, Sturmey P (1991) Staff perceptions of sadness among people with mental handicaps. *Journal of Mental Deficiency Research*, **35**, 147–153

Cooper SA (1997) Learning disabilities and old age. *Advances in Psychiatric Treatment* **3**, 312–320

Cooper S-A, Collacott RA (1996) Depressive episodes in adults with learning disabilities. *Irish Journal of Psychological Medicine*. **13**, 3, 105–113

Department of Health (2001) *Valuing People: a new strategy for learning disability for the 21st century*. London, The Stationery Office

Eisenmajer R, Prior M, Leekman S, Wing L, Gould J, Welham M. Ong B (1996) Comparison of clinical symptoms in autism and Asperger's syndrome. *Journal of the American Academy of Child and Adolescent Psychiatry*, **35**, 1523–1531

Evenhuis H, Kengen M, Eurlings H (1990) Dementia questionnaire for mentally retarded persons. Hooge Burch, PO Box 2027, 2470 AA Zwammerdam, Netherlands

Eysenck MW (2004) *Psychology: An international perspective*, Hove, Psychology Press

Gedye A (1995) *Dementia scale for Down syndrome*. Vancouver, Canada, Gedye Research and Consulting, PO Box 39081

Goldman HH (1992) *Review of General Psychiatry* (3rd edn). London, Prentice Hall

Gross R (2005) *Psychology: The Science of Mind and Behaviour* (5th edn). London, Hodder Arnold

Knussen C et al (1992) The use of the Ways of Coping (Revised) questionnaire with parents of children with Down's syndrome. *Psychological Medicine* **22**, 775–786

Hewitt H (2006) Uncovering identities: the role of life story work in person-centred planning. In Jukes M, Aldridge J (eds) *Person-centred Practices. A therapeutic perspective,* London, Quay Books

Holland AJ (1994) Down's syndrome and Alzheimer's disease. In: Bouras N (ed) *Mental Health in Mental Retardation*. Cambridge, Cambridge University Press

Hussain F, Racza R (1997) Life story work for people with learning disabilities. *British Journal of Learning Disabilities* **25**, 73–76

Klin A, Volkmar F (1995) *Asperger's Syndrome: Guidelines for Assessment and Diagnosis (www.aspennj.org/guide.html)*

Kohlberg L (1963) Development of children's orientations toward a moral order. *Vita Humana* **6**, 11–36

Lazarus R, Folkman S (1984) *Stress, Appraisal and Coping*. New York, Springer

Leff J (2001) *The Unbalanced Mind*. London, Weidenfeld & Nicolson

Lovett H (1985) *Cognitive Counselling and Persons with Special Needs*. New York, Praeger

McClimens A (2005) From vagabonds to Victorian values: the social construct of a disability identity. In: Grant G et al (eds) *Learning Disability: a life cycle approach to Valuing People*. Maidenhead, Open University Press

McConkey R (2005) Promoting friendships and developing social networks. In: Grant G et al (eds) *Learning Disability: a life cycle approach to Valuing People*. Maidenhead, Open University Press

Morgan S, & Wetherell A (2004) Assessing and Managing Risk. In: Norman I, Ryrie I (Eds.) The Art and Science of Mental Health Nursing, Maidenhead, Open University Press

Moss S (2002) Mini PASS-ADD Interview Pack. Brighton, Pavilion

Piaget J (1932) *The Moral Judgement of the Child*. London, Routledge & Kegan Paul

Piaget J (1952) *The Origins of Intelligence in Children*. New York, International Universities Press

Priest H, Gibbs M (2004) *Mental Health Care for People with Learning Disabilities*. Edinburgh, Churchill Livingstone

Ramirez S, Morgan V, Manns R, Welsh R (2000) Are fears in adults with mental retardation adequately represented in fear surveys? *Journal of Developmental and Physical Disabilities* **12**, 1, 1–15

Reed J (1997) Understanding and assessing depression in people with learning disabilities: a cognitive-behavioural approach. In: Stenfert Kroese B, Dagnan D, Loumidis K (eds) *Cognitive–Behaviour Therapy for People with Learning Disabilities*, London, Routledge

Reed J, Clements J (1989) Assessing the understanding of emotional states in a population of adolescents and young adults with mental handicaps. *Journal of Mental Deficiency Research* 33, 229–233

Reiss S, Levitan GW, Syzsko J (1982) Emotional disturbance and mental retardation: diagnostic overshadowing. American Journal of Mental Deficiency 86, 6, 567–574

Rotter J (1966) Generalised expectancies for internal versus external control of reinforcement. *Psychological Monographs* 30, 1, 1–26

Seligman MEP (1974) Depression and learned helplessness. In: Friedman RJ, Katz MM (eds) *The Psychology of Depression: contemporary theory and research*. Washington DC, Winston-Wiley

Simpson N (1995) Applying the Health of the Nation policy to people with learning disabilities. Paper presented at conference *Enabling People with Learning Disabilities*, St George's Medical School

Tsouris JA, Patti PJ (1997) Drug treatment of depression associated with dementia or presented as 'pseudodementia' in older adults with Down syndrome. *Journal of Applied Research in Intellectual Disability* 10, 4, 312–322

Vaughn C, Leff J (1976) The measurement of expressed emotion in the families of psychiatric patients. *British Journal of Social and Clinical Psychology* 15, 157–165

Zubin J, Spring B (1977) Vulnerability – a new view of schizophrenia. Journal of Abnormal Psychology 86, 103–126

Emerging areas of practice in learning disability nursing

CHAPTER 6

Emerging areas of practice
Supplementary nurse prescribing

Caron Thomas

Introduction

The development of nurse prescribing in the United Kingdom has been well documented over the last three decades as a gradual, evolutionary process. The move towards organisations and practitioners embracing the concept of nurse prescribing was an almost inevitable outcome of a predicted skills shortage in the National Health Service (NHS), namely the shrinking number of practising psychiatrists (Gournay & Gray 2001), a reduction in junior doctors' hours, and a way of easing doctors' workloads (Mazhindu & Brownsell 2003). Filling deficits in skills shortages with nurses is not a new concept, and nurses have traditionally been the source from which shortages in health care services have been filled when it is expedient. During the First World War, 200 nursing sisters were specially trained as anaesthetists, and their employment in 1918 released a corresponding number of medical officers for service at the 'front' (Whitehead 1999).

The advent of supplementary prescribing and – more recently – the further development of independent prescribing (DH 2006) needs to be seen as another stage in the evolutionary process, placed in the context of ongoing changes taking place in the modern NHS. The legal basis for supplementary prescribing is identified in section 63 of the Health and Social Care Act (2001), which allowed ministers, by order, to:

- Designate new categories of prescriber
- Set conditions for prescribing,
- Make changes to NHS regulations to allow the introduction of supplementary prescribing, which came into operation in April 2003 *(www.dh.gov.uk)*.

Supplementary prescribing is defined as:

> *'A voluntary prescribing partnership between an independent prescriber and a supplementary prescriber to implement an agreed patient specific clinical management plan with the patient's agreement'* (DH 2003)

Supplementary prescribing presents an opportunity for learning disability nurses to demonstrate the adaptability and flexibility of their roles at a time when recruitment and retention of all professionals, doctors, nurses, allied health professionals, and dentists is a major cause for concern and will continue to be so for the foreseeable future. There is already considerable movement in relation to role redesign for medical consultants and future roles for nurses need to be considered alongside this. In the NHS, supplementary prescribing by nurses and pharmacists has been hailed as a means to ease the burden on doctors and reduce waiting times for patients *(www.dh.gov.uk)*. On a cautionary note, Jukes et al (2004) suggested that the appointment of supplementary prescribers requires a systematic review of roles and responsibilities, coupled with a well designed job description, to develop the role sensitively and effectively.

Training and preparation for nurses to become supplementary prescribers is open to nurses working in any setting, including mental health and learning disability nurses. Supplementary prescribers are required to undertake the course covering the Extended Formulary nurse prescribing and supplementary prescribing, amounting to 26 days, plus clinical practice development *(www.npc. co.uk)*. The intention is to enhance care by providing quicker and more efficient access to health care through the increased and flexible use of the skills of nurses and pharmacists. In this model of prescribing, nurses are not expected to make the initial diagnosis but can prescribe care related to their specialty.

Supplementary prescribing requires learning disability nurses to work in a clinical management plan set up in partnership with doctors, with agreement from people with learning disabilities and/or their carers. The plan will identify the condition to be treated, the aims of treatment, a range of medicines related to the individual needs of the person, instructions for reporting adverse events, and the evidence base for practice in the form of guidance or protocols.

Supplementary prescribers can prescribe all drugs identified on the General Sales List (GSL) and all prescription-only medicines (POMs), with the exception of some controlled drugs and all 'P' category (pharmacy only) drugs, 'off licence' and black triangle drugs.

The drugs in the Extended Formulary (British Medical Association and the Royal Pharmaceutical Society of Great Britain (2005) are related to four areas of care:

- Minor ailments
- Minor injuries
- Health promotion
- Palliative care

Supplementary prescribing may not be appropriate for someone with multiple health needs and multiple professional carers. Supplementary prescribers are not required to enter into a prescribing partnership that would entail prescribing medication they do not feel competent to prescribe.

In the USA, full prescriptive authority for nurses has arguably improved and increased access to health care for many individuals, and enhances the nurse's ability to provide comprehensive care (Plonczynski et al 2003). This practice is restricted however, to advanced practice nurses (APNs) who have worked towards achieving recognition of nurse prescriptive authority for the last 30 years. Much can be learned from the way that prescriptive authority has developed for nurses in the USA, especially in relation to the barriers to prescribing and the variance in legislation from state to state. In contrast, nurses in the UK have not fully explored this model of prescriptive authority at present, despite this being endorsed from the 'top down' – supported by successive governments in its evolution. This includes a perceptibly slow response by practitioners and organisations in England to the Department of Health publication *Improving Patients' Access to Medicines: A guide to implementing nurse and pharmacist independent prescribing in the NHS in England* (DH 2006). The inclusion of pharmacists and other professions as non-medical prescribers *(www.dh.gov.uk)* will herald a change in the profile of health practitioners generally in the NHS as prescribing continues to evolve.

Person-centred planning

At the heart of person-centred planning (PCP) lie the principles of rights, independence, choice, and inclusion (DH 2001a). Person-centred planning is an ongoing process of working together to make changes that the person – and those close to them – agree will significantly improve the quality of that person's life. This will help to facilitate and empower individuals to take control over their lives and make choices by getting to know them, listening to them and helping them to explain their views. Being person-centred also means working in someone's capabilities and achievements rather than their deficiencies, and recognising the need to work outside normal systems or boundaries that may prevent someone from maximising their life opportunities.

As much as possible, person-centred planning offers the service user, carer, and the prescriber a philosophical framework on which to hang prescribing practice. This is achieved by recognition that with supplementary prescribing, the dynamics of the relationship between the prescriber, client, and/or carer change from an arguably paternalistic relationship to a much more egalitarian one. Working in partnership with clients and carers, and gaining agreement with the clinical management plan is a central tenet of supplementary prescribing. There has to be agreement between all parties that the supplementary prescriber will play a key role in managing medicines, and that the clinical management plan is acceptable to the individual. Any concerns the service users or carers may have need to be explored during the consultation so that they gain confidence in both the medication to be prescribed and the prescriber.

In 1992 the Values into Action group, supported by the Joseph Rowntree Foundation, published a report highlighting parents' perceptions of the administration and side effects of drugs prescribed for people with severe learning disabilities (Hubert 1992). The report identified grave concerns among parents with regard to the use of psychotropic drugs for behavioural and social problems, dosage, ongoing monitoring, and side effects of drugs.

The key aim of supplementary prescribing is to meet the health needs of the individual. Prescribing practice should be related to health needs identified in the person's Health Action Plan (HAP), one of the key targets in the *Valuing People* white paper (DH 2001a). However, access to health services has been well documented as being problematic for people with learning disabilities (DH 1998; 1999; 2001b; 2003; van Schrojenstein Lantman-de Valk et al 2000; Brown & Paterson 2003; NHS Health Scotland 2004). Maintaining health and managing treatment regimes against this backdrop is fraught with difficulty for the service users and carers who do not feel empowered to discuss or challenge prescribing decisions. The therapeutic relationship with nurses and patients is well documented, and is characterised by the nurse being approachable, providing reassurance, continuity of care, information giving and providing health promotion details (Brooks et al 2001). Communication skills, an understanding of methods of communication, and providing information in a user friendly, accessible way are essential for effective consultation with people with learning disabilities, and help to facilitate an effective meaningful consultation. For people who cannot communicate verbally, other forms of communication such as the use of the Change Picture Bank *(www.changepeople.co.uk)* may be useful.

Consent issues are paramount in relation to treatment. In the NHS the Department of Health Guidelines offer a framework to assist the practitioner in gaining informed consent (DH 2001b), and more recently the Mental Capacity Act (2005) outlines the legal position related to people who lack capacity, decline or refuse treatment, or wish to make an advanced directive. With regard to people who lack capacity to consent, people with learning disabilities should not be excluded from decision making about their treatment. Rather, a decision may be made in relation to the best interests of the person, perhaps with the assistance of an advocate or carer, which is considered to be a person-centred approach to decision making.

Health psychology models

Health psychology involves:
- Understanding the perceptions of what it means to be healthy
- Belief systems
- Improving compliance or concordance with medication

The aims of health psychology are to emphasise the role of psychological factors in the cause, progression, and consequences of health and illness (Miller & Rollnick 1991; Ogden 2000). A key factor that may influence the prescribing consultation is the nurse's health beliefs. This will need to be considered in terms of ethical issues in prescribing practice, such as the prescriber taking a paternalist stance (Gillon 1997) that may negate the possibility of the service user and/or carer making an informed choice based on the principles of autonomy, justice, beneficence, and non-maleficence (Beauchamp & Childress 1989). To increase concordance and gain continuity when prescribing and monitoring medications, it is important to involve people with learning disabilities and their carers, especially with regard to gaining consent to treatment (DH 2001b).

In relation to gaining concordance with treatment regimes generally, Ley (1988) described a model entitled *Cognitive Hypothesis Model of Compliance,* to help predict whether people may concord with treatment. The model works on the premise that understanding, memory, and satisfaction with the consultation result in concordance with treatment. This is crucial to carrying out individual health promotion programmes with people with learning disabilities. Psychological factors – involving cognition, emotion, and motivation – also affect health behaviours, and this will involve working in the range of reference of the individual in terms of communication methods and language used to assess concordance with treatment.

There is much debate as to where nurses 'fit' into prescribing practice. Supplementary prescribing by nurses may provide the answer to this question through team prescribing, shared decision making, and being seen as a check and balance for the Independent prescriber or doctor, complementing medical practice rather than replacing it. However, good prescribing practice does not always mean that the nurse prescriber will resort to a prescription (While 2002). Alternatives to medication therapy should always be sought first. Although it could be argued that nursing is closely aligned to medical practice, learning disability nurses may be seen to work in multiple frameworks, including psychosocial approaches to care. Medication therapy should be planned alongside other forms of therapy such as behavioural interventions, counselling, and psychotherapy (National Institute for Clinical Excellence 2002; Deb et al 2006).

One way of looking at this issue is to consider the breadth and depth of nursing skills as a 'toolbox'. This toolbox is a means by which the nurse will make a decision as to which course of action needs to be taken, based on an assessment of need. Learning disability nurses will be involved in developing the overall care package for the individual, and in the main this will have significant involvement from carers, and medication will not be the first consideration of treatment for people with learning disabilities. Other forms of intervention such as family therapy or cognitive behavioural therapy may be carried out first before resorting to medication. In some circumstances, however, medication may help the person gain some stability in relation to their illness or condition, relieving them from severe levels of distress to undertake psychological therapies, with the aim of withdrawal once this has been achieved. For someone with severe depression, medication may assist in lifting their mood so that they can participate in other forms of therapy.

Clinical governance issues

As well as person-centred planning and health psychology models, the clinical governance framework is one in which nurses and all other NHS employees are required to sign up and adhere to (National Health Service Executive 1999). Under the 'umbrella' of clinical governance comes clinical decision making, evidence-based practice, training and education, client and carer involvement, and clinical risk issues. Contemporary health care services require practitioners to identify the evidence base underpinning clinical practice. The nurse prescriber will be required to have this underpinning knowledge to practise effectively. Prescribing practice carries with it an increased accountability, requiring effective clinical risk management.

Robust record keeping is essential in the prescribing partnership. As well as ensuring that the clinical management plan contains all relevant information, nurse prescribers are also required to adhere to professional standards for maintaining health records. (Nursing & Midwifery Council 2005). One of the most effective ways of managing risk in clinical practice is through clinical supervision. Jukes et al (2004) recommended Titchen's (1998) critical companionship model as an appropriate means of developing nurse prescribing through the supervisory relationship, using reflection and critical dialogue.

There are also legal and ethical issues to consider in prescribing practice. The nurse prescriber is required to be competent and work in the scope of professional practice (NMC 2001). Undoubtedly there is an increased accountability in these roles, but this should not prevent nurses from moving forward and undertaking prescribing practice, and should be viewed as an opportunity to put extensive knowledge and skills to better use in a better rounded way. Nurse prescribing can be seen as 'closing the loop' with regard to service users' experience:

- Following up care and treatment in a timely manner
- Enabling better concordance with treatment through monitoring side effects
- Reporting problems to the independent prescriber
- Discussing as a team

The Audit Commission publication *A Spoonful of Sugar* (2001) highlights poor concordance with medicines and indeed poor medicines management generally among professionals. The cost to the National Health Service is growing year on year, so much so that NHS organisations are required to consider medicines management in terms of effective risk management processes from an organisational perspective. Khurana (2003) suggested that nurses can make a significant contribution to the management of medicines – especially in relation to the degree of waste – prescribing and helping clients, carers, and clinicians evaluate and tackle concordance issues. This was supported by Nolan et al (2001) in a study that examined mental health nurses' perceptions of nurse prescribing. Nurses in the study identified that nurse prescribing would significantly improve clients' access to medication, improve concordance, prevent relapse, and prove to be cost effective.

Most prescribing errors are due to the prescriber not having access to accurate information about the medicine or its interactions, indications, contraindications, therapeutic dose, or side effects; or full information about the patient's allergies, medical conditions, or the latest laboratory results (Audit Commission 2001). The potential risk to the individual could be catastrophic. The systems in place for supplementary prescribing should alleviate this problem in that the clinical management plan would flag up all of these issues for each individual person, with better communication between prescribers, clients, carers and GPs.

The clinical management plan has been identified as the cornerstone by which supplementary prescribing works (Baird 2003). The person's details are entered on the front of the document and the clinical management plan identifies:

- The condition to be treated
- The details of treatment
- Reduction, titration, or maintenance of dose
- Guidelines to support practice
- What to do in the event of an adverse reaction
- The people involved in the decision making process.

Joseph's case study is an example of a clinical management plan, and highlights the partnership working required between the service user, carer, doctor (the independent prescriber), and the supplementary prescriber, for it to be effective.

Challenges of prescribing practice

Due to the nature of the learning disability there may be difficulties in diagnosing and treating someone for health-related problems, including mental health problems, which may be exacerbated by communication difficulties. Rates of psychiatric disorder seem to increase with the severity of the learning disability (Gillberg 1986). There may also be comorbidity with other conditions, such as epilepsy, autistic spectrum disorders, Down syndrome, tuberous sclerosis, Tourette's syndrome, diabetes, or pain (Clarke 1997) that require caution when prescribing antipsychotic drugs.

People with learning disabilities are generally excluded from drug trials, due to the lack of capacity to consent (Duggan & Brylewski 1999), so it could be argued that the effects of antipsychotics with this group are largely unknown. When introducing antipsychotics to someone with a learning disability, it is advisable to exercise caution in dosing and titration, through prescribing smaller doses with a very gradual introduction over time. This will help to minimise any adverse reactions and interactions. The consultation process should include monitoring for possible side effects of antipsychotic medication by asking the client or carer, as well as using a recognised rating scale such as the Liverpool University Neuroleptics Rating Scale (LUNSERS) (Day et al 1995), or the Abnormal Involuntary Movement Scale (AIMS) (Guy 1976; Munetz & Benjamin 1988). The routine use of these rating scales should be an integral part of ongoing treatment to optimise the health care experiences of the individual.

Awareness of potentially adverse drug reactions (ADRs) is essential for any prescriber, and nurse prescribers have to realise that recognising and reporting ADRs is a key component of practice. The 'yellow card' system to report adverse reaction to medicines has now been extended to include the person taking the medication, and their carers, as well as health care professionals *(www.yellowcard. gov.uk)*. The clinical management plan should clearly state how to report adverse reactions, and supplementary prescribers, doctors, clients and carers agree this at the outset. Kieve (2004) suggested that although therapeutic relationships are of

Case study: Joseph

Joseph is a 41-year-old man with moderate to severe learning disabilities. Joseph lives at home with his father, his mother having passed away nine months ago. Joseph was referred to a consultant psychiatrist Dr Spencer by his GP, following concerns from Joseph's father that since his mother died Joseph has become very anxious, has difficulty in sleeping, and his weight has increased due to him binge eating. Joseph also receives treatment for epilepsy, which he has had since he was a child, and is prescribed sodium valproate 200 mg twice daily to help reduce his tonic clonic seizures.

The clinical management plan for Joseph outlines exactly what should be happening with regard to his medication (Table 6.1). This also reflects the complexity of intervention and that medication plays only one part in Joseph's treatment. An explanation of the purpose of the medication will identify that fluoxetine can be given to relieve anxiety as well as helping with eating disorders, however, caution needs to be exercised with people with epilepsy as this can reduce the seizure threshold (British Medical Association and Royal Pharmaceutical Society of Great Britain 2005).

The supplementary prescriber will play a key role in monitoring and reviewing the effectiveness of the fluoxetine as well as monitoring Joseph's seizures. An increase in seizure frequency would mean that Joseph may need to be referred back to the independent prescriber (Dr Spencer) for a possible increase in sodium valproate as a temporary measure until Joseph's anxiety and sleeplessness decreased as a result of a combination of taking fluoxetine, monitoring of dietary intake, and bereavement counselling. A timely intervention from the supplementary prescriber will ensure that this is referred back to the independent prescriber quickly, with the aim of minimising any possible distress to Joseph.

This case study highlights the complexity of knowledge and skills required by a learning disabilities nurse as a supplementary prescriber. Knowledge of epilepsy, anxiety disorders, nutrition, medication and associated interactions, side effects, and carers' needs, all come into play when considering Joseph's needs and the desired outcomes of care. This is coupled with good interpersonal skills and a willingness to accept the autonomy required to make decisions in prescribing practice.

great importance, a 'therapeutic audit' of medication prescribed for someone may help in discovering symptoms resulting from ADRs. Learning disability nurses have a crucial role to play in this, from discussion with clients and carers to being involved in clinical audit of prescribing practice.

Antipsychotics are also frequently prescribed for behavioural disorders or challenging behaviour with people with a learning disability, even though there is little evidence for the efficacy for this (Brylewski & Duggan 2004). This is usually a clinical decision with varying reports on the benefits of this 'off-licence' prescribing. Clarke (1997) identified that the decision to prescribe will often be based on case reports and personal experience, and that there was often pressure

Table 6.1 Supplementary prescribing clinical management plan: example

Client's name:	Medical sensitivities to medication:
Joseph Woods	Penicillin
Patient identification number:	**Date of birth:** 30/08/64
87632	
Address:	**Telephone number:**
20 'The Mount',	01785 xxxxxx
Ridgeway	
Staffordshire ST30 7BZ	
Carer details	**GP details**
Mr D Woods (Father)	DR MW Poole (GP Code: XXX xxxx)
20 The Mount,	The Valley Practice,
Ridgeway	Ridgeway,
Staffordshire ST30 7BZ	Staffordshire ST30 6BZ
Tel no: 01785 xxxxxx	Tel. no: 01785 xxxxxx
Independent prescriber	**Supplementary prescriber** Mrs C Jones
Dr J Spencer,	The Radleys Clinic
The Radleys Clinic,	Stafford
Stafford ST29 3JB	ST29 3JB
Tel no: 01785 xxxxxxx	Tel. no: 01785 xxxxxx
Condition(s) to be treated:	**Aim of treatment:**
Eating disorder	Reduce anxiety
Anxiety	Assist in increasing sleep
Epilepsy	Reduction in binge eating
	Reduce seizure frequency

Medicines that may be prescribed by supplementary prescriber			
Preparation	*Indication*	*Dose schedule*	*Indications for referral back to independent prescriber*
Fluoxetine	Anxiety and eating disorder	25 mg in 5ml daily, increase to a maximum of 60 mg daily if no improvement in reducing anxiety, increasing sleep and reducing binge eating	12 months or earlier if Joseph has an adverse drug reaction or there is no improvement following increases to maximum dose
Sodium valproate	Tonic clonic seizures	200 mg to be taken twice daily at 08.00 and 18.00	12 months, or earlier if Joseph has an adverse drug reaction or there is an increase in seizure frequency

Table 6.1 continued

Guidelines or protocols supporting treatment plan:	
British National Formulary	
Maudsley Guidelines	
NICE guidance on the use of antidepressants	
Frith Prescribing Guidelines for Adults with Learning Disability	
Review, monitoring and documentation arrangements for independent prescriber:	**Review, monitoring and documentation arrangements for supplementary prescriber:**
Monitor and review at least annually and document in client notes	Monitor weekly and review bimonthly. Next review due April 2005. Document in client notes

Process for reporting adverse drug reactions:
Inform independent prescriber.
Complete Yellow Card system for reporting to the Medicines Control Agency
Follow the Trust's procedure for adverse incident reporting

Additional information/comments (e.g. relevant medical history):
Monitor seizure frequency through seizure diary completed by Joseph's father
Monitor any changes in Joseph's mood to ascertain optimum therapeutic dose of fluoxetine for Joseph
Joseph is currently working with a bereavement counsellor following his mother's death
Liaise with GP and dietician to monitor Joseph's weight and diet
Joseph is not receiving any other prescribed or over-the-counter medication for any other condition

Signature of independent prescriber: Dr J Spencer 25th November 2006
Signature of supplementary prescriber: C Jones 25th November 2006
Signature of client or confirmation of client's involvement: D Woods
Date 25th November 2006

(South Staffordshire Healthcare NHS Trust 2004)

to prescribe especially in situations of aggression to others or self-injurious behaviour.

In an audit of prescribing for people with learning disabilities with challenging behaviour carried out by Marshall (2004), over a quarter of people were prescribed psychotropic medication, with polypharmacy that lasted an average of five years. Other medication prescribed for challenging behaviour included antidepressants and antiepileptic agents. Treatment reviews had been carried out in only 26% of cases, with only 20% asked about side effects, and only 8% had the risks of treatment explained to them. Nurse prescribers do not work in isolation from doctors; the whole concept behind supplementary prescribing is a partnership between the service user and/or carer, the nurse, and the doctor. Regular monitoring and review of treatment is facilitated more easily in a team approach to prescribing – changes to medication can be made in a more timely way rather than having to wait for an outpatient appointment (Thomas 2003).

Clarke (1997) asserted that advances in neurochemistry and psycho-pharmacology opened up the possibility of more rational approaches to treating maladaptive behaviours associated with learning disabilities. These approaches could be based on a knowledge of underlying biological abnormalities, and the action of specific drugs on specific receptors or neuroregulatory systems. This poses one of the key challenges for nurse prescribers and employing organisations in maintaining competency to practise. A key concern will be that nurses will be left to 'get on with it' once they have registered as prescribers with the NMC. Once the initial educational requirements are met to undertake prescribing practice, there is a danger that further education is neglected in terms of prescribing practice. Nolan et al (2001) suggested that nurses are heavily involved with medicines management and the pharmacological components of mental health nursing curricula need to be strengthened to strengthen the knowledge base of nurses.

This applies to all nursing curricula, including learning disability nursing. To address this in the author's employing trust, learning disability and mental health nurses who completed the Independent and Supplementary Prescribing course were encouraged to undertake a neuropharmacology module to further develop knowledge in relation to pharmacokinetics and pharmacodynamics (Allsop et al 2005). Future challenges include the proposed additions to the extended nurse prescribing formulary (Medicines and Healthcare Products Regulatory Agency 2004) including the number of controlled medicines and 'off-licence' prescribing.

Conclusion

The contextual frameworks for supplementary prescribing include person-centredness (DH 2001a), clinical governance (NHSE 1999) and standards for prescribing practice (NMC 2006). In turn these will support the principles of rights, independence, choice, and inclusion for people with learning disabilities (DH 2001a). Supplementary – and now the opportunity to further develop independent – prescribing by learning disability nurses offers an opportunity to enhance and improve the experience of people with learning disabilities in relation to their medication. Knowledge of health psychology, clinical syndromes and associated medical conditions should already be in the repertoire of the learning disability nurse and are essential prerequisites to the prescribing role. Working in a person-centred framework would appear to enhance the therapeutic relationship between prescribers and people with learning disabilities and their carers. Prescribing practice should be based on sound evidence and working in a prescribing partnership, avoiding the pitfall of the practitioner prescribing in isolation.

Nurses of the future, including those who focus on learning disability practice, need to be familiar with the evidence and principles of prescribing and medicines management at a preregistration level to meet the needs of people with learning disabilities in a well-rounded way. This would assist in meeting the future needs of the health service workforce, and ensure that prescribing practice is done as a partnership with clients, carers, and other professionals working as a team in prescribing practice.

References

(websites accessed 7 June 2007)

Allsop A, Brooks L, Bufton L, Carr C, Courtney Y, Dale C, Pittard S, Thomas C (2005) Supplementary prescribing in mental health and learning disabilities. *Nursing Standard* April 6–12 2005, **19**, 30

Audit Commission (2001) *A Spoonful of Sugar: medicines management in NHS hospitals.* London, Audit Commission *(www.auditcommission.gov.uk)*

Baird A (2003) Supplementary prescribing: a review of current policy, *Nurse Prescribing* Feb 2003, **1**, 1

Beauchamp TL, Childress JF (1989) Principles of Biomedical Ethics (3rd edn). Oxford, Oxford University Press

Bhaumik S, Branford, D (2005) *The Frith Prescribing Guidelines for Adults with Learning Disability.* London, Taylor & Francis

British Medical Association and Royal Pharmaceutical Society of Great Britain (2005) *British National Formulary.* London, BMA and RPS

Brooks N, Otway C, Rashid C, Kilty E, Maggs C (2001) The patient's view: The benefits and limitations of nurse prescribing. *British Journal of Community Nursing* **6**, 7, 342–348

Brown M, Paterson D (2003) Addressing inequalities. In: Brown M (2003) (ed) Learning Disability: A Handbook for Integrated Care. Salisbury, APS Publishing

Brylewski J, Duggan L (2004) Antipsychotic medication for challenging behaviour in people with learning disability (Cochrane Review). *The Cochrane Library*, Issue 3, 2004. Chichester, John Wiley & Sons

Clarke DJ (1997) Towards rational psychotropic prescribing for people with learning disability. *British Journal of Learning Disabilities* **25**, 46–52

Day JC, Wood G, Dewey M, Bentall RP (1995) A self-rating scale for measuring neuroleptic side effects: Validation in a group of schizophrenic patients *British Journal of Psychiatry.* **166**, 650–653

Deb S, Clarke D, Unwin G (2006) *Using medication to manage behaviour problems among adults with a learning disability: Quick reference guide.* University of Birmingham

Department of Health (1998) *Signposts to Success.* London, NHSE

Department of Health (1999) *Once a Day* London, NHSE

Department of Health (2001a) *Valuing People: A Strategy for Learning Disability for the 21st Century.* London, The Stationery Office

Department of Health (2001b) *Reference Guide to Consent for Examination or Treatment.* London, The Stationery Office

Department of Health (2003) *Tackling Health Inequalities: A Programme for Action.* London, The Stationery Office

Department of Health (2006) *Improving Patients' Access to Medicines: a guide to implementing nurse and pharmacist independent prescribing in the NHS in England.* London, Department of Health

Duggan L, Brylewski J (1999) Effectiveness of antipsychotic medication in people with intellectual disability and schizophrenia: a systematic review. *Journal of Intellectual Disability Research* **43**, 2, 94–104

Gillberg C, Persson E, Grufman M, Themner U (1986) Psychiatric disorders in mildly and severely mentally retarded urban children and adolescents: epidemiological aspects. *British Journal of Psychiatry* **49**, 68–74

Gillon R (1997) *Philosophical Medical Ethics.* Chichester, John Wiley & Sons

Gournay K, Gray R (2001) Should Mental Health Nurses Prescribe? *Maudsley Discussion Paper 11.* London, Maudsley Publications

Guy W (1976) ECDEU *Assessment Manual for Psychopharmacology* (rev.) Rockville, Maryland, US Dept of Health, Education and Welfare.

Health and Social Care Act (2001) London, The Stationery Office

Hubert J (1992) Too many drugs, too little care: Parents' perceptions of the administration and side effects of drugs prescribed for young people with severe learning difficulties Values into Action, London

Jukes M, Millard J, Chessum C (2004) Nurse prescribing: a case for clinical supervision. *British Journal of Community Nursing* July **9**, 7, 291–297

Khurana V (2003) Maximising effectiveness and minimising cost: improving patients' use of medicines. *Nurse Prescribing* **1**, 4, 161–164

Kieve M (2004) The importance of recognising adverse drug reactions. *Nurse Prescribing* **2**, 6

Ley P (1988) *Communicating with Patients.* London, Croom Helm

Marshall T (2004) Audit of the use of psychotropic medication for challenging behaviour in a community learning disability service. *Psychiatric Bulletin* **28**, 447–450

Mazhindu D, Brownsell M (2003) Piecemeal policy may stop nurse prescribers fulfilling their potential. *British Journal of Community Nursing* **8**, 6

Medicines Control Agency Mental Capacity Act (2005). London, The Stationery Office

Miller WR, Rollnick S (1991) *Motivational Interviewing: Preparing People to Change Addictive Behaviour.* New York, The Guildford Press

Munetz MR, Benjamin S.(1998) How to examine patients using the abnormal involuntary scale. *American Psychiatric Association.* **39**, 1172–1177.

NHS Scotland (2004) *Health Needs Assessment Report: People with Learning Disabilities in Scotland.* NHS Scotland.

National Institute for Clinical Excellence (2002) *Schizophrenia: Core interventions in the treatment and management of schizophrenia in primary and secondary care.* London, NICE

National Health Service Executive (1999) *Clinical Governance and Quality in the NHS.* Leeds, NHSE

Nolan P, Haque SM, Badger F, Dyke, R, Khan I (2001) Mental health nurses' perceptions of nurse prescribing. *Journal of Advanced Nursing* **36**, 4, 527–534

Nursing and Midwifery Council (2002) Circular 25/2002. London, NMC

Nursing and Midwifery Council (2005) *Guidelines for Records and Record Keeping* (Update on previous publication 2004). London, NMC

Nursing and Midwifery Council (2006) *Standards of Proficiency for Nurse/Midwife Prescribing*, London, NMC

Ogden J (2000) *Health Psychology: A Textbook* (2nd edn). Buckingham, Open University Press

Plonczynski D, Oldenburg N, Buck M (2003) The past, present and future of nurse prescribing in the United States. *Nurse Prescribing* **1**, 4, 170–174

Taylor D, McConnell D, McConnell H, Kerwin R (2001) *Maudsley Prescribing Guidelines* (6th edn). London, Martin Dunitz

Thomas C (2003) The nurse consultant and clinical governance. In: Jukes M, Bollard M (eds) (2003) *Contemporary Learning Disability Practice*. Salisbury, Quay Books

Titchen A (1998) A *Conceptual Framework for Facilitating Learning in Clinical Practice*. Centre for Professional Education Advancement, Australia.

Van Schrojenstein Lantaman-De Valk H, Metsemakers JF, Haveman MJ, Crebolder HF (2000) Health problems in people with intellectual in general practice: a comparative study. *Family Practice* **17**, 5, 405–407

While A (2002) Practical skills: prescribing consultation in practice. *British Journal of Community Nursing* **7**, 9, 469–473

Whitehead IR (1999) *Doctors in the Great War.* Barnsley, Leo Cooper, from Macpherson WG (1922) *Official History of the War – Medical Services, Surgery of the War*, **1**, 178–179, London, HMSO

Websites

(accessed 7 June 2007)

Audit Commission: *www.auditcommission.gov.uk*

Change: *www.changepeople.co.uk*

National Prescribing Centre: *www.npc.co.uk*

Department of Health: *www.dh.gov.uk*

Medicines and Healthcare Products Regulatory Agency: *www.mhra.gov.uk*

CHAPTER 7

Emerging areas of practice
Acute liaison nursing

Anne-Marie Glasby

'Good health is important to everyone and we all have the same right to use the NHS. But many people with learning disabilities find it difficult to keep healthy and to get the services they need'

(Department of Health 2002, p4)

'People with learning disabilities and their carers frequently express concerns about the attitude and treatment they experience when using general hospital...services' (NHS Executive 1998)

'I told them how to prevent my son getting bed sores but they ignored my advice and he came home from hospital with the first one he's had since the last time he was in hospital' (Band 1998, p24)

Introduction

It is now widely recognised that people with learning disabilities have higher health needs than the rest of the population (National Patient Safety Agency (NPSA) 2004). In particular, they are more likely to experience mental illness, chronic health problems, epilepsy and physical and sensory disabilities (DH 2001). It is estimated that 26% of people with learning disabilities are admitted to acute hospitals every year (compared with 14% for the general population), and some 79% of people with learning disabilities have been to a hospital at some point in their lives (Band 1998, p23).

Not only is there a range of medical conditions that often accompany learning disabilities (for example, coronary heart disease, obesity, epilepsy and hypertension), but demographic changes and medical advances mean that people with learning disabilities are living into older age and requiring more support from both primary and secondary health services. This trend has also been accelerated by the shift towards community living for those previously living in institutionalised care. This shift has meant that many more people with learning disabilities are exercising their rights as citizens to access generic and community-based health services, rather than receiving their medical care in long-stay hospitals.

Despite their higher health needs, people with learning disabilities often experience greater barriers to health services and poorer quality services. This is the result of a range of factors:

Poor uptake of national screening programmes: For example, a survey by Mencap found that among women over 18 only 3% of those living with their family took part in cervical screening, with the figure slightly higher at 17% for those living in formal care. This compares with 85% of the general population aged 18–64 (Band 1998). Reasons cited for the poor uptake of such services are:

- Lack of awareness by people with learning disabilities of such programmes
- Lack of available accessible information
- Difficulties in carrying out physical examinations
- Assumptions by primary care staff about what screening services people may or may not require (Band 1998)

Problems accessing primary care: Some people with learning disabilities have difficulties in accessing primary care and, despite having higher health needs, access the GP less frequently on average than the rest of the population (Alborz et al 2003). In addition to physical access problems such as lack of transport and lack of communication aids, there are barriers caused by the attitude of primary care staff when dealing with people with learning disabilities.

Missed symptoms: Symptoms of physical illness are often overlooked either by carers (particularly if deterioration is gradual) (Alborz et al 2003), or by GPs who have little training for dealing with people with learning disabilities and can make assumptions that their symptoms are part of their disability (NPSA 2004). People

---

Box 7.1 Hospital services for people with learning disabilities

'*People with learning disabilities and their carers frequently express concerns about the attitude and treatment they experience when using general hospital...services*'

(NHS Executive 1998)

'*I told them how to prevent my son getting bed sores but they ignored my advice and he came home from hospital with the first one he's had since the last time he was in hospital*' (Band 1998, p24)

'*They left John's meal on the bedside table. He could not reach and did not have it, so it was taken away*' (Band 1998, p25)

'*By the time we were seen, he was in such a state that the appointment was almost a waste of time. There was no consideration for C – they could see he was agitated by the wait*' (Band 1998, p24)

'*David was left in a terrible state – they said hygiene wasn't a priority*'

(Band 1998, p26)

'*I sat by my daughter's bed for six weeks and the staff never offered me any respite or support; a few of them expected me to do the dressings too*' (Band 1998, p26)

with learning disabilities themselves are often unable to describe or communicate their symptoms. The NPSA has highlighted such diagnostic overshadowing as a key patient safety issue, which:

> '...could lead to undetected serious health conditions and avoidable deaths' (NPSA 2004, p16)

Lack of professional skills: In hospital, there is growing evidence that many practitioners do not have the appropriate skills and knowledge to deliver high quality care for people with learning disabilities (Box 7.1).

A national study conducted by learning disability charity Mencap found that:

- 50% of those questioned found it difficult to find their way around hospitals.
- 43% of family carers felt that staff were not well informed and that information they gave them about the needs of the person they cared for was not listened to and/or not passed on to other staff.
- Staff in outpatient departments also found that the absence of clear consent procedures led to delays in treatment and raised fears among staff about litigation. Although the Department of Health (2002b) has issued guidance on consent and trusts have been rewriting their own policies, there still seems to be considerable confusion around this issue, with people either being denied treatment or being treated without appropriate consideration of consent issues (see below for further details).
- Hospital staff were felt to lack understanding of learning disability, leading to people not being given the support they needed with personal hygiene, communication, medication and meals.
- Carers often spend most of their time at the hospital either because they are expected to do so by staff (63% of carers said staff expected them to stay) or because they have had previous bad experiences of hospital care. Staff assume that because the carer is there, they are taking care of all the person's needs. There is rarely any provision for carers staying over and they are expected to pay for parking and their own food and drink (Band 1998, Mencap 2004)

Against this background, there have been a number of official calls for an improvement in the quality of health services provided to people with learning disabilities. In 1998, the government set out an action plan for general hospitals in its good practice guidance – *Signposts for Success* (NHS Executive 1998). This recognised that specialist learning disability services should have a:

> '...facilitatory and advisory role in helping other health staff to understand the special needs of people with learning disabilities...
> [and] 'provide direct assistance if commissioned to do so'

This has since been given further impetus by the learning disability white paper *Valuing People* (Department of Health 2001), which emphasises the need for specialist learning disability services to adopt a health facilitation approach – supporting people with learning disabilities to access generic health care services.

As subsequent guidance suggested, health facilitators should:

'...help people access mainstream services [and carry out] development work in mainstream services to help all parts of the NHS to develop the necessary skills, [thus ensuring that] 'good health care is delivered in primary and secondary care' (DH 2002a, p8)

While this has tended to focus on access to primary care services, there are a growing number of acute liaison posts that seek to improve hospital services for people with learning disabilities. The remainder of this chapter describes one such post in Birmingham, highlighting key lessons learned during the project and placing these local developments in a regional and national context. Boxes highlight good practice from around the country, and there is a list of key sources and websites at the end of the chapter.

The role of the acute liaison nurse

The role of the acute liaison nurse has developed over the last 10 years. From isolated areas of good practice in areas such as Lothian, Plymouth, Stoke and Barnet it has spread across the country and National A2A (Access to Acute network for those interested in supporting people with learning disabilities in general hospital) meetings have representation from across the regions.

Although it appears that more and more posts are being created across the country this gives a somewhat false impression of the work that is being done. In areas where there is no dedicated liaison nurse, nurses – often in community nursing teams – work closely with acute hospitals in their area, forging links with specific wards and departments and even offering training to staff. However, dedicated posts continue in the main to be fixed-term secondments for one or two years, with funding frequently being withdrawn or not being renewed. There are very few substantive posts in this area, and some of those that do exist are held by people who also act as health facilitators for primary care.

The role itself can vary significantly from place to place. Nurses whose positions are fixed-term often find themselves seconded by the primary care trust (PCT) into the acute hospital and are based in it. This works when the PCT works primarily with one acute trust. However, other posts are based with community nurses and may cover anywhere from one or two hospitals to seven or eight (Box 7.2).

There are generally three aspects to the role of an acute liaison nurse (although different posts may focus on different elements):
- Clinical
- Strategic
- Educational

Clinical role

Clinical work covers a wide remit and involves working with people with learning disabilities before and during admission, as well as, at times, post-discharge. The work varies but primarily aims at addressing the difficulties and problems experienced by people with learning disabilities shown in Box 7.1). Much time is spent on advising hospital staff on how best to meet someone's needs and

> **Box 7.2** Different models of acute liaison
>
> **Solihull**   The health facilitator for primary care also works closely with the local hospital, linking in with senior nursing staff and offering training to ward staff.
>
> **Shropshire**   The health access nurse is based with a learning disability team on a hospital site. She covers primary care and spends the rest of her time between two local hospitals.
>
> **Birmingham**   The acute liaison nurse is based with a community nursing team, but works across the whole city supporting community nurses to work with people in eight hospitals.

some areas even use support workers to work directly with individual people with learning disabilities during a hospital stay (for example, encouraging them to participate with their physiotherapy exercises or showing hospital staff how someone can best be supported at mealtimes). The role also involves liaising between hospital and community staff and co-ordinating planning meetings to ensure that someone's discharge is both safe and timely.

Strategic role

Although clinical work can make a great deal of difference to individual people with learning disabilities, a more strategic approach is required to try to change hospital care and embed good practice in current services (Box 7.3). The importance of having the ear of someone in a senior management position in the hospital cannot be overestimated. A good relationship with a committed senior member of staff, be they clinical (e.g. matron) or managerial (e.g. director of nursing) can open many doors, leading to openings on existing hospital working groups or committees and senior support for changes required. Such an individual can also act as a contact point for all learning disability issues, disseminating information to staff, advertising training and tackling any concerns or bad practice examples.

The other key allies of the acute liaison nurse are the PALS (patient advice and liaison service) team. While many PALS tend to focus on individual concerns and complaints, a more strategic relationship can be developed which can lead to a more proactive approach. For example, in Shropshire, the health access nurse has an agreement with PALS that, if she is not in the office for the day due to training or leave, the PALS team will visit any people with learning disabilities in the hospital that day to ensure they are not experiencing any difficulties.

Educational role

The final crucial role of the liaison nurse is that of providing education, and this again can vary considerably across the country. Some nurses concentrate on short training sessions in particular areas (for example, in accident and emergency) where they feel it will have the most impact, aiming to ensure all members of staff receive at least some input. Others offer day-long sessions open to any staff,

Box 7.3 The benefits of a strategic approach

Gloucester-shire	A 'traffic light' assessment has been developed for people with communication difficulties in hospital (with a red, yellow and green system to signpost hospital staff to critical, important and useful information about somebody). This short document has been very well received and is currently being used in many areas around the country
Surrey	Surrey Oaklands Trust has produced the Hospital Communication Book for hospital staff, giving guidance on how to communicate with people with learning disabilities.
Shropshire	The Health Access has designed a series of leaflets for people with learning disabilities, explaining various procedures and tests that they may need to undergo.
Sheffield	The Royal Hallamshire Hospital eye department has developed a photo journey for people visiting the department.
Birmingham	An acute liaison nurse has worked with the University Hospital Foundation Trust to develop a poster advising staff on how best to support patients who become agitated, distressed or wander. She has also worked with the Heart of England Foundation Trust to develop a carer's charter. This is a statement of the trust's commitment to carers, recognising their expertise and the vital role they play. It offers advice on where they can get help if they are not happy with the service the person they care for is receiving and offers some practical help for those carers who choose to spend long periods at the hospital (for example, access to food and refreshments).
Chester	The Countess of Chester Hospital has guidance for working with carers of people with learning disabilities. Carers receive a badge that denotes them as carers. The hospital also provides pagers for carers who wish to leave the ward but remain in the hospital, with or without the person they care for. Thus, if they are needed back on the ward (for example, to meet with the doctors or for a test or examination), they can be alerted.
Bristol	In Bristol, a video developed by the British Heart Foundation supports people with learning disabilities who may require heart surgery.
Birmingham	City Hospital Birmingham have developed a website for staff, providing information on learning disability services, training links and other sites that may be of interest.

Plate 15.1 Risk level calculation chart

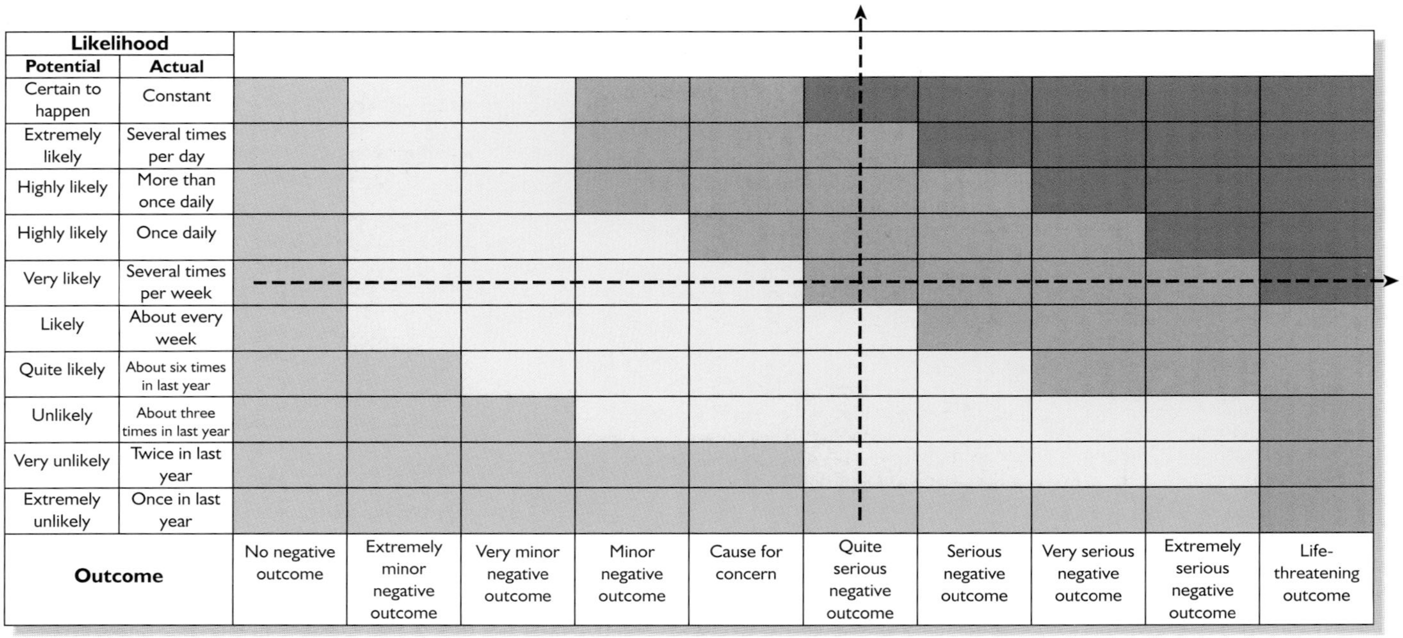

Likelihood

Potential	Actual
Certain to happen	Constant
Extremely likely	Several times per day
Highly likely	More than once daily
Highly likely	Once daily
Very likely	Several times per week
Likely	About every week
Quite likely	About six times in last year
Unlikely	About three times in last year
Very unlikely	Twice in last year
Extremely unlikely	Once in last year

Outcome: No negative outcome · Extremely minor negative outcome · Very minor negative outcome · Minor negative outcome · Cause for concern · Quite serious negative outcome · Serious negative outcome · Very serious negative outcome · Extremely serious negative outcome · Life-threatening outcome

INSTRUCTIONS

Risk = outcome multiplied by likelihood

1. Decide on the Outcome category (horizontal axis) and draw an imaginary vertical line
2. Decide whether to use Potential Risk or Actual Risk to calculate Likelihood
3. Decide on the Likelihood category (vertical axis) and draw an imaginary horizontal line
4. Note where your imaginary lines cross, to give the Risk Level. The dotted lines give an example

Double Red Very high risk	Red High risk	Amber Medium risk	Green Low risk

* I have avoided numerical scores because the risk levels are relatively subjective and are intended primarily to offer a basis for team discussion.
This is not a definitive or absolute measurement of risk and should not be used to compare one individual with another

© John Aldridge

Plate 15.2 A decision making flowchart in safety planning

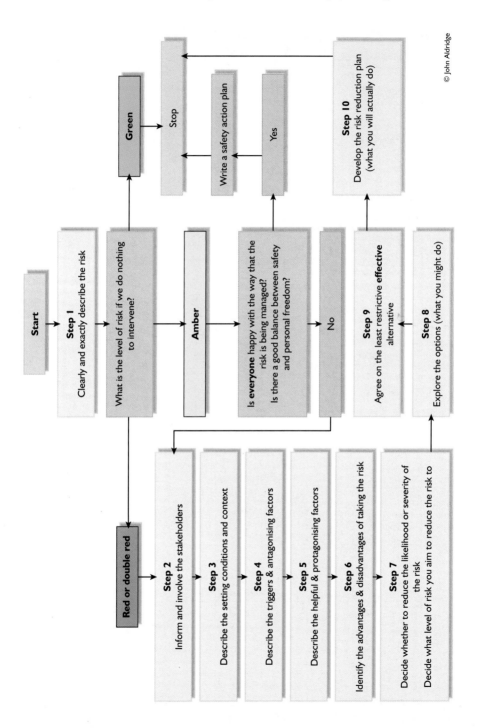

covering a wide range of topics including communication, consent, behaviour and working with carers. Many nurses also involve people with learning disabilities or carers in their training, and this can be particularly effective.

A common difficulty experienced with training in hospitals is ensuring that staff attend. Attendance is often poor, with those booked on the sessions having to cancel at the last minute, as they cannot be released from the ward. This can be both frustrating and time consuming and has forced liaison nurses to be creative about how they get their message across (Box 7.4).

Box 7.4 Training

Birmingham	In Birmingham, the liaison nurse attended ward meetings/handovers on wards where they regularly had people with learning disabilities admitted and delivered short training sessions. Several liaison nurses have gained a short slot on the hospital induction programme, sometimes as part of the disability awareness session.
South Warwickshire	The acute liaison nurse provides regular training in partnership with people with learning disabilities for junior doctors in the hospital as part of their rolling education programme.
Birmingham	The acute liaison nurse in Birmingham delivers a short session on an existing study day on Managing Agitated Patients. She also tries to embed her message in services by teaching on a wide range of courses (for example, for local social workers, for student nurses and for future NHS chief executives).
Hertfordshire	Hertfordshire have developed a training package and video: 'Through Barry's Eyes.' The package comes complete with all the materials needed to run a full day session and explores the issues at stake from the perspective of a person with a learning disability.

The Birmingham story

Having looked at the role of the liaison nurse generally, the chapter now focuses in more depth on the acute liaison model developed in Birmingham. This is a first-hand account, and is designed to highlight a range of good practice, things that could have been improved and lessons learned en route.

In Birmingham, as in other areas, carers of people with learning disabilities have raised ongoing concerns with service providers about the standard of care in hospitals and the lack of understanding shown by hospital staff. As a result of these concerns and in response to official initiatives such as *Signposts for Success* (NHS Executive 1998), a bid was made for funding by Birmingham Specialist Community NHS Trust (now South Birmingham PCT) to the (then) Birmingham and Solihull Education Consortium. This led to two years' funding (from 2001) for a dedicated team to provide an interface between acute services, the adult patient with learning disabilities and his/her family or carers. At this stage, the Acute Hospital Liaison Team consisted of the following experienced learning disabilities staff:

- 1.0 WTE G grade nurse
- 1.0 WTE F grade nurse
- 3.0 WTE B grade support workers

The team offered a service to any adult with a learning disability accessing a Birmingham hospital for a planned or emergency admission, regardless of home setting. The team also provided a service for individuals living in Birmingham who needed to access a hospital outside the area. During the two-year project, the team supported 146 people with learning disabilities across ten hospitals (see Julie's case study for a practical example).

Case study: Julie

Julie is a woman with mild learning disabilities who was referred to one of the local hospitals by her GP for an endoscopy. She lives in sheltered accommodation and is quite independent. Julie is scared of hospitals and was frightened about what might be the matter with her. The hospital sent an appointment but Julie was too scared to attend. The hospital sent another appointment but again Julie felt too nervous to attend.

Julie's social worker contacted the team at this point, as she felt that Julie's health problems needed investigating and she was concerned that the hospital would not send out another appointment.

The nurse from the team visited Julie at home to carry out an assessment. Julie agreed that the nurse could contact the hospital to arrange another appointment. The nurse talked to Julie about her anxieties and tried to reassure her. The support worker from the team began to visit Julie regularly to get to know her. She spent time with her at home and also took her out into the community. On one occasion they went to the hospital canteen for a cup of tea.

The nurse contacted the hospital and explained the situation. The hospital agreed to offer another appointment. The nurse then contacted the endoscopy suite and arranged for Julie to visit the week before her appointment to have a look round and meet the nurses and doctor who would be there on the day.

The nurse met with Julie and discussed the questions that Julie wanted to ask the doctor. The support worker accompanied Julie to the endoscopy suite and supported her to ask her questions.

The following week Julie went for her endoscopy with the support worker. She had the procedure and subsequently received the treatment she required.

The social worker contacted the team some time later and reported that Julie was a 'new woman and very proud of what she'd achieved'. She has also put on weight and is much more confident.

As well as supporting individual people with learning disabilities, the team also began to explore how services more generally could be developed and improved. This included:

- Auditing numbers of people with learning disabilities in hospital departments
- Supporting trusts to develop policies
- Delivering training across acute trusts
- Providing information on available resources
- Supporting trusts to look at how they produce information for people with limited reading skills

From the beginning, this approach was based on ongoing consultation with service users and their carers. A multiagency steering group advised the team, with representatives from the learning disability service, social services, voluntary agencies, carers and the acute sector.

Over time (and particularly after the initial grant funding ran out) the focus of the project has shifted from its initial emphasis on practical and individual support to a strategic initiative, trying to change services more generally. At the same time (and again reflecting the lack of dedicated funding), the project now comprises a senior part-time nurse, covering the whole city and all eight Birmingham hospitals. As these changes have occurred, a number of key lessons have emerged:

Speed: Such was the need for the service that, as soon as the original team leader came into post, referrals were immediately received. This meant that there was very little time to establish links with the hospitals, develop the aims and objectives of the service and advertise it widely, as the team was immediately dealing with people going into hospital on a case-by-case basis.

An initial period of four to six months before referrals were accepted would have allowed for the foundations of the service to be agreed and documentation to be developed. It would have also allowed the hospitals to be contacted before any workers visiting and clear boundaries for the service explained to all stakeholders, preventing any confusion at a later date.

Champions: Throughout the project, the team discovered the importance of having champions in the acute trusts. At times, it was difficult to establish contact at senior level in the hospitals and this has still not been achieved in all the hospitals in the area. Often, the first person approached did not become the link person, but perseverance resulted ultimately in the identification of a committed person to champion the needs of people with learning disabilities in the hospital. The importance of such an individual as a link into the hospital and a force for change cannot be underestimated.

Tip of the iceberg: Although the service was established in response to the concerns of carers about the negative experiences of many people with learning disabilities in acute hospitals, no one realised how endemic these issues were until the team was up and running. There were many examples of people with learning disabilities being denied access to treatment, and receiving very poor quality personal and health care. These are only the people we know about, and those who have used the service so far may well only be the 'tip of the iceberg'.

Consent errors: Despite new Department of Health (2002b) guidance, there are still errors made about the correct procedure for consent. Medical staff continue to ask for the next of kin or main carer to sign consent forms before surgery and appear to assume that because the individual has a learning disability they are unable to give consent. Surgery has often been delayed or even temporarily cancelled when relatives have not been able to sign consent forms. Fortunately, with intervention from the team, these issues have been resolved in individual cases. However, this can only happen where the Team are aware of the situation and are involved early enough to prevent such situations from occurring.

Training: The team has experienced difficulties when organising training. The acute trusts have highlighted the difficulties they have in releasing staff to attend even mandatory training, and this has been reflected in the attendance at learning disability training sessions. Although some sessions have been well attended, as many as four or five full-day sessions have had to be cancelled, either in advance or even on the day, due to poor uptake. It is not clear whether this situation is due to lack of interest on the part of individual staff, a lack of importance attached to it by ward managers or a genuine difficulty with releasing staff for study days (or a combination of all three).

Support: The team received requests from some residential units who wanted support to cover shifts in the hospital when they had someone admitted. Unfortunately, due to the number of people the service worked with – and the size of the team – this level of support was not possible on a regular basis and could only be provided when the needs of the service user demanded it. The team felt that on occasions where these requests for support were turned down, some units did not re-refer and so did not make use of the service the team could provide.

Underlying many of these individual issues is a central and unresolved tension. By intervening in individual cases, an acute liaison team can significantly improve the quality of care provided to that individual. However, this only works on a case-by-case basis when the team is involved at an early stage. It can often remove responsibility from hospital staff for what should be everyday good practice – people with learning disabilities deserve the same access to hospital services as everyone else, and many of the issues at stake (personal care, communication, working in partnership with family members etc.) are not 'rocket science'.

By adopting a more strategic approach, it is possible to have a longer-term impact. This often involves *working with* hospital services (supporting them, helping them to do it themselves) rather than *doing it for them*. This is much less tangible than direct, individual casework, and may not have the same immediate impact for the individual.

When a person with a learning disability receives poor care in hospital, should the nurse intervene to provide care directly and thus improve the quality of care? Or should the aim be to support others to do it better, which may not have such instant effects but might have a bigger impact over time? Several years after the advent of acute hospital liaison, this question is almost impossible to resolve, and working with this ambiguity and tension goes to the heart of the liaison role.

National and regional developments

At a national level, there is a range of new initiatives and opportunities that give grounds for optimism. Since the advent of the Birmingham team, the health care needs of people with learning disabilities have received increasing attention from bodies such as the *Valuing People* Support Team (Department of Health 2002a), the Disability Rights Commission (2004) and the NPSA (2004). While the first two of these might be expected to champion the needs of people with learning disabilities, the research and development work of a mainstream NHS body like the NPSA is a particularly timely and welcome step forward (Box 7.5).

Box 7.5 Key concerns highlighted by the NPSA (2004)

The NPSA has highlighted these patient safety priorities:

- Inappropriate use of physical intervention
- Vulnerability of people with learning disabilities in general hospitals
- Swallowing difficulties
- Lack of accessible information
- Illness or disease being mis- or undiagnosed

In response, the NPSA:

- Has set up a steering group looking at issues for people with learning disabilities in hospital
- Is planning to pilot a number of tools nationally designed to support people with learning disabilities and hospital staff
- Will issue a safety alert on the vulnerability of people with learning disabilities on admission to hospital in 2006

Access to Acute (A2A)

The main national body focusing on these issues remains the A2A (Access to Acute) network. This is a national peer support network, meeting regularly in different locations across the country. The network welcomes anyone interested in the care of people with learning disabilities in hospital and is co-chaired by the lead nurse from Shropshire and a member of the Taking Part self-advocacy group. The emphasis of the group is on sharing good practice and learning from others' experiences. This support is valued by for all those involved but has proved crucial for those seconded into a post for a year or two. Speaking to liaison nurses already engaged with hospitals and learning from their successes and failures can save a great deal of time.

The group also seeks to influence the national agenda and members of the network have been involved in discussions with the NPSA. More recently, the national A2A group has sought to develop a regional structure. This came about due to the number of new people coming into post or taking on acute liaison as an additional responsibility. At a regional meeting, there is more opportunity for these people to receive peer support, meeting with others carrying out this role to share ideas and learn from existing good practice. With demands on time at a premium, it is sometimes difficult for practitioners to be released or arrange time to attend national meetings, with the travelling time and expense involved. This is particularly true of staff working in the acute hospitals who are often given no extra time to carry out this aspect of their work and do so through their commitment to meeting the needs of people with learning disabilities. The peer support provided by such networking is invaluable to practitioners working in what can be an isolating and – at times – misunderstood role. By holding regular regional meetings, it was hoped that at least one or two members from the regional network would be able to attend the national meetings, feed in what is happening in their region and report back to the region on the national picture.

In the West Midlands, each regional meeting has a theme (for example, discharge, dysphagia, carers, admission) selected in advance by the group as being an area where there are particular difficulties for people with learning disabilities. Group members are encouraged to invite colleagues from both community and acute services who have a special interest or expertise in the area to be discussed (for example, discharge liaison nurses, speech and language therapists, dietitians). Such professionals may not be able to attend every meeting, but have a great deal to offer focused discussions on particular issues. The meetings include an opportunity for members who attend the national A2A group to feed back from the latest network meeting and for the regional group to feed into the national network what is happening locally. Details of local and national A2A meetings are available on *www.nnldn.org.uk/a2a*, and this website also contains details of many of the examples of liaison work cited throughout this chapter.

Conclusion

The experiences of people with learning disabilities in acute hospitals can still be negative, with communication difficulties, stereotyping and poor quality care all common occurrences. Despite this, the acute liaison nurse has the potential to make a substantial difference to the lives of people with learning disabilities, and to the confidence and skills of hospital staff. Achieving these benefits takes time, perseverance and considerable motivation – but it can work and it is worth it. With more support available locally, regionally and nationally, there is still much to do, but now more hope than ever that people with learning disabilities will one day be able to access the same health care as everyone else.

References and further reading

Alborz A, McNaily R, Swallow A, Glendinning C (2003) *From the cradle to the grave: a literature review of access to health care for people with learning disabilities across the lifespan.* Manchester, National Primary Care Research and Development Centre

Band R (1998) *The NHS – Health for all? People with learning disabilities and health care.* London, Mencap

Barr O (1997) Care of people with learning disabilities in hospital. *Nursing Standard* **12**, 8, 49–56

Bollands R, Jones A (2002) Improving care for people with learning disabilities. *Nursing Times* **98**, 35, 38–39

Department of Health (2001) *Valuing People*: a new strategy for learning disability for the 21st century. London, The Stationery Office

Department of Health (2002a) *Action for Health:* health action plans and health facilitation. London, The Stationery Office

Department of Health (2002b) *Reference guide to consent for examination or treatment.* London, The Stationery Office

Department of Health (2003) *Discharge from hospital:* pathway, process and practice. London, The Stationery Office

Disability Rights Commission (2004) *You can make a difference:* improving hospital services for disabled people. London, Department of Health

Hannon L (2003) Secondary health care for people with learning disabilities *Nursing Standard* **17**, 46, 39–42

Hannon L (2004) Better preadmission assessment improves learning disability care *Nursing Times* **100**, 25, 44–47

Mencap (2004) *Treat Me Right! Better health services for people with learning disabilities.* London, Mencap

National Patient Safety Agency (2004) *Understanding the patient safety issues for people with learning disabilities.* London, NPSA

NHS Executive (1998) *Signposts for success in commissioning and providing health services for people with learning disabilities.* London, NHS Executive

Websites

(accessed 7 June 2007)
National Network for Learning Disability Nurses: *www.nnldn.org.uk*
Valuing People: *www.valuingpeople.gov.uk*
National Patient Safety Agency: *www.npsa.co.uk*

Regional focus on learning disability nursing

CHAPTER 8

Regional focus
Scotland

Michael Brown

Introduction

This chapter will provide an overview of health of the Scottish general population and outline the key issues impacting on the health and well-being of people with learning disabilities. Legislative frameworks since devolution will be explored and the main policy areas outlined that have been developed specifically with people with learning disabilities in mind detailed. Key organisations with a remit to support wider social inclusion and health improvement will be detailed, their contributions to people with learning disabilities identified and their impact discussed.

Box 8.1 Demographics

Scotland is a country of some five million people situated in Northern Europe. While many of the countries in the European Union have increasing populations, this is not the case in Scotland. The Scottish population is ageing and contrasts with a falling birth rate, suggesting that by 2031 there will be significant population shifts. It is estimated the number of people over 65 will rise from 787,000 to 1,200,000 and those over 85 from 84,000 to 150,000. Included in these estimates will be people with learning disabilities, now living into older age (Public Health Institute of Scotland 2001a, Scottish Executive 2002a).

Geographically, Scotland is a diverse country with two-thirds of the population living in the central belt. The country comprises the lowland areas that border England and comprises towns and village communities such as Dumfries, Stranraer, Selkirk, Melrose, Hawick, Galashiels and Jedburgh, moving onto the more densely populated and industrialised areas with cities and towns such as Edinburgh, Glasgow, Hamilton, Paisley, Ayr, Dundee, Kirkcaldy, Dunfermline, Stirling and Falkirk. The highland areas unfold from the central belt and have major cities and towns such as Inverness, Aberdeen, Pitlochry, Thurso and Wick. There are also a significant number of outer islands which include the Western Isles, Shetland and Orkney, which can only be accessed by ferry or flight. People with learning disabilities live in all parts of Scotland, including the outer islands, and they may have to travel to the mainland for some aspects of their care.

Table 8.1 Scottish population, June 2003

Argyll & Clyde	417,010
Ayrshire & Arran	367,140
Borders	108,280
Dumfries & Galloway	147,210
Fife	351,960
Forth Valley	279,680
Grampian	523,390
Greater Glasgow	866,370
Highland	209,080
Lanarkshire	553,440
Lothian	780,010
Orkney	19,310

The health of the people of Scotland

Scotland's health ranks poorly when compared with most European countries, with higher mortality and morbidity rates. Life expectancy is shorter overall for both men and women and death rates are among the highest in Western Europe. This has not always been the case, and is a phenomenon that has occurred in the past 50 years. The current evidence of the health of the people of Scotland points to the higher prevalence rates in areas such as coronary heart disease, cancers, obesity and mental ill health, with marked variation between areas and communities across Scotland (Public Health Institute of Scotland 2002). To respond, the Scottish Executive established a national working group in 2004 chaired by Professor David Kerr, Rhodes Scholar in cancer therapeutics and clinical pharmacology at Oxford University, with a remit to focus on the health needs of the Scottish population.

The report *Building a health service fit for the future* (Scottish Executive 2005a) made recommendations to the government on the issues that require to be addressed to reduce health inequalities and redesign health services to meet the needs in the future.

The government response to the health inequalities and service redesign issues identified in Kerr's report was *Delivering for Health* (Scottish Executive 2005b). The report identifies and outlines the actions required to redesign health services and reduce the health inequalities.

Broad actions will include:

- A National Health Service that is integrated and available equitably for the whole of Scotland
- Health delivered as locally as is possible
- Systematic management and support for people with long-term conditions
- Reducing the inequalities gap
- Actively managing hospital admissions and discharge

Devolution in Scotland

Many areas of policy are devolved to the Scottish Parliament, a situation that has resulted following devolution in 1999. At this time, the Scottish Parliament assumed responsibility for policy development and implementation in health care, social work, education, transport and a range of other areas. Elections for the Scottish Parliament are held once every four years and in the May 2003 election no single political party obtained an outright majority resulting in a coalition between the Scottish Labour Party and the Scottish Liberal Democrats. As a result of this coalition a joint statement, *A Partnership for a Better Scotland,* outlining the key policy areas was published (Scottish Executive 2003a). The need to form a coalition government may become the norm and it could be that in the future the Westminster Parliament is of one political persuasion and in Scotland another, following different health policy, thereby impacting on the concept of a UK-wide 'National Health Service'. While to date this has not occurred, the possibility is real and could bring yet further differences in health care services in Scotland.

In the May 2007 election the Scottish National Party (SNP) secured 47 of the 129 seats and Labour 46. As in 2003, no single party achieved an outright majority and SNP have not sought to form a coalition administration. This means they will negotiate with other political parties in the Parliament on an issue by issue basis to take forward their policies. This is in contrast to the Westminster Parliament, where a majority is held by a single political party.

As health is a devolved issue in Scotland the administration can adopt different health policies to that of the rest of the United Kingdom, challenging the concept of a UK-wide 'National Health Service'. While to date this has not occurred, the possibility is now real and could result in differences in health care and other services in Scotland.

Since devolution the Scottish Executive has been the administrative body responsible for implementing government policy. The Minister for Health and Community Care is responsible for determining wider health and social care policy, including policy for people with learning disabilities. Learning disability policy implementation sits in the Community Care Division of the Health Department, with the 14 NHS health boards and 32 local authorities responsible for providing health and social care services. Seven special NHS health boards provide countrywide services in areas such as the ambulance service, telehealth, education, quality improvement and health improvement. Services in the NHS in Scotland have been the subject of strategic review and are now going through a process of development and change in keeping with *Delivering for Health* (Scottish Executive 2005b) (Figure 8.1).

Health and social care policy

The health improvement policy focus was articulated in 1999 when the then administrative body, the Scottish Office, published *Towards a Healthier Scotland,* which set out the actions required to address the health needs (Scottish Office 1999). From that policy developed another central theme, partnership working

Figure 8.1 Overview of health and social care services in Scotland

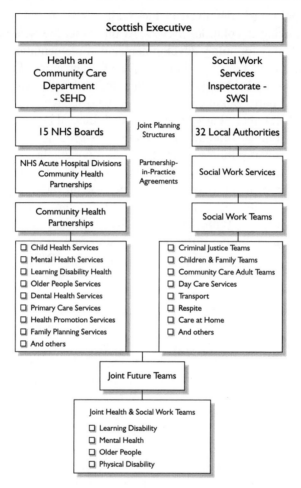

between health services and the Local Authorities (Scottish Executive 2000a). Termed *Joint Future,* the policy centres joint on collaborative working to improve care and focuses on:

- Joint management of health and local authority services in a single structure
- Joint resourcing of services, staff, equipment, finance and premises
- Joint premises for primary care and community care services

These joint activities are set around the structure of a single shared assessment process, aimed at the effective identification of individual need and a plan of care. *Joint Future* initially focused on older people and has now been extended to include all community care groups, including people with learning disabilities.

The government developed the plans further for health care and set them out in the report in *Our National Health: A Plan for Action, A Plan for Change* (Scottish Executive 2000b), which detailed the actions required from government, the NHS and their partners to 'rebuild' the health service in Scotland:

- Improving the care journey
- Meeting specific health needs to address inequalities
- Providing a lifetime of care for those that require it
- Working in partnership with patients and local authorities to improve care

Improving Health in Scotland: The Challenge set out the public health challenges that need to be addressed in Scotland to address health inequalities and improve health (Scottish Executive 2002b).

NHS trusts no longer exist in Scotland and legislative changes were required by way of the NHS Reform (Scotland) Bill 2003 to bring about further developments. The modernisation of services was taken a step further with the publication of Partnership for Care: Scotland's White Paper in 2003 (Scottish Executive 2003a). The report is significant as it sets out the creation of new community health partnerships (CHPs) – an evolvement of local healthcare co-operatives by bringing about further partnership working between health services and local authorities. Community health partnerships were established in 2005 and their core functions are to:

- Support local communities and enable health improvement
- Support partnership working between the NHS and local authorities
- Support the ongoing development of *Joint Future*
- Bring care closer to patients

Community health partnerships will be key organisations in Scotland to support health improvement, and an advice note was issued to all NHS Boards by the Scottish Executive detailing the key issues in relation to meeting the health needs of people with learning disabilities and autistic spectrum disorder (Scottish Executive 2004a). This advice note is important, given the increasing evidence of the health inequalities experienced by people with learning disabilities and the explicit role of the CHP as health improvement organisations. The creation of community health partnerships has the *potential* to offer a vehicle to bring about local action to address the health needs of children, adults and older people with learning disabilities in the future. The key challenge will be recognising the needs and acceptance of the responsibility for group by the community health partnerships and developing working partnerships with specialist learning disability health services in the future, thereby exploiting their knowledge and skills.

The future policy direction in Scotland

Today government public health policy is firmly directed at addressing the health needs of the people of Scotland. However, the longer-term benefits and impact have yet to be determined and will require sustained efforts for years to come. To ensure the NHS continues to address the needs of the people of Scotland, the Scottish Executive commissioned a report, chaired by Professor David Kerr: *Building a Health Service Fit for the Future* (Scottish Executive 2005a). The report sets out a framework to meet the challenges required to address Scotland's poor health, health inequalities and the increasing ageing population.

To achieve this, it is recognised it will be necessary to:

- Ensure local services are sustainable and safe
- Ensure the NHS services are delivered in local communities
- Ensure responses are preventative rather than reactive
- Integrate the whole care systems to respond to the challenges
- Become a modern NHS
- Enable the development of new skills to allow local services respond to need
- Develop options for health service change with patients

Legislation in Scotland

This section provides a brief overview of some aspects of legislation in Scotland with a specific impact on children, adults and older people with learning disabilities. Legislative power for many policy areas rest with the Scottish Parliament, with other areas being reserved issues for the Westminster Parliament. Additionally, European-wide legislation such as the European Convention of Human Rights impacts on all Scottish citizens and is particularly relevant to people with learning disabilities given the nature of various articles contained in the Human Rights Act (1998). Freedom from discrimination, Article 14, is particularly important and may be relevant to care and treatment by health care services.

Another significant piece of UK-wide legislation is the Disability Discrimination Act (1999). The Act has been implemented in three stages, with the last part coming into force in 2004. This part of the Act makes it explicitly illegal for public sector bodies to discriminate on the grounds of disability (including people with learning disabilities), requiring the public sector to make a 'reasonable adjustment' to meet the needs of such people. This legislation may prove to be significant for people with learning disabilities in the future, as some will require reasonable adjustments from both a cognitive and a physical access perspective to enable their needs to be addressed appropriately in health care settings. The potential for a legal challenge is therefore real, should health services fail in their duty.

The Adults with Incapacity (Scotland) Act 2000 provides a clear legal framework in Scotland for gaining consent when an adult is incapacitated or allowing someone to act on the behalf of a person who is incapacitated. The Act is in different parts and relates to:

- Principles
- Powers of attorney
- Accounts and funds
- Residents' finance

Part V of the Act is particularly relevant and relates to medical care and research and includes physical and mental health. The Act is accompanied by a Code of Practice to guide practitioners.

In Scotland there is separate mental health legislation from the rest of the United Kingdom. The Mental Health (Care and Treatment) (Scotland) Act 2003 has brought about significant change in mental healthcare and was implemented

Box 8.2 The Millan Principles

The Millan Principles seek to ensure that care is based on:

- Non-discrimination
- Reciprocity
- Informal care
- Participation
- Protecting child welfare
- Enabling equality
- Respect for diversity
- Respect for carers
- Least restrictive alternative
- Benefiting the individual

in October 2005. The legislation is set around the ten Millan Principles (Box 8.2) that influence and inform how the Act is to be interpreted in practice.

Contained in the Act are safeguards that will protect vulnerable people suffering from mental disorder, including people with learning disabilities:

- The right of appeal to a mental health tribunal
- The right to have a named person
- The right to independent advocacy
- The right to an advanced statement

Previously in Scotland, appeals against detention were dealt with by sheriff courts. Under the new Act, these issues are dealt with by the mental health tribunal, which conducts reviews, considers plans of care and make rulings on compulsory treatment orders. In the Act is the provision of an advanced statement – a written statement made when a person is well that is witnessed and lays out the treatment wishes should they become mentally unwell. A named person concept has been introduced and will allow those over 16 to nominate a person to protect their interests should they become mentally unwell.

The most significant legislation that related to the care of children is the Children (Scotland) Act (1995) which aims to ensure that all children lead ordinary lives and requires that services for children with disabilities act to minimise the effects and impact of the disability. Further legislation that has an impact on the care and education of children with learning disabilities in Scotland are the Special Educational Needs and Disability Act (2001) and Education (Disability Strategies and Pupils' Educational Records) (Scotland) (2002) Act.

The need for additional legislation focusing on the protection of vulnerable adults has been debated and is being taken forward in the Scottish Parliament by way of the Adult Support and Protection (Scotland) Bill. This legislation seeks to ensure there are appropriate frameworks in place to take account of the need to provide protection for vulnerable adults who by virtue of a significant impairment are at risk of harm and exploitation. A Code of Practice will support the implementation of the Bill for practitioners, service users and their carers.

People with learning disabilities in Scotland

There has been considerable activity and interest in the care and support of children, adults and older people with learning disabilities in Scotland following devolution. Since 2000 the government has initiated national work leading to the publication of three major reports:

- *The Same As You?* (Scottish Executive 2003c)
- *Promoting Health, Supporting Inclusion* (Scottish Executive 2002c)
- *People with Learning Disabilities in Scotland* (NHS Health Scotland 2004)

Collectively they signal a sound focus on the needs of children, adults and older people with learning disabilities in Scotland, providing a policy direction on the actions required to ensure the needs of this population are addressed. This is important, as historically people with learning disabilities have not been valued and included as full and equal members of society (Curtice 2003).

The Same As You?

In May 2000 the Scottish Executive published *The Same As You? A review of services for people with learning disabilities,* the first to be undertaken on supports and services for people with learning disabilities in Scotland in over 30 years. The review process was inclusive and took place over a two-year period and involved stakeholder events, reference groups, workshops, conferences, roadshows, specifically commissioned work and other activities across the country to inform and shape the recommendations.

The Same As You? defines learning disability as a significant, lifelong condition that has three facets:

- Reduced ability to understand new or complex information or to learn new skills
- Reduced ability to cope independently
- A condition that started before adulthood (before the age of 18) with a lasting effect on the individual's development

(Scottish Executive 2003c, p103)

The review includes people with autistic spectrum disorder as it is recognised that 70% of them also have a learning disability and may require access to specialist services and support. More detailed work on the needs of people with autistic spectrum disorder has been undertaken in Scotland, with best estimates suggesting the prevalence in children in Scotland is 60 per 10,000 and that the population is increasing (Public Health Institute of Scotland 2001b).

The Same As You? is set in the context of seven core principles that clearly state the intention that people with learning disabilities must be seen as equal citizens who have the right to be included in society. The seven principles state that people with learning disabilities should be:

- Valued
- Treated as individuals

- Asked about what they need and should be involved in choices
- Given the help and support to do what they want to do
- Able to get local services like everyone else
- Able to get specialist services when they need them
- Able to have services that take account of age, abilities and needs

The report contains 29 recommendations which are being taken forward by the Scottish Executive and implemented by *The Same As You* implementation group (SAYIG) which comprises people with learning disabilities, family carers, representatives from social work, health services and key independent sector organisations (Scottish Executive 2003a). In addition, a user and carer reference group brings together representatives from organisations such as ENABLE, People First, Down's Syndrome Scotland, PAMIS and Key Housing.

The full implementation of the recommendations arising from the review is expected to take place over a ten-year period, with some being taken forward by the Scottish Executive and others requiring collaboration between NHS Boards and local authorities to bring about action in the following areas:

- Developing partnership-in-practice agreements (PiPs)
- Developing local advocacy
- The closure of all long-stay institutions by 2005
- NHS boards to develop four assessment and treatment beds per 100,000 population
- NHS boards to develop local community services to avoid unnecessary hospital admission
- The development of support services for people with challenging behaviours
- A national review of speech and language therapy
- The development of local area coordination
- The establishment of the Scottish Consortium for Learning Disability
- A long-term programme to raise public awareness of learning disabilities
- A Scottish service network for autism
- The development of lifelong plans
- Direct payments being available by 2003 for those that wish them
- A change fund to support service developments
- Commissioning research on people with learning disabilities in secure environments
- Training for professionals to recognise early onset dementia

The Same As You? requires partnership approaches to service development and delivery between health services and local authorities with many of the 29 recommendations reflecting a joint approach to implementation. There is a health focus on:

- Primary care
- Mental health
- Challenging behaviour
- Criminal justice
- Profound and multiple learning disability

While there is a focus on some health aspects, a closer analysis demonstrates an absence on other important areas of health care, with no reference or action in the area of health education and health improvement recommended, despite evidence regarding the benefits to inclusion in such activities and more importantly of the impact of their exclusion. There is also a substantial body of evidence regarding the potential benefits of health screening and while *The Same As You?* recognises the difficulties experienced in this area, there is a missed opportunity to recommend national action to address them.

As the evidence base of the health needs of this group evolves, it is now apparent that people with learning disabilities will be high users of all aspects of health service and for many their care needs are significant, yet no action is recommended to ensure that additional support and help are available throughout the healthcare journey – one of the seven principles. A positive focus would have been to require partnership working *in* and *across* all aspects of the health care systems across the lifespan in recognition of the fact that many will be high and frequent attendees and should be able to access local services. Furthermore, no reference is made to the issue of antidiscrimination and equal access to health care in areas such as general hospitals and child and adolescent mental health services, where there is a specific need for development and improvement.

While there are gaps in the review recommendations from a health perspective, there are many positive examples of the developments arising from the implementation of *The Same As You?*

Partnership-in-practice agreements

Partnership-in-practice agreements (PiPs) have been introduced as a result of the review and are developed in collaboration between NHS boards and local authorities in partnership with people with learning disabilities, their families and carers and other key stakeholders. PiPs cover a three-year period and outline the areas of development that will be taken forward in specific areas to improve services and supports for children, adults and older people. The plans include financial commitments, and all PiPs are available for public scrutiny on the Scottish Executive Same as you? website. To share practice and provided a co-ordinated approach to the development and implementation of PiPs, a network of professionals has been established comprising those responsible for the agreements from local authorities and health services, the Director of the Scottish Consortium and Scottish Executive officials.

Change Fund

The Same As You? recognised that to support change and develop services it was necessary to put in place additional finance. Year-on-year, local authorities and their partners can apply to the Scottish Executive Change Fund for funding to support the development of projects and services. For 2001–2002 the Change Fund totalled £8 million, with further funding being made available for the 2002–2003 and 2003–2004 periods. The funding has been used for a range of local developments such as supported breaks, supported employment, advocacy, supported housing, developing accessible information, local needs assessment and the development of local registers of needs.

Scottish Consortium for Learning Disability

The Scottish Consortium for Learning Disability (SCLD) was established as a result of another recommendation in *The Same As You?* The SCLD has people with learning disabilities at the heart of the organisation and works in partnership with carers and other key stakeholders. The Scottish Consortium is a partnership of organisations, funded by the Scottish Executive and comprises ENABLE, ARC, PAMIS (Profound and Multiple Impairment Service), Key Housing Association, Quality Action Group, Scottish Down's Syndrome Association, Badaguish Outdoor Centre, The British Institute for Learning Disabilities (BILD) and academics from the Universities of Abertay, Dundee, St Andrews and the University Affiliated Programme at the University of Glasgow.

The broad focus of the work programme of the Scottish Consortium is on:
* Training
* Information
* Public education
* Research

Hospital closure

In Scotland few people with learning disabilities were resident in long-stay institutions; the majority have always lived in the community, usually with their families or in their own home. Today government policy is that long-stay institutions should not be home for people with learning disabilities. The initial target was for all long-stay institutions to close by 2005, however as this was not achieved in all areas, a revised target was set for the end of 2007. The resettlement and closure programme has been undertaken across Scotland over a five-year period and today sees people with learning disabilities living in community settings. As part of the resettlement programme the Scottish Executive published *Home at Last? a Report of the short-life working group on hospital closure and service reprovision* (Scottish Executive 2003b). The report sets out the recent history of long-stay institutions in Scotland and the issues that need to be taken forward to support and bring about full closure by 2005.

Local area co-ordination and personal life plans

Local area co-ordination is a model of care that was developed in Western Australia to co-ordinate local services; provide information and support individuals and their families. *The Same As You?* recommended that all areas in Scotland develop local area co-ordination, with a specialist worker role developed to work with a small number – around 50 – people with learning disabilities and their families and support them through what can be complex and complicated care systems.

An aspect of the role of local area co-ordinator is to support the development of a personal life plan for those that wish one. The personal life plan sets out how people who support a person with a learning disability and their family will work together to ensure that the needs of the individual can be met in a way that enables personal development building on their strengths and creating opportunities, and help them to make a contribution to the local community and lead fulfilling lives.

A national network for autism

The review identified the need to develop appropriate services and responses for people with learning disabilities who have autism, as currently there is wide variation across the country. Local and national priorities have been identified to improve services and support for people with autism:

- Improve early diagnosis
- Provide professionals with local access to information, specialist knowledge and training
- Develop the range of local support and services available
- Enable people to get specialist services when needed

Additionally, a national service network for children and adults with autistic spectrum disorder has been established, with NHS boards and local authorities identifying a named professional to lead on local service improvement and link with the national network.

Support in secure environments

There has been a limited strategic focus in the past on the needs of people with learning disabilities with forensic and offending behaviours in Scotland. To address this issue the Health and Community Care Social Research Unit of the Scottish Executive commissioned the Scottish Development Centre for Mental Health to undertake more detailed work and *On the Borderline? People with Learning Disabilities and/or Autistic Spectrum Disorders in Secure, Forensic and Other Specialist Settings* was published in 2004 (Scottish Executive 2004b). The work looked at The State Hospital, a national secure resource serving Scotland and Northern Ireland, the 16 prisons in Scotland, six secure units for looked after children and 24 secure-type units for adults with learning disabilities. The report highlights the challenges in identifying and meeting the needs of people with learning disabilities and autistic spectrum disorder in secure settings – suggesting that some fall between services, with no organisation taking responsibility, which points to an under-identification of the true prevalence.

People with learning disabilities are also thought to be disadvantaged in the criminal justice system by virtue of their cognitive and developmental delay and the associated impact on comprehension and ability, with many having comorbid mental health and other needs. There is acknowledgement of the limited understanding of the needs of people with autism and the suggestion that further work needs to be done in this area.

The nursing and midwifery contributions in Scotland

In 2000, the Scottish Executive published *Caring for Scotland: The strategy for nursing and midwifery in Scotland* (Scottish Executive 2000d). The report recommends that the Scottish Executive undertake a review of the contribution of nurses and midwives to the care of people with learning disabilities, in recognition of the changing care arrangements for this group. In 2002, *Promoting Health, Supporting Inclusion: The national review of the contribution of all nurses and midwives to the care and support of people with learning disabilities* was published (Scottish Executive 2002c) detailing the actions required for all nurses and midwives, whatever their area of clinical practice, to improve the health and well-being of children, adults and older people with learning disabilities The report identified five core areas:

- The current nursing and midwifery contributions across the lifespan of children, adults and older people with learning disabilities
- The areas of best nursing and midwifery practice
- The education needs of nurses and midwives
- The nursing and midwifery contributions required in the future
- The practice development and research needs of nurses and midwives

From this work the message is clear – all nurses and midwives in Scotland have important contributions to make to address the health needs of all children, adults and older people with learning disabilities in Scotland. Since the launch of the report there has been considerable activity to implement the 24 recommendations, which can be grouped in five broad areas:

- Health improvement
- Nurse education
- Co-ordination of care
- Practice development
- Joint working

Work has been taken forward across Scotland to implement the recommendations from the review, developing and enhancing the contributions made by nurses and midwives, whatever their area of clinical practice. The review recognises the important role of children's and learning disability nurses and the central part they need to play in promoting and improving the health and well-being of children and adults with learning disabilities as part of the contribution towards enabling social inclusion and community participation.

A different health profile

People with learning disabilities comprise a sub-population of the general Scottish population with distinct needs, many of which will be lifelong. All have a range of health needs that require care and support from primary care, secondary care and some will require specialist child health and learning disability health services. With the shift in policy emphasis away from long-stay institution care, it is important to recognise that few people with learning disabilities overall were resident in these care settings – most have always lived in their communities – yet there has been a limited focus and allocation of resources directed at their health needs (Scottish Executive 2003b). This point is significant and when considered in the context of the wider health inequalities, helps in part to contextualise their poor health status.

As the evidence base evolves and is better understood nationally and internationally, it is apparent that people with learning disabilities have a *different* pattern of health disease from the general population, have higher levels of health needs, with many going unrecognised, undiagnosed and therefore untreated (Beange 1995; van Schrojenstein Lantman-de Valk 1997; Webb & Rogers 1999; Cooper et al 2004). This situation is now viewed as unacceptable, and addressing their health disparities is therefore a wider public health responsibility that requires sustained effort and investment to effect change and bring about improvement. This is important – unlike the general population, which is decreasing, the learning disability population is increasing, a situation that is expected to continue (Hollins et al 1998). The effect of this phenomenon will be more people with learning disabilities living into older age and will include those with more complex care needs, with many having a clear health care component. These health components will result in an increase use of all aspects of the healthcare system (Brown et al 2005). This is new – in the past few people with learning disabilities lived into older age, so a clear focus on recognising and responding to the health needs of this group of the Scottish population is needed.

To address this issue, the Public Health Institute of Scotland assessed the health needs of children, adults and older people with learning disabilities at the request of the Scottish Executive. This work commenced in 2002, with the final report *People with Learning Disabilities in Scotland: The Health Needs Assessment* being published in 2004 (NHS Health Scotland 2004). The Health Needs Assessment is a major review of the evidence of the health needs of children, adults and older people with learning disabilities, with the key issues identified in the health needs assessment report concluding that:

- The demographics of the learning disability population is changing, with an overall increase that is expected to continue
- Life expectancy is increasing
- The learning disability population is ageing
- There will be more people with complex needs living into older age
- People with learning disabilities experience significant health inequalities when compared to the general population and have higher health needs
- Their health profile differs from the general population
- The health needs of people with learning disabilities need a range of responses from health services from primary care to specialist health services
- The cause of death differs from the general population, with respiratory and cardiovascular disease being highest for people with learning disabilities
- Many health needs of people with learning disabilities go unrecognised and therefore unmet, impacting on life expectancy and quality of life

- Some people with intellectual disabilities would benefit from a targeted health screening programme
- People with learning disabilities experience significant barriers to accessing health care appropriate to their needs
- The cancer pattern differs from the general population, with oesophageal, stomach and gall bladder cancers being more prevalent
- Scottish health policy must take account of the different health profile of people with learning disabilities to reduce the health inequality gap, not widen it
- People with learning disabilities experience institutional discrimination in health care systems, despite legislation aimed at eliminating discrimination against vulnerable groups

From a learning disability perspective, there is no national system of identifying the total population in Scotland at present. Data does exist for some populations, such as children and young people with learning disabilities attending special schools, who have their needs recorded on a special needs system. However, this work is not continued at present across the lifespan and there are no accurate figures available for adults and older people. Based on prevalence studies, it is estimated that there are 120,000 children and adults with learning disabilities in Scotland, with about one-third being in contact with health and social care services (Scottish Executive 2000c).

Scotland is responding to the need for accurate data of prevalence and support needs by the development of local Registers, the e-SAY project, part of the Scottish Executive national e-Care projects. The e-SAY project is being taken forward by the Scottish Consortium for Learning Disability and has seen the development of a dataset that will be used by NHS boards and local authorities to support the collection of information. This local data will be used to create a national database, ensuring that across Scotland information is recorded in the same way. Over time this will build a picture nationally of the needs being met, as well as areas of unmet need for people with learning disabilities and their families, thereby enabling appropriate responses.

Key Scottish organisations

In Scotland there are organisations with key strategic roles in meeting health and social care needs. Their remits impact on the support of people with learning disabilities, whose needs are central to their work programmes.

The Care Commission

The Scottish Commission for the Regulation of Care (The Care Commission) is a national organisation established under the Regulation of Care (Scotland) Act (2001). The Care Commission was formed in 2003 with the remit to regulate and inspect independent care providers, including private hospitals and clinics and their statutory powers relate to regulation in the areas of registration, inspection, complaints and enforcement. These functions were previously undertaken locally in each area of Scotland by inspection units located in NHS boards and social work departments.

Today the term 'care home' is used in Scotland to include all settings subject to formal inspection and registration by the Care Commission, replacing such terms as 'nursing home'. This change recognises the importance of ensuring that – as part of the inspection process – care homes are in a position to meet the potential changing needs of their residents, requiring the organisation to respond rather than require the resident to move care settings. To support this, national care standards have been developed, with specific standards relating to the care needs of people with learning disabilities in addition to other care standards that may also apply, such as day care or respite.

The Mental Welfare Commission

The Mental Welfare Commission is an independent organisation set up by Parliament to protect people with mental disorder and includes people with learning disabilities and those with dementia (Mathieson 2005). The Commission has a duty to anyone with a mental disorder, irrespective of whether they are in hospital, in local authority care, the independent sector or their own home. The Commission is required to visit people with mental disorder in hospital and the community and to investigate cases where there are concerns about care or treatment.

The work of the Commission is to:
- Undertake visits in hospital and the community – both announced and unannounced
- Undertake inquiries into issues of care and treatment
- Review requests for discharge of detention orders
- Visit people on welfare guardian orders
- Monitor intervention orders and visit as appropriate
- Undertake suicide and accident reviews
- Provide information and advice

In Scotland the changes in The Mental Health (Care and Treatment) (Scotland) Act (2003) have specific implications for the Commission and their enhanced powers under the Act will enable the development of their role in protecting people with mental disorder.

Under the Act the Commission has responsibility to:
- Monitor the operation of the Act
- Promote best practice in mental health care
- Carry out visits to patients, undertake investigations and interviews and where necessary medical examination
- Inspect and review records
- Publish information and guidance on mental health issues
- Bring issues and concern to the attention of the mental health legal system

NHS Health Scotland

NHS Health Scotland was formed in 2003 by the government with the merger of the Public Health Institute of Scotland and the Health Education Board for Scotland. It is charged with supporting the improvement of the health of the people of Scotland, and has these core functions:

- Deliver health improvement programmes to improve Scotland's health
- Use knowledge about the determinants of health to influence policy and practice to improve health in Scotland
- Support the implementation of programmes of health improvement

One strand of the work has been the publication of needs assessments in a range of health and health improvement areas that aim to promote evidence-based services in Scotland. All the needs assessments are relevant to people with learning disabilities, with some having particular relevance, given their needs. Examples of needs assessments with particular relevance to children, adults and older people with learning disabilities are:

- People with learning disabilities in Scotland – the health needs assessment
- Oral health in primary care
- Needs assessment of dementia and older people in Scotland
- Risk factors for dementia and cognitive decline
- Child and adolescent mental health NHS audiology services in Scotland
- Liaison psychiatry and psychology
- Autistic spectrum disorders

NHS Quality Improvement Scotland

NHS Quality Improvement Scotland was established in 2002 when organisations across Scotland with a quality improvement function were brought together. The function of the organisation today is to promote and support improvements in the quality of care throughout the NHS in Scotland, which:

- Sets standards
- Monitors performance
- Provides advice, guidance and support to NHS in Scotland on effective clinical practice and service improvements

Health improvement visits are undertaken with a national learning disability inspection programme having been established that centres on quality standards against which services and care are evaluated (NHS Quality Improvement Scotland 2004). Each NHS board area is visited and inspected by a team of trained peer reviewers, drawn from health care, social care, the independent sector and users and carers. The quality indicators have been developed and structured around the tiered model of care outlined in *Promoting Health, Supporting Inclusion* –ensuring that all aspects of health care across the lifespan are included.

As part of the recommendations from *Promoting Health, Supporting Inclusion*, a number of other areas of work have been progressed by NHS Quality Improvement Scotland that focus on service improvement for people with learning disabilities.

A national database of nursing and midwifery practice in learning disabilities across the lifespan has been developed, along with a national mapping exercise to identify the practice development needs of all nurses and midwives. A national Best Practice Statement aimed at frontline staff, detailing the actions required to ensure that people with learning disabilities receive equitable access to mainstream healthcare was published in 2006.

NHS Education for Scotland

NHS Education for Scotland is responsible for supporting the development and education of nurses, midwives and public health nurses, medicine, clinical psychology, pharmacy, the allied health professions, dentistry and health care scientists in the NHS in Scotland.

Four recommendations arising from *Promoting Health, Supporting Inclusion* were directed at NHS Education for Scotland, inviting them to take forward developments in undergraduate education for *all* nurses and midwives on the needs of people with learning disabilities. Further recommendations required a review of the learning disability and child health undergraduate nursing programmes to ensure they produce practitioners competent and fit for practice in the future. The final area of development is continuing professional development opportunities in learning disability practice. These developments focus on five areas of practice:

- Health promotion
- Autistic spectrum disorder
- Challenging behaviours
- Complex care needs
- Person-centred planning

The education opportunities are all delivered by accessible learning methods, enabling a wide range of practitioners from any discipline to access and continue their education and development in this area. The achievements have been significant, and NHS Education for Scotland published Getting *it Right Together* outlining the education developments and progress on implementation of their recommendations to ensure the health needs of people with learning disabilities are addressed in the future (NHS Education for Scotland 2004). Building on *Getting it Right Together,* NHS Education for Scotland worked with higher education institutions who provide the branch programme to develop a national framework for learning disability nurse education in Scotland. *The Right Preparation: The Framework for Learning Disability Nurse Education in Scotland* was published in February 2005 and will support a national approach to the theory and practice components of the branch programme, ensuring that practitioners are skilled to meet the needs of children and adults with learning disabilities in the future.

Conclusion

The evidence points to the poor health record of the people of Scotland and it is important to recognise the impact of this on people with learning disabilities and to appreciate that many present with a range of layered, complex needs. To address their health inequalities, the people in Scotland require a sustained focus to bring about long-term improvement, with government policy clearly directed towards this end.

The evidence base of the disparities experienced by people with learning disabilities is clear and is now a policy area that is receiving attention. Today in Scotland there are legislative and policy frameworks that focus on the needs of children, adults and older people with learning disabilities. This is important given their complex care needs and the increasing numbers living into older age and the range of health, social care, housing, education and independent sector organisations that need to respond. Since government devolution in Scotland there have been significant changes and developments with clear policies directed at improving health and social inclusion. Key national organisations have been developed to support the initiatives required, thereby ensuring the foundations are in place to address the needs of the Scottish population and sub-populations.

In recognition of the many challenges ahead, ensuring these organisations work for and meet the health needs of people with learning disabilities will be the test. Ensuring government policy and strategy are fully implemented in a political and changing culture of service delivery is the real challenge – the vision set out by the Scottish government generally receives support and builds aspirations. As part of any policy implementation, national monitoring needs to be in place and be sustained over time. For people with learning disabilities, this is vital to ensure they are included in wider public health activities aimed at the general population and are also the focus of population-specific health improvement initiatives; action is required on both fronts if their health needs are to be addressed.

The Scottish government views joint working between health and local authorities as the way forward and the policy framework reflects this. The key challenge will be to ensure that the service developments that are taking place work effectively for all people with learning disabilities and take account of their specific needs. National work needs to be undertaken to detail the health improvement indicators necessary to support sustained and focused improvement over time. Without such indicators on which changes and improvements can be measured, there is the distinct possibility that people with learning disabilities become 'lost' as a care group, leading to yet another form of institutional neglect. Identifying the key workforce needs will be central to this as there is a clear need to ensure there is a range of professionals available with an interest in – and knowledge of – the care needs of children, adults and older people with learning disabilities in the future.

References

Adults with Incapacity (Scotland) Act (2000) Edinburgh, The Stationery Office

Beange H, McElduff A, Baker W (1995) Medical disorders of adults with mental retardation: a population study. *American Journal on Mental Retardation* **99**, 6, 595–604

Brown M, MacArthur J, Gibbs S (2005) *A New Research Agenda: Improving General*

Hospital Care for People with Learning Disabilities. Edinburgh: NHS Lothian

Children (Scotland) Act (1995) Edinburgh, HMSO

Cooper S, A, Melville C, Morrison J (2004) People with intellectual disabilities: Their health needs differ and need to be recognised and met. *British Medical Journal* **239**, 414–415

Curtice L in Brown M (2003) *People with Learning Disabilities: A Handbook of Integrated Care*. Wiltshire, APS Publications

Disability Discrimination Act (1999) London, HMSO

Education (Disability Strategies and Pupil's Educational Records) (Scotland) Act (2002) Edinburgh, The Stationery Office

Hollins S, Attard M, T, von Fraunhofer N, McGuigan S, Sedgwick P (1998) Mortality in people with learning disability: risks, causes, and death certification findings in London. *Developmental Medicine and Child Neurology* **40**, 1, 50–56

Human Rights Act (1998) London, HMSO

Mathieson A (2005) Scotland the Brave. *Learning Disability Practice* **8**, 1, 8–9

Mental Health (Care and Treatment) (Scotland) Act (2003) Edinburgh, The Stationery Office

NHS Education for Scotland (2004) *Getting it Right Together*. Edinburgh, NHS Education for Scotland

NHS Education for Scotland (2005) *The Right Preparation: The Framework for Learning Disability Nurse Education in Scotland*. Edinburgh, NHS Education for Scotland

NHS Health Scotland (2004) *People with Learning Disabilities in Scotland*. Glasgow, NHS Health Scotland

NHS Quality Improvement Scotland (2004) *Quality Indicators for Learning Disabilities*. Edinburgh, NHS Quality Improvement Scotland

NHS Quality Improvement Scotland (2006) Best Practice Statement. Promoting access to healthcare for people with a learning disability - A guide for frontline staff. Edinburgh, NHS Quality Improvement Scotland.

NHS Reform (Scotland) Bill (2003) Edinburgh, The Stationery Office

Public Health Institute of Scotland (2001a) *Chasing the Scottish Effect. Why Scotland needs a step-change in health if it is to catch up with the rest of Europe*. Glasgow, Public Health Institute of Scotland

Public Health Institute of Scotland (2001b) *Autistic Spectrum Disorder: Needs Assessment Report*. Glasgow, The Public Health Institute of Scotland

Public Health Institute of Scotland (2002) *Health Inequalities in the New Scotland*. Glasgow, Public Health Institute of Scotland

Regulation of Care (Scotland) Act (2001) Edinburgh, The Stationery Office

Scottish Executive (2000a) *A Joint Future – Report of The Joint Future Group*. Edinburgh, The Stationery Office.

Scottish Executive (2000b) *Our National Health: A Plan for Action, A Plan for Change*. Edinburgh, The Stationery Office

Scottish Executive (2000c) *The Same As You? A review of services for people with learning disabilities*. Edinburgh, The Stationery Office

Scottish Executive (2000d) *Caring for Scotland: The strategy for nursing and midwifery in Scotland*. Edinburgh, The Stationery Office

Scottish Executive (2002a) *Adding Life to Years. Report of the expert group on the healthcare of older people.* Edinburgh, The Stationery Office

Scottish Executive (2002b) *Improving Health in Scotland: The Challenge.* Edinburgh, The Stationery Office.

Scottish Executive (2002c) *Promoting Health, Supporting Inclusion: The national review of the contribution of all nurses and midwives to the care and support of people with learning disabilities.* Edinburgh, The Stationery Office

Scottish Executive (2003a) *A Partnership for a Better Scotland.* Edinburgh, The Stationery Office

Scottish Executive (2003b) *Home at last? Report of the short-life working group on hospital closure and service reprovision.* Edinburgh, The Stationery Office

Scottish Executive (2004a) *Improving the health and wellbeing of people with learning disabilities and/or autistic spectrum disorder.* Edinburgh, The Stationery Office

Scottish Executive (2004b) *On the Borderline? People with Learning Disabilities and/ or Autistic Spectrum Disorders in Secure, Forensic and Other Specialist Settings.* Edinburgh, The Stationery Office

Scottish Executive (2005a) *Building a Health Service Fit for the Future.* Edinburgh: The Stationery Office

Scottish Executive (2005b) *Delivering for Health.* Edinburgh: The Stationery Office

Scottish Office (1999) *Towards a Healthier Scotland. A White Paper on Health.* Edinburgh, HMSO

Special Educational Needs and Disability Act (2001) Edinburgh, The Stationery Office

van Schrojenstein Lantman-de Valk HM, van den A, Maaskant M, Haveman M, Urlings H, Kessels A, Crebolder H (1997) Prevalence and incidence of health problems in people with intellectual disability. *Journal of Intellectual Disability Research* **41**, 42–51

Webb O, Rogers L (1999) Health screening for people with intellectual disability: the New Zealand experience. *Journal of Intellectual Disability Research* **43**, 497–503

Websites

(accessed 7 June 2007)

The Same As You? Implementation site: *www.scotland.gov.uk/Topics/Health/care/ VAUnit/SAYIG*

NHS Education for Scotland: *www.nes.scot.nhs.uk*

NHS Quality Improvement Scotland: *www.nhshealthquality.org*

NHS Health Scotland: *www.healthscotland.com*

Scottish Consortium for Learning Disabilities: *www.scld.org.uk*

Mental Health Tribunal for Scotland: *www.mhtscot.org*

Mental Welfare Commission for Scotland: *www.mwcscot.org.uk*

The Care Commission: *www.carecommission.com*

The Scottish Executive: *www.scotland.gov.uk*

CHAPTER 9

Regional focus
Northern Ireland

Maurice Devine and Owen Barr

Introduction

Northern Ireland, although part of the island of Ireland, is a constituent part of the United Kingdom (consisting of Northern Ireland, Scotland, England and Wales) and has a population of approximately 1.7 million. The capital of the country, and its administrative base for health and social care, is Belfast.

The health and social care system in Northern Ireland is linked to the United Kingdom National Health Service, with medical, health and social services being free to every citizen at the point of delivery. However, Northern Ireland's health service is organised very differently from that in the rest of the United Kingdom.

A frustrating aspect of being part of the Health and Social Services machinery in Northern Ireland is that, at times, legislation brought in to other parts of the UK did not immediately apply in Northern Ireland. Due to the arrangements under 'direct rule' the extension of such legislation required an 'Order in Council' to be extended to Northern Ireland, a process that often took several years to complete. However, this process will change if the Northern Ireland Legislative Assembly is successfully reconstituted and maintained following the elections in March 2007.

As a key purpose of this book is to integrate the development of practice with variations in policy, demography and local structures, the focus of this chapter is to consider these issues from a Northern Ireland perspective. It will outline some of the key messages and recommendations arising from a review of policy and services for people with a learning disability in Northern Ireland, contained within the report *Equal Lives* (DHSSPS 2005).

In line with government policy and new and emerging demographic trends, there is a need for learning disability services to further develop, reshape, and adapt, in order that successful implementation of the *Equal Lives* review takes place and that people with a learning disability receive high quality, safe and effective care from the range of qualified and unqualified staff that are employed in this area in collaboration with mainstream services.

Nursing is a central component of these service delivery systems in hospitals, community settings, day care, education, and independent sectors. Although this chapter provides a direction for nursing, it should be considered in the multidisciplinary context of the setting the nurse is working in, such as the hospital-based team, the community learning disability team or the primary care team.

The structure of service provision

Unlike the rest of the United Kingdom, Health and Personal Social Services in Northern Ireland has been provided as an integrated service since the 1970s. Before 1st April 2007 the structure consisted of one overall Department of Health, Social Services and Public Safety, four health and social services boards and 19 health and social services trusts.

These previous structures have been reviewed as a result of the Review of Public Administration in Northern Ireland, which was instigated in June 2002 by the Northern Ireland Assembly. In November 2005, far-reaching revised structures for the future of local government, education and health and social services structures were announced. These new structures will replace the previous arrangements and will involve a smaller Department of Health and Social Services, the setting up of a Health and Social Care Authority, which will replace the four health and social service boards and one Patient and Client Council to replace the previous four health and social services councils. Seven local commissioning authorities will be responsible for commissioning local services and five health and social care trusts will replace the previous 19 trusts and be responsible for the delivery of services.

These new structures came into being on 1 April 2007 *(www.rpani.gov.uk/index.htm)*. It is envisaged that the revised structures will build further on the integrated health and social services structures and seek to build on this to provide a more co-ordinated and effective service to the people of Northern Ireland. Time will tell how much this restructuring improves services and outcomes for people in Northern Ireland.

From a learning disability nursing perspective, representatives of learning disability nurses in Northern Ireland regularly meet through the Department of Health, Social Services and Public Safety (DHSSPS) endorsed Regional Professional Development Forum for learning disability nurses (PDF). This body was formally established during 2004–05, and is representative of learning disability nurses working in hospital, community, independent and education settings across Northern Ireland.

The forum aims to promote practice improvement and development initiatives that can support regional consistency and best practice, and its main objectives are:

- To maintain a strategic view of developments in services for people with learning disability and their families, with a view to how these relate to developments in learning disability nursing
- To provide a co-ordinated regional representation of informed views from nurses in statutory, independent and nurse education providers involved in the

delivery of learning disability services across Northern Ireland
- To provide considered views, working papers and contribute to relevant discussions on learning disability and related policy development at a strategic and regional policy level

The prevalence of people with learning disabilities

The numbers of people with learning disabilities in the total population have been estimated on the basis of prevalence rates identified in each country. Prevalence rates in Scotland and England have been reported as 3–4 people with profound and severe intellectual disabilities among 1,000 people in the general population, and between 20–25 people with mild/moderate intellectual disabilities per 1,000 of the population (Scottish Executive 2000; Department of Health 2001). In Northern Ireland a combined prevalence of all people with intellectual disabilities has been reported as 9.7 people per 1,000 people in the population. This ranges from an overall prevalence of 16.3 for people 19 years old or less, 10.2 is the rate for people aged 20–34 years, and 7.0 for those between 35–49 years, with the rate dropping to 4.5 for those people aged 50 years or older (McConkey et al 2003). Of the identified 16,366 people with learning disabilities, 85.5% live with family carers or in their own home, and 11.6% live in community-based residential or nursing home accommodation. The remaining 3% (approximately 400 people) continue to reside in learning disability hospitals, of which there are three in the country (McConkey et al 2003).

People with learning disabilities are living longer, and as a result there will continue to be an increasing number of older people with learning disabilities. The numbers of people with learning disabilities are expected to continue rising by 1% every year over the next 10–15 years (SE 2000: DH 2001). This will result in a greater proportion of younger people and older people with learning disabilities who will present with complex health needs. Both these groups of people will present challenges to adult services as to date, they have limited experience in supporting younger adults and older people with such complex needs. The increasing life expectancy of people with learning disabilities will also lead to a greater proportion of people with learning disabilities living with older parents and family carers, or outliving their parents and carers. This trend has already been reported in Scotland with a quarter of people with learning disabilities living with a family carer over 65 years of age; 20% of people with learning disabilities have two carers aged 70 or over, and 11% have one carer over 70 years of age.

A time of change in services

In the other three countries of the United Kingdom there have been a number of policy reviews (Scottish Executive 2000, DH 2001, Welsh Office 2001) that have acted as drivers to reshape the direction of learning disability service provision – and ultimately nursing – in the respective countries.

Health and social care professionals in Northern Ireland have at times been able to use the 'being behind' scenario in relation to policy development, in a very positive and considered way, as it has allowed us – with hindsight – to learn the lessons from the successful and not-so-successful policy-driven developments in other parts of the UK and further afield.

The Review of Mental Health and Learning Disability (Northern Ireland) and the associated Learning Disability review *Equal Lives* (DHSSPS 2005) sought to use this hindsight to best effect. The Review of Mental Health and Learning Disability (Northern Ireland) was initiated by the Minister for Health, Social Services and Public Safety in October 2002, before the suspension of the Northern Ireland Assembly. The intention of this Review was to:

- Examine law, policy and service provision in mental health and learning disability services
- Consider, and learn from evidence based best practice developments in service provision regionally, nationally and internationally
- Propose a range of recommendations regarding future policy, strategy, service priorities and legislation, that reflect the current and emerging needs of users and carers *(www.rmhldni.gov.uk* – look under published reports for Equal Lives Learning Disability Report)

The review of learning disability service provision in Northern Ireland has been undertaken in the wider Review of Mental Health and Learning Disability. In this review, the learning disability element was constituted as one of ten working committees listed below, with links to the other committees, and forms an integral part of the overall review process (Box 9.1).

Unlike Scotland (*Same As You* 2000) and England (*Valuing People* 2001), this is not a standalone review of learning disability services, and has resulted in some concern being expressed that a separate review would have been more appropriate and beneficial in ensuring that the needs of people with a learning disability, and their families, were not compromised in the larger review of mental health.

One strategy to reduce some of the concerns expressed about learning disability issues not being adequately addressed has been the decision that the Learning Disability Committee will produce a separate report specific to learning disability services under the title of *Equal Lives*. However, all the other expert working groups had a clear remit to consider issues related to people with learning disabilities in their discussions. To produce the *Equal Lives* report, six task groups of this Learning Disability Working Committee were established to examine the key areas of:

- Accommodation and support
- Day opportunities
- Children and young people
- Ageing
- Mental health
- Physical health

The active involvement of people with learning disabilities and carers was one of the key principles underpinning the *Equal Lives* review. From the outset,

Box 9.1 Working committees and sub-groups set up in the overall Review of Mental Health and Learning Disability in Northern Ireland

- Adult Mental Health Working Committee
  - Severe Mental Illness Sub-Group
  - Community and Primary Care Sub-Group
- Social Justice and Citizenship Working Committee
  - Human Rights and Equality Sub-Group
  - Promoting Social Inclusion Sub-Group
- Legal Issues Working Committee (four sub-groups)
- Learning Disability Working Committee
  - Children and Young People Task Group
  - Day Opportunities Task Group
  - Mental Health Task Group
  - Physical Health Task Group
  - Ageing Issues Task Group
- Child and Adolescent Mental Health Working Committee
- Forensic Services Working Committee
- Mental Health Promotion Working Committee
- Needs and Resources Working Committee
- Dementia and Mental Health Issues of Older People Working Committee
- Alcohol and Substance Misuse Working Committee

the family carers group and the *Equal Lives* group, (consisting of people with learning disabilities), have been extremely active in producing their own reports, and commenting on, advising and guiding the work and progress of each task group, and ultimately the final report. All of the above reports are accessible via the review website *(www.rmhldni.gov.uk)*

The review also commissioned an audit of research in learning disability in Northern Ireland, which resulted in:

- A directory of research studies into learning disability that have been undertaken in Northern Ireland
- A strategic review of learning disability policy and service provision (including comparisons with current international thinking).
- A literature review on each of the six 'task group' topics mentioned above.
- A study of current organisational arrangements and how they may look in the future (McConkey et al 2004)

The full audit report is also accessible via *www.science.ulster.ac.uk/inr/ddch/audit.html*.

This chapter will focus on the main thrust of the *Equal Lives* report and the anticipated overall direction of future services for people with learning disabilities, with particular reference given to the implications for learning disability nursing.

Key principles, objectives and messages

The learning disability working committee has recognised that progress has been made over the last decade. However, it is also quite emphatic in its message that there is much to be done and that there is a need for major co-ordinated developments in support, attitudes and services over the next 15 years, if the stated values for people with a learning disability are to be achieved (DHSSPS 2005):

- Inclusion
- Citizenship
- Empowerment
- Partnership
- Individual support

Box 9.2 summarises the 12 core objectives that *Equal Lives* states must be driven by all future policy that aims to improve the lives of children and adults with a learning disability. To achieve these core objectives, 75 recommendations were made.

Equal Lives suggests a number of key messages for service provision into the 21st century, and identifies many current and emerging trends in the learning disability population. It shows that learning disability nurses are very well placed to play significant – if not lead – roles in service provision. These include:

- Co-ordinating early intervention services for children with a learning disability and their families
- Improving models of service provision around meeting the physical and mental health needs (including challenging behaviour) of people with a learning disability. Similar to *Valuing People* (DH 2001), the document has recommended the introduction of health facilitation and health action planning, but has recommended that these processes are introduced in the context of a regional framework that will ensure that health facilitation and health action plans are applied in a consistent and similar fashion throughout the province, with clear targets and parameters around their introduction and responsibilities.
- There is a very strong push in the review of the need to facilitate increased access to mainstream health, social services and education for children and adults with a learning disability
- Increasing numbers of technologically dependent children
- Inadequate service provision for parents with a learning disability
- Increasing numbers of older people with actual or suspected Alzheimer's disease
- Increasing numbers of school leavers with learning disability and an autistic spectrum disorder
- The apparent lack of mental health provision and expertise that is available to children and adults with a learning disability
- The level of complexity that is now becoming apparent in the adults with learning disabilities who use day care services.

Box 9.2 Core objectives for future policy and services that support people with learning disabilities

1   To ensure that families are supported to enjoy seeing their children develop in an environment that recognises and values their uniqueness as well as their contributions to society

2   To ensure that children and young people with a learning disability get the best possible start in life and access opportunities that are available to others of their age

3   To ensure that the move into adulthood for young people with a learning disability supports their access to equal opportunities for continuing education, employment and training and that they and their families receive continuity of support during the transition period

4   To enable people with a learning disability to lead full, meaningful lives in their neighbourhoods, have access to a wide range of social work and leisure opportunities and form and maintain friendships and relationships

5   To ensure that all men and women with a learning disability have their home in the community, the choice of whom they live with and that, where they live with their family, their carers receive the support they need

6   To ensure that an extended range of housing options is developed for men and women with a learning disability

7   To secure improvements in the mental and physical health of people with a learning disability through developing access to high quality health services that are as locally based as possible and responsive to the particular needs of people with a learning disability

8   To ensure that men and women with a learning disability are supported to age well in their neighbourhoods

9   To enable people with a learning disability to have as much control as possible over their lives through developing person centred approaches in all services and ensuring wider access to advocacy and direct payments.

10 To ensure that health and social services staff are confident and competent in working with people with a learning disability

11 To ensure that staff in other settings develop their understanding and awareness of learning disability issues and the implications for their services

12 To promote improved joint working across sectors and settings in order to ensure that the quality of lives of people with a learning disability are improved and that the *Equal Lives* values and objectives are achieved

(DHSSPS 2005)

We view the *Equal Lives* messages and proposals as a challenge to – and an opportunity for – the nursing profession. The document has created an opportunity for the profession to reinvent its future, but to do so, practitioners and their managers must have the foresight and the courage to grasp this opportunity, and recognise that, although the role that they have undertaken to date has been largely valued, this may not be what is required in future services.

The nursing context

Learning disability nurses are a significant workforce group in Northern Ireland, represented in a wide variety of settings and environments. Figures calculated in 2004 showed that there were 817 nursing staff working in learning disability services in Northern Ireland of which 440 are qualified (407.61 WTE) and 377 unqualified (353.18 WTE). A gender analysis of these figures revealed that 22.2% are male and 77.8% female. Qualified nurses make up 53.1% (53.6% WTE) of the total workforce.

Another point of note is the age profile of learning disability nurses, and the demographic breakdown of qualified nursing staff. The age range of qualified staff varies from 21 years to 65 years. Further analysis of the age of qualified nursing staff showed that 38.4% were 39 years of age or less, and 61.6% were 40 years or above. Of these 22% were 50 years and over. This is a key concern when considering the implications of mental health officer status (enabling a number of qualified staff to retire at 55 years) and special retirement options for female staff. Up to 20 staff are eligible for retirement each year over the next five years (approximately 12% of the total workforce).

The workforce of learning disabilities nurses provides services across a range of hospital and community facilities. Most learning disability nurses work in hospital services. Three hospital settings for people with learning disabilities remain in Northern Ireland services, at the time of writing this chapter these hospitals were Muckamore Abbey Hospital, Tower Hill Hospital and Lakeview. Presently these facilities provide inpatient support for people with complex needs, including people with challenging behaviour, people with complex health needs, and people with a history of or risk of offending behaviour. Major redevelopments are under way to further reduce the size of the hospitals and refine the specialist services they will provide.

The remaining learning disability nurses work in a variety of learning disability facilities in statutory and independent sectors. In the statutory services, community nurses for people with learning disabilities are employed in all community trusts in Northern Ireland and are integral members of community learning disabilities teams. These teams are joint health and social services teams, and exist in the joint health and social services trust structure in Northern Ireland. This is different from the emerging structures in other parts of the United Kingdom in which nurses are moving to work in social services structures in so-called 'integrated teams'. Recent developments have also seen learning disability nurses employed in nursing roles in daycare facilities and special schools. Over the past 10 years, the independent sector has also been a consistent employer of learning disability nurses, both in nursing and residential home services.

A small – but growing – number of nurses work in specific emerging community-based services, including behaviour support and epilepsy services for people with learning disabilities. Others have completed a course in meeting the mental health needs of people with learning disabilities. At present this course meets the Nursing and Midwifery Council requirements for a specialist practitioner course. It is estimated that up to 20 nurses currently work in community-based behaviour support services, and two have a specific role working with people with learning disability who have epilepsy.

Northway (2004) says that the learning disability nursing profession should never rest on its laurels, and in Northern Ireland, the *Equal Lives* agenda demands that once again, some professional introspection is required, if we are to enter into the post *Equal Lives* era:

> '...with a renewed sense of purpose, devoid of confusion and
> ambiguity associated with the legacies of the past'(Jukes 2003, p3)

We suggest that there are four key issues that the learning disability nursing profession in Northern Ireland particularly needs to consider in the direction of future services as outlined in *Equal Lives* (DHSSPS 2005). These relate to:

- Working with children
- The social model of disability
- Realignment with the core values of nursing, and with the wider nursing 'family'
- Recruitment of nursing students

Working with children

Few, if any, would disagree with the fact that children with disabilities should be treated as children first, disabled second. All too often the care provided to children with disabilities and their families is fragmented and uncoordinated. There is no doubt that a range of disciplines, both generic and specialist, have an important role to play in improving the situation, but there is a growing sense of frustration that the skills, knowledge and experience of learning disability nurses are not always used to best effect with children and their families (Northway 2004).

In a review of the caseloads of community learning disability nurses throughout Northern Ireland, Barr (2006) found that there has been a considerable reduction of contact with children (from 8% of caseload numbers to 1.5%) when compared with a similar review carried out 11 years earlier (Parahoo & Barr 1996).

This is in part due to the development of 'teams' in children's services that have often excluded nurses for people with learning disabilities from full team membership. Many children with learning disabilities only gain access to learning disability qualified professionals after the failure of other local services to successfully meet the needs of the child and their family – during which time the difficulties for the child and other family members have increased. Learning disability nurses need to develop more successful links with staff in children's services and other professionals who work with children, so that they can be involved more effectively and use nurses at an earlier stage, reducing the chances of escalation in the child's problems.

> 'Learning disability nurses do have skills, knowledge and experience
> that can assist children and young people with learning disabilities
> and their families and carers. We need to make sure that they get
> access to such support and that learning disability nurses are
> available right from the start'   (Northway 2004, p3)

The social model of disability

A full debate of the issues associated with a social model of care is beyond the scope of this chapter. However, it requires some attention, as in the review of policy and service provision in Northern Ireland this issue has become very prominent for nurses and for other specialists working in the field of learning disability.

First, it is important that the nursing profession and others more aligned towards a social care approach to care provision, recognise and understand that using the art and science of nursing for people with a learning disability does *not* equate to the adoption of a medical or sickness model. Nor is it in contravention of the social model of disability. The false dichotomy at times presented between the so-called medical and social models as competing and incompatible approaches has been quite divisive – in particular, the erroneous view that the social model of disability is synonymous with a social services approach, whereas attention to health needs is necessary a 'medical' approach (Thomas & Woods 2003).

Evidence submitted to the Learning Disability Working Committee by the Regional Professional Development Forum for Learning Disability Nurses in Northern Ireland (PDF) during the consultation on *Equal Lives*, suggested that such an approach, if adopted unilaterally, has not always served people with a learning disability well. For example, if one considers the experience in Victoria, Australia, where, in the mid 1980s, employment of specialist staff (including nurses) was abandoned in the provision of services to individuals with a learning disability. Only 20 years later has it become recognised that such a philosophy has resulted in serious health deficits and inadequate service provision for many. Consequently, there has been a drive towards the re-establishment of specialist services (Davis et al 2002). These concerns have been echoed by Rob Greig, the regional director of the *Valuing People* Support Team:

> 'The trouble with the move to a social model of disability is that it has
> led many people to think that they don't have to concern themselves
> with learning disability any more'   (Carlisle 2004)

Following consultation to the draft *Equal Lives* report (DHSSPS 2004) the Committee responsible for the final draft of the document, accepted the need to move away from the previous distinctions between traditional (medical) and social models. The review team recognised that:

> 'People with learning disabilities are not a homogenous groups,
> and that the needs of individuals can vary considerably... all

services, across all sectors, should aspire towards a holistic, or bio-psycho-social model, encapsulated by inclusive and person-centred approaches. The model allows for the holistic view of an individual's needs' (DHSSPS 2005, p18)

A model of this nature, by definition, is non-discriminatory, will be less divisive, and is inclusive of all mainstream service providers. It would have as a central theme the right of people with a learning disability to access expertise and resources that are available to the rest of society.

Realignment with nursing

It could be argued that the emphasis given to the social model of disability has resulted in some learning disability nurses having lost – or no longer seeing themselves as having an association with – the wider 'family of nursing'. Some nurses have aligned themselves and their interventions more closely with other professional groups working in social care systems.

A recent consensus statement by the North West Learning Disability Nursing Network (Unpublished Feb 2005) has focused on the role and contribution of community learning disability nursing in integrated health and social work teams in England, and emphasises how essential it is that learning disability nurses are enabled to deploy their specialist health knowledge, skills and experience, and do not simply slip into or be pushed into 'pure' care management roles or functions, while retaining the title of 'nurse'. Integrated teams have been in existence in Northern Ireland since the late 1980s. It is clear that some nurses have been inappropriately diverted away from their specialist roles and functions and have aligned themselves and their interventions more closely with other professional groups working in social care systems (Barr 2006).

This has not been helped by some individuals who perceive learning disability nursing as part of the problem faced by people with a learning disability in achieving true inclusion (Turnbull 2004). It is definitely not a purpose of this chapter to dismiss the vital importance of good professional team working, but rather to encourage the profession to have the insight and confidence to realign themselves with the 'family of nursing', and to recognise and value that it is by using our unique nursing skills, knowledge and expertise that we will help achieve the aspirations and vision of *Equal Lives*.

For example, in *Equal Lives* there is a major drive towards increased access to, and use of mainstream services, such as those provided in primary care. GPs are most often the first point of contact for individuals with a learning disability, who to date have been poorly served by the primary care sector (Stein 2000; Gill et al 2002). If one considers the high levels of physical and mental health needs among people with learning disabilities (McConkey et al 2004), it is clear that much improvement is required in this sector in relation to accessibility for people with a learning disability and increased understanding of their health needs and vulnerability. Learning disability nurses have a crucial role to play in improving this situation and will be expected in the future to align themselves more closely with the range of primary care and acute care colleagues.

Key responsibilities will be to:

- Educate and support mainstream colleagues
- Develop health facilitation roles
- Implement health plans
- Improve access to primary care and acute services (e.g. acute liaison role)
- Incorporate a more preventive, downstream and public health approach to casework
- Improve and develop interventions to improve the health status of children and adults with a learning disability

However, learning disability nurses will also increasingly be expected to be available to – and facilitate access to – other specialist services such as mainstream mental health, forensic services and child and adolescent mental health services (CAMHS). Indeed, in many areas of the United Kingdom learning disability nurses have been employed to work full time in positions such as acute care liaison, primary care liaison, and in dual diagnosis services (children and adult teams) to facilitate access, and add their specialist skill base to these mainstream services.

The specialist knowledge and skills possessed by learning disability nurses will be a central requirement of smaller, locally based community assessment and treatment facilities. It is expected that such facilities will be established as alternatives to hospital admissions, and as step-up and step-down facilities to reduce the need for, and the length of, hospital stays. As a result, the clientele of such services are likely to be those individuals with the most complex needs, incorporating people with challenging behaviour needs, forensic needs and/or dual diagnosis needs.

Evidence suggests that people with learning disabilities who have coexisting difficulties are often detained in hospital longer than they should because of inadequate community-based services or buildings, receive inadequate therapeutic interventions or talking therapies, are often crisis-managed, and that very few have had access to preventive or early intervention approaches (Taggart 2003).

The skills, knowledge and expertise of learning disability nurses will be key to ensuring an effective, workable, and robust community infrastructure that has a focus on preventive work, early intervention, improved therapeutic interventions, and community-based crisis response and by so doing, preventing hospital admissions and facilitating earlier hospital discharge.

However, we also believe firmly that learning disability nurses must adopt a more proactive involvement in wider nursing developments. This includes involvement in aspects such as nurse prescribing, practice development, care pathways, encouraging specialist and advanced practice, clinical supervision, and increased use of evidence-based practice. The profession also needs to become more active in generating new knowledge through increased participation in research. By becoming active in these areas it is argued that learning disability nurses will be less marginalised, develop a stronger identity, become more confident and articulate about what it is they do, and ultimately help others to recognise the 'added value' of nursing to the lives of people with a learning disability.

Recruitment of nursing students

Similar to other parts of the United Kingdom, applicants to the learning disability branch of nursing have been reducing, and some thought needs to be given as to why this is so. The 'stigma' and 'negative images' of learning disability are often cited as a primary difficulty, with other branches of nursing being promoted as being more attractive, and with a wider range of future career pathways (Mitchell 2000). But more than ever before, learning disability nursing has a central role to play in future service provision in Northern Ireland. This will provide increased opportunities for new recruits to work in a wide diversity of roles, and will offer a wide range of career pathways following registration.

A number of approaches need to be considered in developing the recruitment of students to learning disability nursing.

Recognition: The distinct identity and recognition of the role of learning disability nursing requires marketing as a positive and secure career choice with the endorsement of the DHSSPS. Media campaigns, and other means of promoting learning disability nursing as a positive career choice should be used.

Commitment: A statement of commitment to the future of the profession in the post-*Equal Lives* world would provide a much needed morale boost and have an indirect but positive effect on the recruitment of nursing students, by reducing current uncertainty about the future and the value of the role.

Strategy: It would be easy to suggest that there should be an increase in the number of student nurse places commissioned for learning disability nursing. However, to predict future numbers accurately there is a need for a more planned and strategic approach with some form of regional review commissioned to inform future recruitment. At the moment it seems that there is a 'best guess' and 'ad hoc' approach to student nurse recruitment into learning disability.

However, current numbers of commissioned places are likely to fall short of the growing demands for the skills and knowledge base possessed by learning disability nurses, in the ever-increasing variety of settings. The availability, recruitment and retention of the necessary numbers and grades of skilled and knowledgeable nursing staff is central to the effective provision of current, emerging and future changes and will provide a stable platform for forward planning and service development. In developing recruitment and retention strategies, careful attention needs to be given to the age profile and likely retirement ages of current staff.

Recruitment: a number of other practical suggestions should be considered in seeking to enhance recruitment of student nurses to learning disability in Northern Ireland. At the time of preparing this chapter, recruitment into this branch only takes place in March of every year, whereas other branches start their programmes in September and March. This means that school leavers have to wait for several additional months after finishing the secondary education before they can enter learning disability nursing. We believe that this is a significant issue in terms of recruiting school leavers who are likely to want to start their chosen career immediately. Further steps could also be taken to encourage nursing and care assistants to enter nurse training. Open University preregistration training programmes have been used to train this group of staff in the fields of adult and mental health nursing.

Consideration should be given to developing a similar path for learning disability nursing. We believe it would also aid recruitment if a similar arrangement could be applied to nursing, as that used in social services, where care assistants are seconded for social work training and their posts backfilled for the period(s) of time out.

Short programmes: Consideration should also be given to the development of a 'shortened branch programme', similar to those available in other areas of nursing, so that nurses from other branches have the opportunity to move to the learning disability branch. Anecdotal evidence suggests that a number of nurses from other branches would be eager and happy to undertake a shortened learning disability branch if this was available.

Conclusion

To deliver a contemporary learning disability nursing service for the 21st century, the profession must consider the objectives and recommendations arising from the review into learning disability policy and practice in Northern Ireland. This chapter has provided an overview of the *Equal Lives* paper (DHSSPS 2005), and a number of issues that have the potential to impact on the practice of learning disability nurses.

Although the emphasis of future service provision for people with a learning disability is increasingly on improving access to mainstream and generic services, it is vital to acknowledge that learning disability nurses and other specialists have a crucial role to play in achieving this vision of real citizenship. In Northern Ireland, as throughout the other countries in the United Kingdom, it also recognised that specialist nursing services will continue to be required to support people with learning disabilities.

We hope that the vision for learning disability policy and service provision as presented in *Equal Lives* (DHSSPS 2005) will be the impetus for the profession to have the courage to inspect and examine itself. Then, where necessary, that it can take the necessary steps to ensure that the learning disability nursing workforce has the appropriate knowledge skills and competencies to meet the needs of people with a learning disability, regardless of the environment of care.

By doing so, the necessary nursing contribution to learning disability services regionally will be secured, which will advance and improve the quality of nursing care offered to people with learning disabilities, their families and carers.

References

Barr O (2006) The evolving role of community nurses for people with learning disabilities: changes over an 11-year period. *Journal of Clinical Nursing* **15**, 1, 72–82

Carlisle D (2004) DH warns against new long stay institutions. *Health Service Journal* Nov 25

Davis R, Phillips A, Nankervis K (2002) *Service delivery to people with an intellectual disability in Victoria and Australia: A report to the Scottish National Review of the contribution of nurses to the care and support of people with a learning disability.* Australia, Monash University

Department of Health, Social Services and Public Safety (2005) *Equal Lives: Draft report of Learning Disability Committee.* Belfast, Department of Health, Social Services and Public Safety

Department of Health, Social Services and Public Safety (2004) *Equal Lives: Review of policy and services for people with a learning disability in Northern Ireland.* Belfast, Department of Health, Social Services and Public Safety *(www.rmhldni.gov.uk)*

DHSS (1995) *Review of policy for people with a learning disability.* Belfast, Department of Health and Social Services

Department of Health (2001) *Valuing People: A new strategy for learning disability for the 21st century.* London, The Stationery Office

Gill F, Stenfert-Kroese B, Rose J (2002) General practitioners' attitudes to people who have a learning disability. *Psychological Medicine* **37**, 1445–1455

Jenkins J, Johnson B (1991) Community nursing learning disability survey. In: Kelly P (ed) *The Community Mental Handicap Nurse-Specialist Practitioner in the 1990s.* Penarth, Mental Handicap Nurses' Association, pp39–54

Jukes M (2003) Towards practice development in contemporary learning disability nursing. In: Jukes M, Bollard M (eds) *Contemporary Learning Disability Practice.* Salisbury, Quay Books, pp 3–19

McConkey R, Slevin E, Barr O (2004) *Audit of Learning Disability in Northern Ireland.* University of Ulster

McConkey, R Spollen M, Jamison J (2003) *Administrative Prevalence of Learning Disability in Northern Ireland. A Report to the Department of Health, Social Services and Public Safety.* Belfast, DHSSPS

Mitchell D (2000) Parallel stigma? Nurses and people with learning disabilities. History of learning disability nursing and the shared stigma between the nurses and people with learning disabilities. *British Journal of Learning Disabilities* **28**, 2, 78–81

Northway R (2004) Right from the start. *Learning Disability Practice* **7**, 7, 3

North West Learning Disability Nurses Network (2005) *Consensus statement: The Role and Contribution of Community Learning Disability Nursing in Integrated Health and Social Work Teams* Unpublished paper, Feb 2005

Parahoo K, Barr O (1996) Community mental handicap nursing services in Northern Ireland: a profile of clients and selected working practices *Journal of Clinical Nursing* **5**, 211–228

Scottish Executive (2000) *The Same as You? A review of the services for people with learning disabilities.* Edinburgh, Scottish Executive

Stein K (2000) Caring for people with a learning disability: A survey of GPs attitudes in Southampton and South-West Hampshire. *British Journal of Learning Disabilities* **28**, 1, 9–15

Taggart L (2003) *Service provision for people with a learning disability and mental health problems.* PhD Thesis, University of Ulster

Turnbull J (2004) Discovering learning disability nursing. In: Turnbull J (ed) *Learning Disability Nursing.* Oxford, Blackwell Science, pp 1–12

Thomas D, Woods H (2003) *Working with people with learning disabilities. Theory and practice.* London: Jessica Kingsley Publishers

Welsh Office (2001) *Fulfilling the Promises.* Cardiff, Welsh Assembly

CHAPTER 10

Regional focus
Wales

John Boarder and Brian Jones

Introduction

The aim of this chapter is to convey an impression of learning disability services in Wales with a particular focus on health care and learning disability nursing. Before doing this, the geographic and linguistic situation of Wales will be introduced, followed by some background about policy and service development, leading on to a consideration of some aspects of learning disability health care and nursing.

Wales and its language

Wales is a small country (population around 3 million) on a western peninsula of Britain. It is arguably on the Western end of English consciousness. (Dr Who suggested that Westminster would not notice if the whole of South Wales disappeared into the sea as a result of alien activity – so it must be true).

The centre of the country is highland. 60% of the land is above 700 feet (Black 2000), rising to 3000 feet in Snowdonia and the Brecon Beacons. This land is wet, infertile and sparsely populated. Transport is made difficult by the geography. East–West travel is often easier than North–South. Transport links are often easier between Wales and England than between North and South Wales. As a result loyalties historically have been arguably local rather than national and have meant that Wales had no natural capital city. Cardiff the capital city is a modern creation, dating from 1955 (Davies 1994).

Like most of Western Europe, Welsh history has been influenced by successive waves of peoples and cultures. During the first millennium BC came the Celts. These tribes brought over the ancestor of the modern Welsh language. Brittonic was spoken in Britain and Gaul (modern France). Though the Roman invasion of 43 AD introduced Latin as the official language, Brittonic was the language used by the masses. It was the invasions by the Germanic tribes, the Anglo-Saxons, which led to the dominance of Old English. Gradually the Celtic languages retreated to the Western fringes of Britain. It was some time between 400 and 700 AD that the transition from Brittonic to Welsh took place (Davies 1999).

The survival of the Welsh language through to the modern day is a minor miracle in the face of dominant English, Norman and American cultures. However, there was a severe decline in the number of Welsh speakers during the 20th century. Although concentrations of Welsh speakers were to be found in areas such as North West Wales, the existence of the language was under threat. Pressure groups such as Cymdeithas Yr Iaith Cymraeg (The Welsh Language Society) campaigned for the official status of Welsh to be placed on a par with English. The Welsh Language Act (1993) established the principle that in the conduct of public business in Wales the Welsh and English languages should be treated on the basis of equality (Davies 1999). This and other factors such as the formation of the Welsh language TV channel (S4C) in 1982 and the development of Welsh medium schools have worked to halt the decline of the language. A sea of change has now occurred where the number of children speaking Welsh has begun to increase.

What this means to the health service and to learning disability nursing, is that there are many people in Wales whose choice of language when receiving a service is Welsh. Most people in Wales have a good grasp of English language and culture. However, in times of stress people are much more comfortable discussing issues in their first language. For an increasing number of people in Wales this language will be Welsh. This means that sensitivity to culture and language must be an integral part of nurse training and development. Likewise, whenever possible people are offered the chance to communicate through the medium of Welsh. This is especially important for people with learning disability whose first language is Welsh and whose communication difficulties may make speaking in English even more difficult.

Devolution and the all-Wales approach

In 1997 the Welsh people voted narrowly in a referendum for the creation of a Welsh Assembly. This met for the first time in 1999:

> '...the first democratically elected assembly in Welsh history'

> (Black 2000, p 233)

The National Assembly for Wales did not originally have law-making or tax-raising powers (National Assembly for Wales, 2004), but the Government of Wales Act, 2006 does give some law making powers to the Assembly. The Welsh Assembly Government (WAG) does have financial, policy and political control over, amongst other areas, Health and Social Services.

This inevitably means differences in policy from the rest of the UK, with perceptions that the Assembly in Wales is currently aligned politically further to the left than the Westminster Parliament. One statement of intent was to have one minister over both social services and the health service. The first such minister, Jane Hutt, was a strong advocate of a 'joined-up' approach to health and social care. She was replaced by Dr Brian Gibbons in 2005, but the work to create close links continues. Unified assessment, a commitment to joint initial assessment by health and social services has been in place for elderly services from April 2005, and since April 2006 for learning disability services.

The Welsh Assembly Government has produced a number of policy documents related to health and social care in Wales, which impact on learning disability services. These include:

- *Fundamentals of Care* (Welsh Assembly Government 2003)
- *Health Care Standards for Wales* (Welsh Assembly Government 2005a)
- *Designed for Life* (Welsh Assembly Government 2005b)

For learning disability services, the white paper *Valuing People* (Department of Health 2001) applies to England but holds no policy status in Wales. Although the evidence base used in forming the policy can inform services in Wales, the policy can not.

It is suggested that the structures in Wales and its size can support networking in a way which is very much more difficult in a country the size of England. For example, preregistration nurse training and education in Wales has been structured at an All-Wales level. Following *Fitness for Practice* (UKCC 1999), a series of meetings was held between NHS trust representatives and higher education providers. The result was a unified approach to standards and structures. A key element was – and remains – the notion of partnership between NHS trusts and higher education institutions.

Similarly strong links are to be found at a NHS trust level in learning disability health services. The All Wales Senior Nurse Advisory group (AWSNAG) for learning disability training meets quarterly and enables the most senior nurse from each trust in Wales to meet with officers from the Assembly to guide learning disability nursing Practice. This allows an unprecedented opportunity for networking and sharing. The group aims to inform and guide policy and practice across Wales. Liaison groups for learning disability services held in North and South Wales develop links between education and service and act as regional sub-groups of the AWSNAG. In relation to clinical specialisms, clinical interest groups have been set up, with a range of groups established in North Wales. This will enable practice developments, protocols, problems and solutions to be shared widely, avoiding duplication of effort. (Box 10.1).

In North Wales there is also a Learning Disability Network with members from the three NHS trusts and local health boards. The Network which co-ordinates a North Wales perspective in service provision, development and planning. In addition, a *Clinical Interest Directory* (NW Wales, Conwy and Denbighshire and NE Wales NHS Trusts 2004) has been produced with the aim of promoting and disseminating good practice through enhancing communication between learning disability nurses. Those with specialist interests and expertise are listed so that people can be contacted. This has enabled staff to support each other and share knowledge and information, as well as being a useful source of facilitators for training and education purposes. It is proposed to extend this to include other professionals working in learning disability. Likewise, highly successful conferences have been organised, which have enabled learning disability nurses across Wales to share good practice and disseminate to others the importance and practical value of their role in supporting people with learning disability and their carers (Fisher 1997).

Box 10.1 Learning disability clinical interest groups in North Wales

- Sexuality and personal relationships
- Forensic
- Epilepsy
- Challenging behaviour
- Autism
- People with multiple and profound disability
- Primary health care
- Older people
- Mental health

Examples of group aims

- Producing standards
- Providing peer group and clinical support
- Opportunity to network
- Sharing and disseminating information, research findings and good practice
- Problem solving
- Developing service development proposals
- Supporting professional development
- Developing consistent approaches to care delivery
- Training and education
- Multiagency working
- Producing newsletters
- Acting as a source of advice

What emerges, then, is a learning disability service in Wales that is fairly joined-up. The services do benefit from the relatively small size of the service (with an estimated population of people with severe learning disability of 10,830 (Learning Disability Advisory Group 2001). However, considerable time and effort is put into creating these networks in a country where physical geography still makes travel between the different Welsh regions a time-consuming affair.

The All Wales Strategy

The All Wales Strategy (AWS) for people with learning disability in Wales was launched and funded by the Welsh Office in 1983 (Welsh Office 1983) with the aim of accelerating the development of community care for people with learning disability in Wales. In the foreword to the Strategy, Nicholas Edwards, then Secretary of State for Wales, wrote that there had been:

*'...too little progress made since the publication in 1971 of
the Government White Paper Better Services for the Mentally
Handicapped with a continuing dependence on institutional care and
insufficient support for people living in their own homes'*

The aim was to redress this to:

*'...effect the transition from a largely hospital based service to
community-based one'* (Welsh Office 1983, p(i))

This new service was based on what may have been considered – at the time of the launch of the AWS – to be a quite a radical view of community care based on the vision of full community integration, achieved, for example, through ordinary housing and integrated work settings. These principles from the Strategy continue to underpin the work of services and learning disability nurses in Wales:

- People with learning disability should have a right to normal patterns of life in the community
- People with learning disability should have a right to be treated as individuals
- People with learning disability require additional help from the communities in which they live and from professional services if they are to develop their maximum potential as individuals   (Welsh Office 1983, p1–2)

Resources earmarked for learning disability were made available across the 10-year period of the All Wales Strategy (AWS) from 1983 to enable these principles to be put into practice, with

> '...especially intensive development in vanguard areas to test the viability and self-sufficiency of the new patterns of services'

> (Welsh Office 1983, p (ii))

The elements of a comprehensive service for people with learning disabilities and their families identified in the AWS are based on the promotion of *Ordinary Living* (King's Fund 1980) and reflect principles of normalisation (Nirje 1980; Wolfensberger 1980). Ordinary housing was used:

> '...new purpose built hostels, hospitals or units should not form part of the new patterns'   (Welsh Office 1983, p 6)

and integration into local communities, using ordinary community services and employment opportunities, was facilitated. Joint planning teams were established in each county to ensure interagency cooperation, to include service users, family representatives and voluntary agencies.

Social services was identified as the lead agency, but with consultation with all those bodies providing services for people with learning disability, including housing, education and health services. At the local level co-ordinated community mental handicap teams were set up to share a single base, with its work co-ordinated around the individual through individual plans and key workers. The work in a given locality was to be overseen by a 'co-ordinator of local services' who might be a community learning disability nurse or a social worker.

It is widely recognised (Welsh Office 1994; Learning Disability Advisory Group 2001; Learning Disability Implementation Advisory Group 2006) that the AWS made progress in developing learning disability services in line with its principles. For example, the numbers of those in hospital reduced from 2,089 in 1983 to 1,058 in 1993 (Welsh Office 1994) with 366 identified on 31 March 2000 (Learning Disability Advisory Group 2001). In June 2006, the number of those in hospital care in Wales was approximately 70 and it is envisaged that all hospital residents requiring social care will have left Welsh hospitals by the end of 2007. Hensol Hospital in South Wales closed officially in 2004 (UDID 2004) and Bryn y Neuadd in North Wales is due to close by the end of 2007.

The widespread development of small, staffed ordinary housing options mainly for a group of up to three people with learning with disability has been an important measure of the success of the Strategy, with the development of:

> '...staffed support in ordinary community housing for more than two-and-a-half thousand people'... 'one of the Strategy's enduring achievements'   (Felce 2003, p1)

Likewise, the AWS has led to a diverse range of work opportunities across Wales, including work experience, supported employment and community projects and flexible one-to-one arrangements around individual needs. Family-based care has expanded with, for example, family-based respite care for children and respite in local staffed housing for adults (Felce et al 1995).

Another key element of the AWS has been the development of multidisciplinary/ agency community learning disability teams and joint service development teams, including advocacy and service representatives (Todd et al 2000).

In 2003 the Welsh Assembly Government established a Learning Disability Implementation Advisory Group to oversee the implementation of its responses to *Fulfilling the Promises*. This led to the further endorsement of the 1983 principles and their update by the Welsh Assembly Government in 2007:

The Welsh Assembly Government's vision for the future is based on the following statement of principles:

'All people with a learning disability are full citizens, equal in status and value to other citizens of the same age. They have the same rights to:

- Live healthy, productive and independent lives with appropriate and responsive treatment and support to develop their maximum potential.
- Be individuals and decide everyday issues and life – defining matters for themselves joining in all decision-making which affects their lives, with appropriate and responsive advice and support where necessary.
- Live their lives within their community, maintaining the social and family ties and connections which are important to them.
- Have the support of the communities of which they are a part and access to general and specialist services that are responsive to their individual needs, circumstances and preferences' (para 2.5)

Implications of the Strategy for learning disability nursing

During the 1980s, the AWS was seen as a leading example of good practice in the UK. However, where did learning disability nursing fit into a service based on a quite radical model of social care with its strong commitment to the principles of social role valorisation (Wolfensberger 1983) for people with learning disabilities, and with social services identified as the lead agency?

There were those in Wales, as elsewhere, who saw the existence of learning disability nurses as ideologically unsound, with the use of the word 'nurse' suggestive of an institutional, medical model of care. However, in the same year as the Strategy was launched, the new learning disability nursing syllabus (Welsh National Board 1983) was introduced, which itself embraced the AWS principles and so promoted an approach fully in line with the All Wales Strategy. The commitment to the AWS principles and the emphasis in training and education on psychological, social and educational aspects of nursing care enabled learning disability nurses in Wales to contribute proactively to the development and delivery of the Strategy. There was a rapid expansion of the number of community learning disability nurses appointed during the 1980s and 1990s, with many posts funded through AWS monies.

During this time, the idea of the community nurse working in a multidisciplinary core team (comprising a community nurse, a social worker and sometimes a clinical psychologist) (NDG 1977; Simon 1983) was strongly promoted as the preferred way of working across the UK. In Wales, community learning disability nurses were firmly embedded in multidisciplinary community mental handicap teams, with particularly close working relationships with social service staff. The All Wales Community Mental Health Team (CMHT) survey carried out in 1988 (McGrath & Humphries) demonstrated how extensive this way of working was by then in Wales.

A new role for learning disability nurses in the AWS working in community settings had thus been created and was generally recognised, while those working in hospital settings continued to facilitate resettlement and the maintenance of a good quality of life for those remaining in hospital.

The move towards a more social, educational role and the close working with social workers and others meant that there was scope for role overlap. This was seen as largely a positive development in the All Wales CMHT Survey

> *'A degree of overlap or 'blurring' of tasks and roles has taken place,*
> *but by and large the pattern is one where the task of one group is*
> *supplemented or complemented by that of another, and this, where it*
> *exists is undoubtedly one of the key strengths of the teams'*

(McGrath & Humphries 1988, p187)

However, some staff working at the time reported that this led to concerns about the professional identity of learning disability nurses (Boarder 2002). This point is made by Bollard and Jukes (1999) about services in the UK generally. They state that before the NHS and Community Care Act (1990) the community learning disability nurse

> *'...had traditionally held a core member role in multidisciplinary*
> *teams , where specialist knowledge and skills base were difficult to*
> *identify and resulted in a blurred and often ill-defined role expectancy'*

(Bollard & Jukes 1999, p12)

Certainly, after the implementation of the Act we believe that the role of the learning disability nurse in Wales was generally clarified and strengthened.

Effects of the NHS and Community Care Act

The *Caring for People* white paper (1989), which led to the NHS and Community Care Act (1990), highlighted the important role of the community nurse in learning disability in the 'mixed economy of care'.

> *'The mental handicap nursing profession plays a particularly important role in providing treatment, care and support to people with a mental handicap, both in hospital and in a range of community settings. Nurses' skills and experiences are highly valued and will continue to be needed as part of the new forms of service'*

(*Caring for People* para 2.17)

However, the distinction between health and social care identified by the Act, and the idea of community nursing input being 'purchased' alongside other 'competitors' meant that roles and services offered had to be very clear. Too much overlap was no longer viable and the health elements of the work had to be emphasised. It had to be made very clear what was being offered. This applied to Wales as to the rest of the UK, with documents appearing that highlighted the health needs of people with learning disability in Wales (Welsh Health Planning Forum 1992) and emphasised the role of the nurse in meeting such needs (All Wales Nurse Group for People with a Mental Handicap 1992).

Community learning disability nurses had, like others, to stake their place strongly in the new 'marketplace' of care. However, care management – with its separation of purchasers and providers – and the need for more distinct roles in service provision were seen by some as harmful to the working together ethos that had arisen during the period of the AWS:

> *'The then Welsh Office insistence on the creation of a single joint agency plan at county level, although creating a challenge to all concerned, eventually produced a distinctive level of joint agency collaboration. However, reforms of recent years have not helped to further this. The separation of purchasers from providers divided the interests of newly established collaborators both between the statutory agencies and between statutory agencies and voluntary bodies'*

(Learning Disability Advisory Group 2001, p40)

It is suggested that while close working and collaboration across learning disability services continued, the reforms led to health and social service teams working to develop clearer and more separate identities. This may be seen as a positive development for learning disability nursing, because it ensured the forging of a clearer and stronger health related role for learning disability, more congruent with the title 'nurse'.

Current policy on service integration

It was planned that the ringfenced funding of the AWS would come to an end in

1993 (ongoing discussion about the equalisation of funds across Wales continued after that date). Although it was intended that the principles of the AWS would continue to be implemented, there was some concern as to whether this would happen, with new priorities perhaps now taking precedence over learning disability services (Welsh Office/SCOVO 1998).

However, in recent years there has been a fresh impetus towards service integration and partnership with social services, with a pooling of funds enabled by the Flexibility arrangements (National Assembly for Wales 2000) and the All Wales Health, Social Care and Well-being Strategies (Welsh Assembly Government 2003). The latter was:

> '...an integrated and multidisciplinary approach to local authority
> and NHS strategic planning for health, social care and well-being'

(Welsh Assembly Government 2003, p1)

The implementation of this policy is building on the original aspirations and achievements of the All Wales Strategy. Initiatives across Wales integrate health and social care for people with learning disabilities with, for example, joint operational managers and unified assessments. This thrust towards a more unified approach is promoted in *Fulfilling the Promises* (Learning Disability Advisory Group 2001) with shared goals for learning disability services for each of the service elements identified in Box 10.2.

Learning disability nursing in Wales

During the 1980s, the emphasis was on ensuring the contribution of learning disability to the achievement of the principles of the AWS, in a primarily social model of care. In the 1990s, the role of the learning disability nurse in meeting health needs has been more strongly emphasised. This reflects the increased recognition of the health-related needs of people with learning disability (NHS Cymru Wales 2001).

One element of this emphasis is the need for nurses to:

Box 10.2 Key service elements in *Fulfilling the Promises*

- Individual planning (person-centred planning)
- Information provision and advocacy
- Partnership in planning
- Children and families
- Transition planning
- Community living
- Employment, further education and day activities
- General health needs
- Complex health needs
- Severe challenging behaviour

*'...further develop their roles in primary care services to influence
positive outcomes for the service users in the provision of integrated
health and social care'* (Welsh Assembly Government 2002, p5)

and to

'...develop effective health screening programmes in GP surgeries'

(NHS Wales 1997 p4)

Certainly, this is an area of work that has received increased attention in Wales, with links being made with primary health care teams to ensure the health needs of people are both assessed and addressed. Initiatives include creating posts for learning disability nurses to take on specific responsibilities in developing links and setting up systems to help ensure this takes place.

Likewise, there has been a trend to further develop areas of expertise in more health specific areas, such as dysphagia and epilepsy. This development has been supported by developments in training and education at both pre- and postregistration levels.

The need for learning disability nurses to promote:

*'...positive relationships to a range of other health and social service
providers'* [and to ensure] *services for this client group continue to be
rooted in an ethos of partnership and equity'*

are identified by the Assembly's *'Framework for Realising the Potential of Learning Disability Nursing Wales (Inclusion, Partnership and Innovation)'* (Welsh Assembly Government 2002, p5). Link learning disability nurses work with mental health services and general hospitals to help enable better access. Close working with social services continues, with learning disability health and social service teams based together across Wales to deliver services and meet client needs.

The role of the health services

In Wales during the 1990s and onwards there has been a clarification and development of more health-specific work in learning disability services, reflected, it is suggested, in a clearer and stronger health-orientated identity for learning disability.

The *Protocol in Health Gain* (Welsh Health Planning Forum 1992) identified health needs for people with learning disability with targets as to when and how they should be met. Likewise, *Challenges and Responses* (Welsh Office 1992) examined and made recommendations for people with learning disabilities with challenging behaviours, including mental health difficulties. More recently the papers *Fulfilling the Promises* (Learning Disability Advisory Group, 2001), the *Learning Disability Strategy Guidance* (Welsh Assembly Government 2004) and the *Statement on Policy and Practice for Adults with Learning Disability* (Welsh Assembly Government, 2007) identify health recommendations as part of an overall framework for learning disability services.

General health needs are identified with the service principles focused on health needs defined as the:

> 'co-occurrence of physical disabilities, hearing/eyesight problems, epilepsy, chest problems, swallowing problems and other chronic medical conditions' (Learning Disability Advisory Group 2001, p80)

The aim is, where necessary, to offer 'specialist arrangements' to ensure that such needs:

> '...are met effectively and safely while still enabling the individuals to enjoy an ordinary life in their local communities'

> (Learning Disability Advisory Group 2001, p80)

Residential care, including specialist treatment and assessment units, for those with more complex needs, including challenging behaviour, have been set up or are planned. The aim is to ensure that fully comprehensive services are provided after the closure of the learning disability hospitals in Wales. When commissioning services, local health boards need to be sure that local services are robust enough to meet those with the most complex health needs.

Running parallel to such documents highlighting the role of the Health Service in meeting the needs of people with learning disability in Wales, papers explaining and promoting the role of community learning disability nurses (CLDNs) have been published and of highly successful conferences held to share the work of CLDNs across Wales. A *Learning Disability Nursing Agenda for Wales* was published in 1997 (NHS Wales), which sought to clarify and promote the roles of learning disability nursing. Part of this was the specification of roles around health promotion, specialist health care, and accessing primary health care teams and general health services. In 2002 the document *Inclusion, Partnership and Innovation* (Welsh Assembly Government) was published as a part of the *Realising the Potential* initiative (National Assembly for Wales 1999) for nursing. In its Preface, Jane Hutt, Welsh Assembly Government Minister for Health and Social Services at the time, strongly reiterates the backing of the Welsh Assembly Government for learning disability nursing:

> 'Since the publication, in 1983, of the Learning Disability Strategy for Wales, huge strides have been made towards improving the care of people in our country who live with a learning disability. I would like to take this opportunity to declare my recognition of the central role that learning disability nurses have played in the success of that strategy.' (Welsh Assembly Government, 2002, pi)

The document established a framework that identified key aims for learning disability nursing (Box 10.3).

Training and education

From 2004 the preregistration training in Wales has been offered at degree level. The two schools that provide learning disability preregistration training in Wales

Box 10.3 Aims for learning disability nursing

- All registered learning disability nurses will have a theoretical and clinical base to their practice, which enables them to create environments of care that promote health, growth and opportunity for the individual client.
- In partnership, all learning disability nurses will work effectively with their clients and their clients' families to provide high quality, inclusive and measurable care.
- All learning disability nurses will develop their practice in a reflective and evidence based manner. Their practice will be founded on a standard of education, which enables them to function as equal partners with other health care professions, supported by continued professional development and clinical supervision.
- Existing career paths for learning disability nurses in Wales will be enhanced, and new ones developed. Such career paths should allow senior staff to remain clinically involved if they so wish. They should also break down unhelpful barriers between education, research and practice, as well as between learning disability nursing and the wider health and social care context.
- The unique value of the learning disability nurse will be recognised and appropriately used to meet the holistic needs of people with a learning disability.   *(Welsh Assembly Government, 2002, pp7–11)*

are the University of Wales (Bangor) and the University of Glamorgan. Between the two, approximately 34 nurses a year enter learning disability nurse training.

Higher education institutions, in partnership with Health Care Inspectorate Wales (HIW), (which replaced the Welsh National Board and Health Professions Wales) have established a flexible modular approach to post-qualification education, which has been very useful in developing courses around specific areas of practice that are responsive to client and service needs.

Currently, postregistration modules are drawn together to enable nurses to acquire diplomas and degrees, with specialist practice awards in learning disability combined with BSc (Hons) Health Studies. Masters programmes are being developed and offered in Wales. Because all preregistration education is now at degree level, there will be a need to offer more courses at postgraduate level, although qualified staff are also looking for other more practical-based courses to consolidate and develop practice.

Each module has a planning team drawing together practitioners and service managers who can contribute to the planning and teaching of the modules from across different localities and disciplines. With students from different areas and disciplines coming together to explore particular topic areas, these planning teams are a powerful catalyst contributing to service and practice development.

Current trends in learning disability nursing

Learning disability nurses in Wales are an integral part of learning disability services in Wales, in terms of resettlement, and developing and maintaining ongoing community services. Support is offered to people with learning disability and their families, as well as people living on their own or in staffed or supported housing. Learning disability nurses are an important part of the support services to those living in ordinary housing community living and their staff, especially for those with health needs and challenging behaviours. Work is being done to ensure sufficient services for people with more complex needs who are moving into community settings. In some areas, learning disability nurses manage houses where people require continued health care. In South Wales NHS Trust, assessment and treatment units have been set up, and in North Wales these are being planned. Pembrokeshire and Derwen NHS Trust run a specialist unit for people with autism.

While there have been numerous discussions and recommendations about the role of the CLDN, there are currently only a few research papers into what is happening in practice, even fewer studies focusing just on Wales. Mansell and Harris (1998) surveyed different professionals working in community learning disability support teams in South Wales and identified the key roles of CLDNs (Box 10.4)

Box 10.4 Key roles of community learning disability nurses

- Client based interventions (direct contact)
- Co-ordination and planning of care
- Training
- Care management
- Health promotion   *Mansell & Harris 1998, p 192)*

Boarder (2002) interviewed 20 experienced CLDNs across North Wales, who reported the main roles shown in Box 10.5.

Boarder's study identified group work and health promotion work as being very important, along with the time spent in supporting and training support staff and the complexity of the extensive liaison necessary with other agencies and professionals.

Conclusion

Learning disability nurses in Wales are well integrated with – and contribute to – a wide range of community services to people with learning disability. There is flexibility in focusing the role around the individual needs and circumstances of each client. Because learning disability encompasses such a wide diversity of need, the roles of the learning disability nurse are varied and can be difficult to define precisely. They undertake a breadth of roles and activities ranging from medically and health-related ones to social and educational aspects of care, demonstrating a

Box 10.5 Main roles of community learning disability nurses

- Health maintenance
- Care planning
- Health promotion
- Group work
- Teamwork
- Assessment
- Staff and carer training and support
- Advocacy
- Supporting community living (residential projects)
- Maintaining place in the community
- Service development
- Challenging behaviour
- Playgroups and work with schools
- Client living skills development
- Sex education and counselling
- Personal relationships
- Bereavement counselling
- Working with clients with specifically identified difficulties (such as autism, learning disabilities and mental health, sensory and communication difficulties)
- Research   *(Boarder 2002, p288)*

strongly holistic approach to care.

While more focused areas of expertise and specialist practice are being developed to ensure a diverse skill mix in teams, learning disability nurses continue to be involved in learning disability generally. Likewise, while a more targeted approach is apparent, with shorter and more focused episodes of care, this is not always considered appropriate for those with multiple lifelong needs, who may need more long-term involvement. This is also the case for preventive work and health promotional activities.

Holistic approach: A greater health focus and definition of their work in health terms has taken place in recent years. However, a strongly holistic approach to care remains a key feature of the work of learning disability nurses, and skills (developed over years) in such areas as challenging behaviour and the development of skills in daily living continue to be practised and developed.

Case management: The co-ordination role and the complexity of the liaison work with other professionals and agencies means that learning disability nurses need good case management skills. However, there is a danger that the health focus of their work may be compromised when the formal role of case manager is combined with that of learning disability nurse and this could lead to role confusion and workload difficulties.

Working with others: Multidisciplinary and multiagency working continues to be central to the work of the learning disability nurse. While working to forge stronger links with the PCT (for example, to carry out health screening), there is also continued effective close working with social services and other agencies.

Advocacy: Although learning disability nurses cannot be seen as independent advocates, an important part of their roles is to act as advocates, working on behalf of people with learning disability to help them access health, social and other services available to the community as a whole.

Education: The role of educator and advisor is an important role, with learning disability nurses commonly contributing to staff training and support across agencies.

This chapter has given a view of what is happening in Wales and emphasises the developing role of learning disability nurses in their contribution to a multiagency and multidisciplinary pattern of service for people with learning disability. The recent restating of commitments to the principles of the All Wales Strategy with services responsive to local needs, culture and language means the further development of learning disability services with a distinctly Welsh character.

The size of Wales and the Welsh Assembly means that a unified approach to learning disability service development can continue to be developed, with health and social care organisations in Wales working in close partnership. In doing so, services can further build on the firm base of the achievements of the All Wales Strategy. However, practitioners and service providers need to continue to be open to innovation and good practice from outside as well as inside Wales. There is no doubt that services can gain a great deal in terms of good practice, innovation and improved service delivery, if experience, practice and successful service delivery are shared across all four principalities of the UK.

References

All Wales Senior Nurse Advisory Group (Learning All Wales Nurse Group for People with a Mental Handicap (1992) *A Statement for the Future: Mental Handicap Nursing in Wales*

Black J (2000) *A New History of Wales*. Stroud, Sutton Publishing

All Wales Senior Nurse Advisory Group (Learning Disability) (1997) *Learning Disability Nursing Action Plan*. All Wales Nurse Advisory Group

Boarder JH (2002) The perceptions of experienced community learning disability nurses of their roles and ways of working. *Journal of Learning Disabilities* **6**, 3, 281–296

Bollard M, Jukes M (1999) Specialist practitioner in community learning: disability nursing and the primary health care team. *Journal of Learning Disabilities for Nursing Health and Social Care* **3**, 1, 11–19

Davies J (1994) *A History of Wales*. London, Penguin Books

Davies J (1999) *A Pocket Guide to the Welsh Language*. Cardiff, University of Wales Press

Department of Health (1990) *NHS and Community Care Act*. London, HMSO

Department of Health (1995) *The Future of Learning Disability/Mental Handicap Nursing CNO PL(94) 7*. London, DH

Department of Health (2001) *Valuing People: A New Strategy for Learning Disability for the 21st Century, Cmnd 5086*. London, The Stationery Office

DHSS (1971) *Better Services for the Mentally Handicapped Cmnd 4683*. London, HMSO

Felce D (2003) Does size matter? – or staffing levels and costs? *Llais* **67** (Winter), 3–6

Felce D, Beyer S, Todd S (1995) Policy and Progress of the All Wales Strategy. *The Welsh Centre for Learning Disabilities: Research Highlights* No 3 (May)

Fisher M (1997) The specialist learning disability nurse in Wales. *International Journal of Nursing Practice* **3**, 188–190

Government of Wales Act (2006) HMSO

King's Fund Centre (1980) *An Ordinary Life: Comprehensive Locally-based Residential Services for Mentally Handicapped People.* London, King's Fund Centre

Learning Disability Advisory Group (2001*) Report to the National Assembly for Wales Fulfilling the Promises: Proposals for a framework for services for people with learning disabilities.* National Assembly for Wales

Learning Disability Implementation Advisory Group (2006) *Proposed Statement on Policy and Practice for Adults with a Learning Disability.* Welsh Assembly Government

Mansell I, Harris P (1998) Role of the registered nurse learning disability in community support teams for people with learning disabilities. *Journal of Learning Disabilities for Nursing, Health and Social Care* **2**, 4, 190–194

McGrath M, Humphries S (1988) *The All Wales CMHT Survey.* University of North Wales Centre for Social Policy Research and Development

National Assembly for Wales (1999) *Realising the Potential: a Strategic Framework for Nursing, Midwifery and Health Visiting in Wales into the 21st Century.* The National Assembly for Wales

National Assembly for Wales (2000) *Flexibilities for Joint Working Between Health and Local Government – Guidance Document.* Cardiff, National Assembly for Wales

National Assembly for Wales (2004) *Your Guide to the Assembly.* Cardiff, National Assembly for Wales

National Development Group (1977) *Mentally Handicapped Children: A Plan of Action.* London, DHSS

NHS Cymru Wales (1997) *Caring for the Future: The Nursing Agenda: Learning Disability Nursing Action Plan.* NHS Cymru Wales

NHS Cymru Wales (2001) *Health Evidence Bulletins Wales: Learning Disabilities (Intellectual Disability).* NHS Cymru Wales

Nirje B (1980) The Normalisation Principle. In: Flyn RJ, Nitsch KE (eds) *Normalisation, Social Integration and Community Services.* Baltimore, University Park Press

North-West Wales NHS Trust, Conwy and Denbighshire NHS Trust and NE Wales NHS Trusts (2004) *Clinical Interest Directory*

Simon G (1983) *Local Services for Mentally Handicapped Children.* Kidderminster, British Institute of Mental Handicap

Todd, S, Felce D., Beyer S, Shearn J, Perry J, Kilsby M.(2000) Strategic Planning and Progress Under the All Wales Strategy: Reflecting the Perceptions of Stakeholders, *Journal of Intellectual Disability Research* **44**,1, 31–44

Unit for Development in Intellectual Disabilities (UDID) (2004*) Fact Sheet: Vision, Mission Statement and Aims* University of Glamorgan / Bro Morgannwg NHS Trust

Unit for Development in Intellectual Disabilities (UDID) (2004) *Newsletter* Issue 2: Autumn, University of Glamorgan / Bro Morgannwg NHS Trust

UKCC (1986) *Project 2000: A New Preparation for Practice.* London, UKCC

UKCC (1999) *Fitness for Practice: The UKCC Commission for Nursing and Midwifery Education.* London, UKCC

Welsh Assembly Government (2002) *Realising the Potential Briefing Paper 3: Inclusion,*

Partnership and Innovation: A Framework for Realising Potential of Learning Disability Nursing in Wales. Welsh Assembly Government

Welsh Assembly Government (2003) *Fundamentals of Care: Guidance for Health and Social Care Staff.*Welsh Assembly Government

Welsh Assembly Government (2003) *Health, Social Care and Well-Being Strategies Guidance.* NHS Wales, GIG Cymru

Welsh Assembly Government (2004) *Learning Disability Strategy Section 7 Guidance on Service Principles and Service Responses.* Welsh Assembly Government

Welsh Assembly Government (2005a) *Health Care Standards for Wales.* NHS Wales GIG Cymru

Welsh Assembly Government (2005b) *Designed for Life: Creating World Class Health and Social Care for Wales in the 21st Century.* NHS Wales, GIG Cymru

Welsh Assembly Government (2007) Statement on Policy and Practice for Adults with a Learning Disability, Welsh Assembly Government.

Welsh Office NHS Directorate: The Welsh Health Planning Forum (1992) *Protocol for Investment in Health Gain: Mental Handicap (Learning Disabilities).* Welsh Office NHS Directorate

Welsh Language Act (1993) HMSO Welsh National Board (1983) *Syllabus for Training: Professional Register Part 5 Registered Nurse for the Mentally Handicapped.* London, English and Welsh National Boards for Nursing, Midwifery and Health Visiting

Welsh Office/Standing Conference of Voluntary Organisations for People with Learning Disability in Wales (1998) *Conference Report: Moving Forward to a Better Future.* Cardiff, Welsh Office/SCOVO

Welsh Office (1983) *The All Wales Strategy for the Development of Services for Mentally Handicapped People.* Cardiff, Welsh Office

Welsh Office (1994) *The Welsh Mental Handicap Strategy Guidance.* Cardiff, Welsh Office

Williams GA (1985) *When was Wales.* London, Penguin Books

Wolfensberger W (1980) A brief overview of the principles of normalisation. In: Flyn RJ. Nitsch KE (eds) *Normalization, Social Integration and Community Serv*ices. Baltimore, University Park Press

Wolfensberger W (1983) Social role valorisation: a proposed new term for the principle of normalization *Mental Retardation* **21**, 6, 234–239

CHAPTER 11

Regional focus England

John Turnbull

Introduction

The aims of this chapter are threefold. Firstly, the chapter will provide a brief overview of the commissioning and providing structure in which services for people with learning disability are delivered in England. Secondly, the chapter will turn to the Government's white paper on learning disability, *Valuing People* (Department of Health 2001a) and discuss the challenges and opportunities that this presents to learning disability nurses. The key issue here will be whether *Valuing People* itself has been responsible for bringing about change or whether there are broader trends in process that influence learning disability nursing. Finally, the chapter will discuss some of the factors that contribute to an English approach to supporting people with learning disabilities.

Although the discussion will make use of statistical information and will refer to experts in the field, it is important to point out that this chapter is essentially a personal viewpoint. However, it is a view informed by someone who has practised in a variety of roles as a learning disability nurse, including a period at the Department of Health, 13 years as a Director of Nursing with a specialist learning disability NHS trust and combining this with experience in an academic environment.

Commissioning services

Health and social care services for people with learning disabilities in England are commissioned through primary care trusts (PCTs) and local authority social services departments respectively. In October 2006 the Department of Health reduced the number of PCTs from 302 to 152 as part of a plan to make them more co-terminus with social service departments whose number currently stands at 150 (DH 2006). This policy change is yet another move aimed at promoting partnership and co-ordinated services for everyone.

Previous initiatives include flexibilities offered by the Health Act 1999 (DH 1999) which allowed for a range of collaborative arrangements at a local level, including the 'pooling' of budgets. Although accountability for expenditure ultimately remains with the NHS or local authority for their proportion of the budget, the 1999 Act also allows for either the PCT or social service department to be the lead commissioner and act on behalf of both organisations.

Most people would agree that the 'joined-up' approach to commissioning introduced by the 1999 Act represents a major step forward for partnership working as well as a potentially more efficient use of budgets. However, this sentiment has not been converted into action as often as anticipated and the use of Health Act flexibilities has been patchy across the country. The reasons for this are unclear. However, it could be imagined that, where there is little history of joint working or good relationships between agencies, they are unlikely to take the significant step to pool their resources and share decision making.

Some people also predict significant risks in pooling money, even in areas where relationships have been positive. For example, if one agency is the lead commissioner, the other partner could find their commissioning gaze gradually being diverted to areas other than learning disability. Although commissioners would hope that this would not happen, it is a genuine risk considering the proportion of NHS and local authority budgets that are set aside for learning disability. In the year 2004/05 the NHS spent £2.5 billion on specialist health services for people with learning disabilities that represented 3% of its total budget (*www.performance. DH.gov.uk* 2006). Comparable figures for local authorities for the same year are unavailable but those for 2000/01 show that their expenditure for learning disability social care services stood at £1.75 billion (*www.performance.DH.gov. uk* 2006) which is 12% of its total budget. Therefore, although the NHS spends more on people with learning disabilities than local authorities, its expenditure represents a relatively minor proportion of the total NHS bill. When put in this way, it confirms an often felt view that learning disability is a 'Cinderella' service but makes it more remarkable that ministers felt that it warranted a white paper in 2001 (Department of Health 2001a).

Although the statistics suggest that the local authority stands a better chance of prioritising learning disability services, future changes might alter this assumption. The latest imperative from government is for the new PCTs and local authorities to produce joint commissioning plans across a range of care groups (Department of Health 2006). Given these additional responsibilities, there is a risk that learning disability could fall even lower down the local authority agenda as the scale of their tasks and their budgets increase. There must also be a concern about the distance between the level at which commissioning strategies will be developed and the level at which those with any knowledge of learning disability will find themselves in the new structures. There has been a trend in NHS services that began with the introduction of NHS trusts in 1990 (Department of Health 1990) that has seen the gradual disappearance of senior learning disability posts in trusts. This has widened an 'influence gap' and is a challenge to which learning disability nurses and others will need to apply themselves seriously if they are to maintain any profile for learning disability.

Providing services

Turning from the commissioning of services to their provision, Emerson (2006) has provided a useful snapshot that has important implications for learning disability nurses. Emerson showed that private, not-for-profit and independent sector services now provide up to 78% of all forms of residential accommodation for people with learning disabilities in England (2006, p117). Emerson's figures show the effects of policy over the previous three decades that has sought the closure of long-term NHS residential provision, whether long-stay hospitals or community-based facilities. It also reflects the policy of transferring responsibility for providing residential services from both NHS and social services towards the independent sector. It would be fair to assume that many learning disability nurses have found employment in the independent sector, although probably not as many as the figure of 50% of the total profession that is estimated by some (Northway et al 2006). It is a testament to the versatility and adaptability of learning disability nurses that they have been able to transfer their knowledge and skills to a range of health and social care environments. However, this has come at a price for the profession. For example, for some, nurses' ability to work successfully in social care environments simply confirms that they should not be health care professionals. Also, some nurses have felt exploited by a rigid health and social care divide which has taken advantage of nurses' training and their competence but has denied them their identity as health care professionals in social care settings (Turnbull & Timblick 1998).

There has yet to be a comprehensive survey of learning disability posts in the NHS, although it is fair to assume that they occupy posts such as community nurses or working with people with more specialist needs, perhaps in specialist assessment and treatment or forensic services or as part of specialist community teams. Although this specialist provision has remained in NHS hands, there have still been changes in how it has been provided, not all of which have been positive for people with learning disabilities. When NHS trusts were created by the 1990 NHS and Community Care Act (Department of Health 1990), there were 14 specialist learning disability trusts in 1993. Today just two remain. Like many other NHS learning disability services, the 12 specialist trusts have been assimilated into larger mental health or community-based trusts that provide services to a range of people. It is impossible to say which configuration of health services works in the best interest of people with learning disabilities. One of the key issues is whether there is sufficient critical mass of expertise in a trust to think critically about services and to plan for their development and keep them running effectively on a day-to-day basis.

With the disappearance of specialist trusts, learning disability nurses in particular have seen their career opportunities curtailed. True to their innovative and creative heritage, many learning disability nurses have taken the chance to think differently and develop other careers in health, social care and beyond. Given the intention of the Labour government under Tony Blair to develop opportunities for different types of organisations such as social enterprise companies to provide health and social care (DH 2006), nurses will need to continue to think broadly about their contribution to the lives of people with learning disabilities. In the next 10 years there will be a need for more and more learning disability nurses to develop a social entrepreneurial outlook and skill base to build as well as work in these new types of organisation.

The impact of *Valuing People*

Valuing People (Department of Health 2001a) was a much anticipated and, at the time, a much welcomed addition to policy on learning disability in England. Based on four key principles of rights, independence, choice and inclusion, the white paper aimed at correcting many of the problems that prevent people with learning disabilities from accessing their rights as equal citizens. These problems included:

- Poor co-ordination between services
- Poor transitional planning from child to adult services
- Poor choice of housing
- Limited opportunities for employment
- A general feeling among people of a lack of control over their daily lives

Six years on from its publication, it is fair to say that *Valuing People* has probably had a mixed impact on the lives of people with learning disabilities and the services they use. At a general level, it has certainly succeeded in re-energising and refocusing the efforts of those supporting people with learning disabilities. Many of the structural changes called for in the document have also been put in place such as partnership boards, health action plans, funding for advocacy and a learning disability task force. The benefits of initiatives such as these may only become apparent in the decades to come.

Apart from the early successes, those supporting the implementation of *Valuing People* face significant challenges, principally because of the scope of the white paper itself. For instance, Styring and Grant (2006) observed that *Valuing People*'s strategy was based around concepts such as citizenship and inclusion rather than targets for services to achieve. They suggested that it might have been better for *Valuing People* to have become one of the Government's national service frameworks (NSF) or to have published a NSF as an appendix to the white paper. If this had happened, it would have been more likely that many of the targets and initiatives in *Valuing People* would have appeared in the NHS' performance indicators for NHS trusts. As things stand, the NHS' planning and priorities framework contain no reference to learning disability services.

Another problem facing the learning disability community is that the partnership boards that were created by *Valuing People* have no statutory role in commissioning or providing services, making it difficult for them to effect change. Finally, *Valuing People* probably missed the opportunity of bringing into being a national quality strategy for services in which benchmarks could be established and measured. Considering the fact that just over £4 billion of public money is spent on learning disability services, there is very little accountability demanded in terms of meeting quality targets. This should be of concern to both the Audit Commission and the general public alike.

Valuing People and learning disability nurses

Assessing the impact of *Valuing People* on learning disability nurses is a difficult task, mainly because there may have been trends and developments already in progress that would have influenced nursing practice whether or not the white paper was published. Nevertheless, before getting into more detailed description, it would be fair to say that *Valuing People* has given some nurses a glimpse into their future in terms of where they will be practising and the aims they will need to pursue. If the previous white paper on learning disability (Department of Health and Social Security 1971) acknowledged that people with learning disabilities had rights, then *Valuing People* aimed to take this on by acknowledging that many people needed extra help to access their rights. This means working to change society as well as to change people with learning disabilities. On a general level, nurses need to work for social change and develop their social entrepreneurial skills and qualities. If nurses are to work for social change, they will also need to prepare themselves to work with people in a variety of settings. Nurses in the future could be employed by a range of organisations to bring about communities that are more supportive to people with learning disabilities.

On a specific level, *Valuing People* has given community learning disability nurses a focus for their practice with the introduction of health facilitation and health action planning, although this must be seen in the context of a trend that has gradually clarified a health care role for nurses. During the 1980s and early 1990s, learning disability nurses became wary of linking their practice explicitly to health care concepts and practices. This was in part due to the emphasis on a social model of learning disability in which specialist health care practitioners were seen by some as part of a problem for people with learning disability, rather than part of a solution to their difficulties (Goble 1998). By the mid 1990s it was fully apparent that the mechanisms that had been employed to try to transform the lives of people with learning disabilities were not sufficient to effect change. For example, de-institutionalisation had almost been completed and much had changed in the lives of people. However, it could not be said that the majority of people living in the community were better off than before (Emerson 2004). In some respects, people with learning disabilities seemed worse off. For example, for some people who were relocated into small homes, their challenging behaviour presented greater risks to others and staff were left unsupported and isolated. The 1990s also marked the beginning of a succession of studies that showed that people with learning disabilities faced considerable barriers to accessing the health care they needed.

In response to these developments, the future for learning disability nurses was firstly seen as making their most significant contribution as specialists in areas such as challenging behaviour (Four Chief Nursing Officers 1991). Later, the Learning Disability Nursing project, initiated by England's Chief Nursing Officer in 1994, encouraged learning disability nurses to incorporate health models into their practice to make a difference in the lives of people with learning disabilities (Kay et al 1995). Whether as a result of these reports, a growing body of research, developments in health services or other factors, journal articles written by learning disability nurses in recent years reflect an increasing focus on health topics. The introduction of health facilitation by *Valuing People* seemed to arrive at an appropriate time for learning disability nurses, to confirm their current practice and open future opportunities for their development.

The key issue about health facilitation is that learning disability nurses should not see it simply as a task or an end in itself. Rather, health facilitation should be seen by nurses as an opportunity to develop a conceptual framework for their practice. One of the persistent criticisms of learning disability nursing is that it has lacked a model or conceptual framework for its practice (Aldridge 2004). Some would argue that this has made nurses feel uncertain about their role and unable to make finer choices in their day-to-day work. Although nurses would claim that their practice has been built on sound principles of promoting the rights and autonomy of people with learning disabilities, these are both too broad and not unique to learning disability nursing. A good conceptual framework is not an abstract, academic artefact but something drawn from practice that provides a clear statement about the goals of a particular profession. Conceptual frameworks can lead to more efficient and effective practice, and provide a benchmark against which to audit and evaluate practice (Meleis 1991, p21). Health facilitation is not a conceptual framework in itself, but it has links to a public health model of practice. There is the potential for learning disability nurses to shape and adapt this model to reflect their distinctive contribution to the lives of people with learning disabilities.

In its broadest sense, public health can be seen as a collection of initiatives aimed at promoting people's health and preventing ill health but it is also a philosophy which is aimed at creating healthy, inclusive and supportive communities through the empowerment of people and groups (Baggot 2004, p336). Box 11.1 shows an extract from a strategy for community learning disability nurses developed by nurses in the Ridgeway Partnership NHS trust. The strategy incorporates three elements of a public health model:

- A **strategic aim** of reducing health inequalities and improving the health of people with learning disabilities
- A **reconceptualised role** for nurses, with three distinct but inter-related functions that provide, support and influence
- An emphasis on the use of **systematically derived information** about the population of people with learning disabilities to inform practice, while not diminishing more traditional nursing skills of relationship building, partnership working and empowerment

The incorporation of a public health model into a conceptual base for practice should not come as alien to the way learning disability nurses have been practising. For example, nurses work with people to assess their health needs and promote their health, which includes working with groups of people with learning disabilities, for

Box 11.1 Extract from a strategy for community nursing*

Strategic aim: The aim of community nursing within the Trust is to reduce health inequalities and maintain and improve the health of people with learning disabilities. This will be achieved by developing the role of the community nurse in the following three areas and implementing and reviewing the following strategic objectives:

Elements of role	Strategic objectives
Provide specifically designed plans to maintain or improve the health of people or groups of people with learning disabilities	• Increase the proportion of group and sessional work undertaken by nurses • Adapt health information and health assessments for use with people with learning disabilities • Where appropriate, become health facilitators • Adapt and develop health promotion resources • Adapt and develop nursing practice to be more sensitive to cultural needs • Maximise the use of assistive technology • Analyse, interpret and communicate information to identify key trends in the population • Identify groups of people at risk • Develop health impact assessments • Promote the use of health action plans • Develop competencies for continuing health care assessments
Support others to enhance their roles in providing services and support to people with learning disabilities	• Raise awareness and transfer knowledge about people with learning disabilities, their lifestyles, wishes and needs to staff in key services • Provide education and training for appropriate services and individuals • Develop partnerships with appropriate services • Ensure that other services incorporate people with learning disabilities into their work on national service frameworks • Ensure that services are supported to include people with learning disabilities as part of national health screening programmes • Support others to meet any relevant recommendations in Disability Rights Commission Report on unequal treatment

Box11.1 continued

Elements of role	Strategic objectives
Influence others to create communities that are supportive and inclusive of people with learning disabilities	Develop a public health action learning network in learning disability • Increase community nurses' knowledge of health and social care policy and legislation • Develop and share an understanding of local political issues and their potential influence on health and social care practice • Increase networking amongst community nurses • Conduct and update community profiles that includes identifying people of influence • Where appropriate, make contact with local media

*Ridgeway Partnership, formerly the Oxfordshire Learning Disability NHS Trust

example, to focus on topics such as male health or sex and personal relationships. In pursuit of improved access to mainstream health services, learning disability nurses have also learned how to work with general practitioners and other members of the primary health care team to help them to adapt and improve the services they offer. In these respects, learning disability nurses would have few problems in linking these aspects of their practice with standards for public health nursing (Nursing and Midwifery Council 2004). However, the issue for learning disability nurses is which of these standards they would emphasise as being representative of what they do.

Nurses would also need to look ahead to the future context of service provision and support for people with learning disabilities to identify any public health approaches that would be particularly useful. It seems that an element of public health practice that has not been as well developed as others among all nurses is the use of political skills to influence the wider community. This would make sense at a conceptual as well as a practical level. For instance, if disability is predominantly a social construct, then it makes sense to seek to alter the perceptions and actions of society to create more supportive communities for people. Learning disability nurses would probably say that they have tried to accomplish this in a very small way in the past but they might not have associated it with a public health model. However, social change to achieve social inclusion for vulnerable people has been a key element in public health approaches for decades (Dalziel 2002).

A public health model would match the aspirations of learning disability nurses and have the potential to resolve some long standing issues for the profession, namely their relationship with other branches of nursing and how to communicate their concept of health. For example, the concept of 'health' has traditionally proved difficult for learning disability nurses. When health was seen simply as the absence of disease and health care became concerned with ill health, learning disability nurses could see little connection between their practice and other health care professionals, especially fellow nurses in the adult branch. As Mitchell (1998) pointed out, since the adult branch has always been seen as the epitome of nursing, it is not surprising that learning disability nurses have felt marginalised.

This picture may be set to change. The government white paper on health *Your Health, Your Care, Your Say* (DH 2006) highlights the changes that have been taking place in the general population and, in particular, the profile of health needs. Essentially, now that people are living longer they are also living with long-term conditions such as arthritis, diabetes, asthma and heart disease. A priority for the Government is to reduce dependence on expensive hospital admissions by ensuring that people are supported adequately in community settings. The emphasis in health care is shifting from ill health to poor health and with it has come a need to change nursing practice. Nursing will need to focus on more efficient and effective ways of supporting people in their own homes. Preliminary research on ways to support people with long-term conditions highlights some critical success factors that would be familiar to learning disability nurses:

- A good relationship
- Bringing specialist knowledge closer to the person
- Making information more accessible to people (Corben & Rosen 2005)

The move to supporting people with long-term conditions and the need to prevent ill health imply a change towards a model of health that takes into account a full range of personal, social, economic and environmental factors. This may align the work of learning disability nurses with that of their nursing colleagues from other branches and, one hopes, mitigate any feelings of marginalisation.

Valuing People has helped learning disability nurses to provide a vehicle for their expertise in health facilitation and health action planning. They could use this experience to help them develop a new conceptual model for their practice and become credible public health practitioners. However, *Valuing People* also contains a potential barrier to this happening. *Valuing People* called for a review of community teams for people with learning disabilities. The hope was that community teams could become a focal point or, to use the jargon, a 'front door' for people and their families to access health and social care services. For many existing teams, their review has resulted in greater levels of collaboration and, in several areas in England, community teams have become joint health and social care teams under a single management structure that is usually provided by social services. Although this level of partnership can serve as an example to other types of community services, there has been a worrying trend in some community teams that has resulted in community nurses carrying out care management functions as well as spending an inordinate amount of time in assessing people who have been referred against increasingly stringent eligibility criteria.

The move towards care management is not worrying simply because it is care management but because of the way that care management is currently implemented. For example, learning disability nurses would bring a great deal of expertise to the care management function. However, the learning disability nurses are health care practitioners whose role it is to change people with learning disabilities or their circumstances, or both, in order for them to lead healthier and more valued lifestyles. It feels as if somewhere since its inception in 1990 and today, care management has lost its energy and capacity to transform people's lives. Instead of assessment there is measurement, and instead of supporting choice there is placement. The pressures on learning disability nurses to become complicit in this process should not be underestimated and strong leadership will be necessary if current community nursing is to transform itself into community public health nursing for people with learning disabilities.

As far as more specialist practice in learning disability nursing is concerned, *Valuing People* had little to say, except to entreat them to work in different ways. This vague statement had less to do with the needs of people with learning disabilities but probably more to do with the Department of Health's ambitions for all health care professionals (Department of Health 2001b) in its search for greater efficiency. Nevertheless, some general points can be made. A key initiative in the white paper, such as person-centred planning, can be seen as posing challenges to many specialist nurses, especially those working with people who have offended or those with mental health issues or severe challenging behaviour. Here, the particular challenge is how to practise in person-centred ways for people whose freedom has been restricted by the law or by others in an effort to manage the risk they pose to themselves or others. There is emerging evidence of how nurses are meeting this challenge (Riding 2004) that includes attempts to fuse person-centred planning with the Care Programme Approach so that it becomes an enabling rather than a controlling process.

Again it is easier to point towards general trends than to specific statements in *Valuing People* as a reason for changes in the way nurses practise. For example, Barr (2006) showed that referrals to community teams in a previous 10-year period have become more focused on the need for specialist support in areas such as challenging behaviour and mental health. In response to this, and given the previous discussion about community nurses, it would be disappointing if community teams simply turned themselves into repositories for specialist nurses in the future. This would impair the development of community learning disability nursing and back nurses into the health care cul-de-sac that Brown (1994) warned against. This is not to say that specialist practitioners should not be part of the community teams of the future. On the contrary, many of the issues involved in developing a public health focus for community nursing could equally apply to specialist nurses. For example, the findings from research into how best to support people with long-term health conditions (Corben & Rosen 2005) has highlighted several issues that could equally apply to people with learning disabilities with more specialist needs. One of the key findings was that people valued having specialist knowledge brought closer to them by meeting with specialists in their local surgeries. Learning disability nurses in many areas have already implemented this approach but the opportunity exists to be even more creative about transferring specialist knowledge. For example, specialist nurses could use information technology to offer more advice via text messaging or e-mail to parents or staff or people with learning disabilities. Specialist nurses could also become involved in developing online resources and e-learning materials. Whatever the specific initiative, the overall challenge for nurses is how specialist practice can be deployed closer to people and the community.

Services in England

At the time of writing, the population of England was 50,431,700 (*www.statistics. gov.uk* 2006). At 83.8% of the United Kingdom population, this makes England by far the largest country in terms of inhabitants among its UK neighbours. The size of the country and, therefore, the huge volume of service provision for people with learning disabilities in England inevitably mean that there will be variation in both the quality and characteristics of services: this is in spite of common legislation and policies. The size of the country is inevitably a weakness when it comes to learning disability services because they are so rarely in the public or even managerial gaze. This may go part of the way in explaining why services in some areas can spectacularly fail (Healthcare Commission 2006). On the other hand, size could be a factor in driving innovation and diversity. Certainly, different areas in England have demonstrated that there are many ways of providing services and the important issue is for these experiences to be shared and learned from.

The great size and scope of health and social care commissioning and provision is certainly an issue for Government. At the current time there seems to have been a realisation among ministers that perhaps the country really is too big for them to be trying to reach into every corner and run the nation's health and social care services. Diversity and local accountability are likely to be a growing trend in which learning disability nursing and services will need to adapt. For nurses in particular, this could see different approaches to education and continuing professional development where the challenge will be to balance public protection and national standards of competence with the need to meet local competencies. Local services may need to prepare for this by ensuring that the quality of their practice-based education and mentoring is on the agendas of managers.

This parochial focus may prove to be the 'default' position for much of the provision in England not just because of ministers' problems in leading innovation and change but because it feels like an essentially English approach. Isolating a set of common values and distilling a sense of identity for people living in England always seems to present difficulties and the English often prefer to align themselves to factors in their local area. Whether this is a problem for those commissioning or providing services is a different matter and the answer is probably that they would prefer to develop services in line with local needs. At the same time, there is a need to make use to all means to share experiences and spread good practice. For learning disability nurses, their relatively small number makes it imperative that they share knowledge if they are to continue to feel a sense of being a profession.

Conclusion

One of the aims of this chapter was to explore whether there is such a phenomenon as an English approach to services for people with learning disabilities. The answer is probably not – although the size of England relative to its neighbours has affected the perspectives of people working in those services. The other two aims of the chapter were to describe the context of service provision, especially in a post-*Valuing People* period and explore the challenges that this presents to learning disability nurses. The brief response to this is that *Valuing People* has probably brought into focus the need for community nurses in particular to evolve into public health practitioners for people with learning disabilities; and for specialist practitioners to develop ways of bringing their skills and knowledge even closer to where they can be most effective. This is not a radical departure from current practice. Rather, it could be seen as a rediscovery of traditional nursing values that emphasise personal and social change.

References

Aldridge J (2004) Learning disability nursing: a model for practice. In Turnbull J (ed) *Learning Disability Nursing*. Oxford, Blackwell Publishing

Baggott R (2004) *Health and Health Care in Britain*. Basingstoke, Palgrave

Barr O (2006) The evolving role of community nurses for people with learning disabilities: changes over an 11-year period. *Journal of Clinical Nursing* 15, 72–82

Brown J (1994) *The Hybrid Worker*. University of York, Department of Social Policy and Social Work

Corben S, Rosen R (2005) *Self-management for long-term conditions: patients' perspectives on the way ahead*. London, King's Fund

Dalziel Y (2002) Community development as a public health function. In: Cowley S (ed) *Public Health in Policy and Practice*. London, Baillière Tindall

Department of Health (1990) *NHS and Community Care Act*. London, HMSO

Department of Health (2001a) *Valuing People: a new strategy for learning disability for the 21st century*. London, The Stationery Office

Department of Health (2001b) *Investment and reform for NHS staff – taking forward the NHS Plan*. London, The Stationery Office

Department of Health (1999) *Health Act*. London, The Stationery Office

Department of Health (2006) *Your health, your care, your say*. London, The Stationery Office

Department of Health and Social Security (1971) *Better Services for the Mentally Handicapped*. London, HMSO

Emerson E (2004) Deinstitutionalisation in England. *Journal of Intellectual and Developmental Disability* 29, 17–22

Emerson E (2006) Models of service delivery. In: Grant G, Goward P, Richardson M, Ramcharan P (eds) *Learning Disability: a Life Cycle Approach to Valuing People*. Maidenhead, Open University Press

Four Chief Nursing Officers (1991) *Mental Handicap Nursing in the Context of Caring for People. The Cullen Report*. London, Department of Health

Goble C (1998) 50 years of NHS involvement in the lives of people with learning difficulties: a cause for celebration? *Disability and Society* 13, 5, 833–835

Healthcare Commission and Commission for Social Care Inspection (2006) *Joint investigation into the provision of services for people with a learning disability at Cornwall Partnership NHS Trust.* London, HC and CSCI

Kay B, Rose S, Turnbull J (1995) *Continuing the Commitment: the report from the Learning Disability Nursing Project.* London, Department of Health

Meleis AI (1991) *Theoretical Nursing: Development and Progress* (2nd edn). New York, Lippincott

Mitchell D (1998) The origins of learning disability nursing. *International History of Nursing Journal* **4**, 1, 10–16

Northway R, Hutchinson C, Kingdon A (2006) *Shaping the Future: A Vision for Learning Disability Nursing.* United Kingdom Consultant Learning Disability Nurses Network

Nursing and Midwifery Council (2004) *Standards of Proficiency for Specialist Community Public Health Nurses.* London, NMC

Riding T (2004) Getting the balance right: the issue of rights and responsibilities in learning disability. In: Turnbull J (ed) *Learning Disability Nursing.* Oxford, Blackwell

Styring L, Grant G (2006) Maintaining a commitment to quality. In: Grant G, Goward P, Richardson M, Ramcharan P (eds) *Learning Disability: a Life Cycle Approach to Valuing People.* Maidenhead, Open University Press

Turnbull J, Timblick D (1998) Residential care homes: challenges for nurses. *Learning Disability Practice* **1**, 2, 10–13

Websites

(accessed 7 June 2007)
Department of Health performance data: *www.performance.doh.gov.uk*
National Statistics: *www.statistics.gov.uk*

CHAPTER 12

Regional focus
Éire Ireland

Paul Keenan

Introduction

The purpose of this chapter is threefold. Firstly, the chapter will outline the philosophies, policies, and provisions underpinning and responding to the needs of people with intellectual disabilities in Éire Ireland. Secondly, the chapter will explore the current role of registered intellectual disability nurses in this continually changing and highly complex context and finally, the chapter will discuss how the role of the registered intellectual disability nurse may develop in Éire Ireland in the foreseeable future.

'Intellectual disabilities' is currently the preferred term in Éire Ireland and will be used throughout this chapter. It is used in current legislation such as the Disability Act (Government of Ireland (GOI) 2005a) and nurse registration (An Bord Altranais/The Irish Nursing Board (ABA/IRB) 2006). Other terms, such as 'mental handicap' and 'learning disability', are still evident in Éire Ireland, but less so.

Éire Ireland

The island of Ireland is politically divided into a sovereign state, the Republic of Ireland (Irish: *Poblacht na hÉireann*. From 1st January 2007 it has been referred to as *'Éire Ireland'* at European level) and Northern Ireland, which is part of the United Kingdom. However, the island operates as one entity at a number of all-Ireland levels, for example:

Sport: Special Olympics Ireland (SOI) provides year-round sporting activities for 35,000 people with intellectual disabilities (SOI 2003, 2006; NDA 2005a).

Health: The Éire Ireland Department of Health and Children (DOHC) and the Department of Health, Social Service and Public Safety, Northern Ireland (DHSSPS) have responsibility for the continued implementation of the co-operation agenda decided by the North-South Ministerial Council under the auspices of the Good Friday Agreement 1998 (HSE 2006). Nursing initiatives in this framework include *A Nursing Vision of Public Health* (DOHC/DHSSPS 2001) and *From Vision to Action* (DOHC/DHSSPS 2003).

The population of Éire Ireland is 4.2 million, an increase of more than 8% since 2002, and the highest since 1861. It is expected to increase to over 5 million by 2016. While the population is relatively young – just 11% are over 65 – this is expected to double in the next 30 years and 40% are expected to be over 50 (GOI 2006).

The structure of health and social care provision

The Irish Constitution *Bunreacht na hÉireann* (GOI 1937) takes precedence over all other sources of law, with the exception of European Community law. While it provides a constitutional right for education to children, it does not provide a constitutional right to health and personal social care (Quinlivan 2004). However a quality health service, similar to the UK and the rest of Europe is provided for under a complex legislative and policy framework. Children and those on low incomes receive free health care, with the remainder of citizens paying for health care, normally through private health insurance (GOI 2004a).

Recent social policy in health and personal social care has lead to fundamental changes to the national structure of health and personal social care provision and is based on the principle of inclusive citizenship for all (DOHC 2006).

Before the implementation of The Health Act (GOI 2004a) in 2005, health and personal social care were delivered through hundreds of different public and private agencies, each of which were independently answerable to the Department of Health and Children (DOHC). It was recognised that reform was required to address the inconsistencies in care nationally as a result of this complex structure. There was concern that existing services in terms of structure and resources would not be able to manage the needs of the increasing ageing population in 20–30 years' time (HSE 2006).

Since 1 January 2005, health and personal social care is structured as follows:

Department of Health and Children (DOHC): responsible for strategically managing the health service, developing policy and ensuring the quality performance of the service delivery system (DOHC 2006).

Health Service Executive (HSE): responsible for managing and delivering, or arranging for the delivery of, health and personal social services, a key function is integrating the delivery of health and personal social services (HSE 2006; GOI 2004a Part 7).

The HSE is the largest employer in the state, directly employing more than 65,000 staff, and funding a further 35,000 staff employed by hundreds of voluntary hospitals, parents' groups, etc. The current budget is almost €12 billion, a threefold increase in funding in less than ten years (HSE 2006; DOHC 2006).

The HSE aims to put patients and clients at the centre of the organisation. Health and Personal Social Services are divided into three service delivery units (Figure 12.1):

- Population Health promotes and protects the health of the entire population
- Primary, Community and Continuing Care (PCCC) delivers health and personal social services in the community and other settings

Figure 12.1 Organisational structure of Health Service Executive

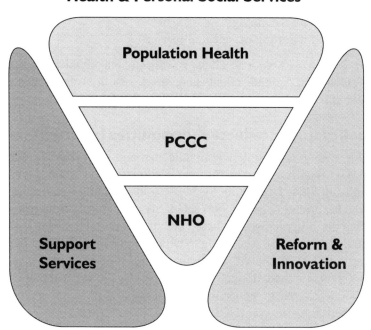

Health & Personal Social Services

- National Hospitals Office (NHO) provides acute hospital and ambulance services throughout the country

The services delivered by PCCC, NHO and Population Health are organised through four administrative areas:

- HSE West
- HSE South
- HSE Dublin North East
- HSE Dublin Mid Leinster

Health Information and Quality Authority and Office of the Chief Inspector of Social Services

The Health Information and Quality Authority (AnTúdarás um fhaisnéis agus cáilíocht sláinte (HIQA)) and the Office of the Chief Inspector of Social Services /Oifig an Phríom-Chigire Seirbhísí Sóisialacha (OCISS) were established under the Health Act 2007 (GOI 2007a) to ensure that the care provided by HSE and HSE-funded services, as well as the voluntary and private sectors, are of high quality and based on 'evidence supported best practice'. This is the first time that all services will be periodically and regularly inspected against agreed national standards (HSE, 2006; GOI, 1990 & 2007b).

The key responsibilities are:
- Developing health information systems
- Promoting and implementing structured programmes of quality assurance
- Overseeing accreditation
- Developing health technology assessment
- Reviewing and reporting on selected services

HIQA is expected to work in alliance with key stakeholders and recognised authorities, including patients, clients and carers, health professionals, academic institutions and international bodies (HSE, 2006 & GOI, 2007).

Social policy and intellectual disabilities in Éire Ireland

Policy and provision for people with intellectual and other disabilities have long been viewed as requiring serious reform (Commission on Nursing 1998; Quinn 2002; Quinlivan 2004; DOHC 2006). In 1996 the Commission on the Status of People with Disabilities (CSPD 1996) set out its blueprint *A Strategy for Equality* for reforming disability legislation based on citizenship grounded in human rights (Quinn 2002; NDA 2003a). According to Quinlivan (2004), this signified the shift from a charity to a rights-based paradigm of care. *A Strategy for Equality* made more than 400 recommendations (CSPD 1996; NDA 2003a), many of which have been incorporated in recent legislation, including:
- Employment Equality Act (GOI 1999a)
- National Disability Authority Act (GOI 1999b)
- Comhairle Act (GOI 2000a)
- Equal Status Act (GOI 2000b)
- Mental Health Act (GOI 2001)
- Health Act (GOI 2004a)
- Education for Persons with Special Educational Needs Act (GOI 2004b)
- Disability Act (GOI 2005a)
- Health and Social Care Professionals Act (GOI 2005b)

Further related legislation was due in 2007 on advocacy and quality.

Comhairle Act

The Comhairle Act (GOI 2000a) established a new body Comhairle (now called the Citizens' Information Board) and repealed the National Social Service Board Act (GOI 1984). The functions of the Comhairle Board are stated in Section 7–1 of the Act. They are to:
- Support the provision of directly, independent information, advice and advocacy services to ensure that individuals have access to accurate, comprehensive and clear information relating to social services and are referred to the relevant services
- Assist and support individuals, in particular those with disabilities, in identifying and understanding their needs and options and in accessing their entitlements to social services
- Promote greater accessibility, co-ordination and public awareness of social

services and of information, advice and advocacy services provided in relation to such services – whether by a statutory body or a voluntary body
- Support, promote and develop the provision of information on the effectiveness of current social policy and services and to highlight issues which are of concern to users of those services
- Promote and support the development of voluntary bodies providing social services

National Disability Act

The National Disability Act (GOI 1999b) established the National Disability Authority (NDA), an independent public body, to promote and secure the rights of people with disabilities. The NDA's function is to inform the Minister for Justice, Equality and Law reform and keep him or her up to date on disability-related issues that may affect policy and practice.

The work of the NDA is to (NDA 2006a, p2):
- Assist the Minister to develop policy on issues concerning people with disabilities
- Research, collect and analyse information on issues related to disability and services for people with disabilities
- Advise on standards and quality of services for people with disabilities
- Prepare codes of practice that will help achieve high standards and good quality in services for people with disabilities
- Monitor the establishment and use of standards and codes of practice
- Acknowledge when services have achieved high standards and good quality. This will include an award system.

In relation to standards, codes of practice, examples of best practice and research the NDA has funded and published a number of research projects, including:
- Person-centred planning (NDA 2005b)
- Review of research into disability in Ireland (NDA 2002)
- Best practice in the provision of further education, employment and training (NDA 2003a)
- Review of access to Mental Health Services for people with intellectual disabilities (NDA 2003b)
- Code of Practice on Accessibility of Public Services and information provided by Public Bodies (NDA 2006b) (in response to the requirements of the Disability Act (2005b) (Part 3, Section 30)

The Code of Practice has not yet been approved, amended or rejected by government. A decision was expected in 2007. The NDA's primary focus in research for 2007 is the needs of children with disabilities.

Mental Health Act

The Mental Health Act (GOI 2001) provides for the involuntary admission to approved centres of people suffering from mental disorders, to provide for the independent review of the involuntary admission of such persons and, for those purposes, to provide for the establishment of a Mental Health Commission and the appointment of Mental health tribunals and an inspector of Mental Health Services, to repeal in part the Mental Treatment Act (GOI 1945).

Section 3 (1) defines 'Mental disorder' as mental illness, severe dementia or significant intellectual disability where:

- Because of the illness, disability or dementia, there is a serious likelihood of the person concerned causing immediate and serious harm to himself or herself – or to other persons
- Because of the severity of the illness, disability or dementia, the judgment of the person concerned is so impaired that failure to admit the person to an approved centre would be likely to lead to a serious deterioration in his or her condition, or would prevent the administration of appropriate treatment that could be given only by such admission
- The reception, detention and treatment of the person concerned in an approved centre would be likely to benefit or alleviate the condition of that person to a material extent.

In Section 3 (2) *subsection (1)*

- *Mental illness* means a state of mind of a person which affects the person's thinking, perceiving, emotion or judgment and which seriously impairs the mental function of the person to the extent that he or she requires care or medical treatment in his or her own interest or in the interest of other persons
- *Severe dementia* means a deterioration of the brain of a person which significantly impairs the intellectual function of the person thereby affecting thought, comprehension and memory and which includes severe psychiatric or behavioural symptoms such as physical aggression
- *Significant intellectual disability* means a state of arrested or incomplete development of mind of a person that includes significant impairment of intelligence and social functioning and abnormally aggressive or seriously irresponsible conduct on the part of the person.

Little is known about the mental health needs of people with intellectual disabilities in Ireland as service provision in this area at primary care and specialist mental health care level is limited (Irish College of Psychiatrists 2004; DOHC 2006). The National Intellectual Disability Database Committee (HRB 2006) should undertake a detailed national prevalence picture yearly, so that sufficient services can be developed carefully (DOHC 2006).

When the Mental Health Act (GOI 2001) is fully enacted, people with intellectual disabilities who are subject to detention, seclusion or restraint in an approved, annually inspected, centre will be afforded a level of legal protection not granted to those individuals with intellectual disabilities subject to detention, seclusion and restraint in intellectual disability services which are not approved centres and therefore not protected by the Mental Health Act (GOI 2001).

There is a need for a legislative enactment to address the whole issue of consent and detainment. The Law Reform Commission consultation paper *Vulnerable Adults and the Law: Capacity* (2005) recommends the enactment of capacity legislation, that emphases capacity rather than lack of capacity and should be enabling rather than restrictive in nature. It also recommends that a functional approach should be taken to the issue of legal capacity, i.e. consideration of capacity in relation to a particular decision at a particular point in time (The Law Reform Commission 2005; DOHC 2006).

Education for Persons with Special Educational Needs Act

The Education for Persons with Special Educational Needs Act (GOI 2004b, p1) sets out to:

- Provide for the education of people with special needs, wherever possible, to take place in an inclusive environment with those who do not have such needs
- Ensure that people with special educational needs shall have the same right to use – and benefit from – appropriate education, as do their peers who do not have such needs
- Assist children with special educational needs to leave school with the skills necessary to participate, to the level of their capacity, in an inclusive way in the social and economic activities of society and to live independent and fulfilled lives
- Provide for the greater involvement of parents in the education of their children
- Establishes the National Council for Special Education and an Appeals board

Disability Act

The Disability Act (GOI 2005a) enables:

- The independent assessment of health and education needs of people with disabilities
- Government ministers to make provision for meeting the assessed needs of people with disabilities in allocated resources
- People with disabilities to appeal if they believe their needs are not being fully met
- The promotion of equality and social inclusion
- Better provision in respect of disabled people using public buildings and working in the public sector

The Disability Act (GOI 2005a Section 2 (1)) defines disability as:

> '...a substantial restriction in the capacity of the person to carry on a profession, business or occupation in the Irish State or to participate in social or cultural life in the Irish State by reason of an enduring physical, sensory, mental health or intellectual impairment'

While the definition is very broad, and does not list specific disabilities but instead states areas of impairment i.e. physical, sensory, mental health or intellectual, this should be viewed as a positive aspect of the Disability Act (GOI 2005a). It provides scope for disability to be described primarily in person-centred terms rather than by rigid, standardised diagnostic subcategories.

The definition of disability contains the concept *substantial restriction* – this is seen as a restriction which:

> '(a) is permanent or likely to be permanent, results in a significant
> difficulty in communication, learning or mobility or in significantly
> disordered cognitive processes, and (b) gives rise to the need for
> services to be provided continually to the person whether or not a
> child or, if the person is a child, to the need for services to be provided
> early in life to ameliorate the disability' (GOI 2005a, Section 7 [2])

Most of the issues on the definition of *disability* contained in the Disability Act (GOI 2005a) are likely to centre round interpretations of the adjectives *'substantial'*, *'significant'* and *'enduring'*. There are likely to be borderline issues that will lead to conflict between assessment and liaison officers and service users, as well as disputes between professionals, and between service providers and service statement expectations. For example, when does each of these adjectives stop being their respective antonyms? These three measurement terms are likely to lead to debate and conflict.

Similar to the NHS and Community Care Act (DH 1990) in the United Kingdom, Éire Ireland's Disability Act (GOI 2005a) does not define precisely what constitutes health and personal social services. Neither act indicates how *need* should be defined, nor does it state what standard of service should be provided by agencies carrying out its responsibilities. These areas are likely to lead to dispute in Éire Ireland and could lead to various interruptions of the act and in turn for service eligibility criteria. Similar to the 1997 UK House of Lords ruling in the 'Gloucestershire case' (Mencap 2001), the Éire Ireland Disability Act (GOI 2005a) states that resources need to be taken into account when deciding which services will be provided. Assessment of needs does not in any way guarantee that services will be provided. However, unlike the UK's NHS and Community Care Act (DH 1990), Éire Ireland Disability Act (GOI 2005a) does provide for a national system for assessment.

For a more detailed analysis of the Disability Act (GOI 2005a) and its potential impact on people with intellectual, and other disabilities see Keenan (2007a–f).

Health and Social Care Professionals Act

The Health and Social Care Professionals Act (GOI 2005b) provides for the establishment and functions of the Health and Social Care Professionals Council and of registration boards for twelve designated health and social care professions (Box 12.1)

Similar to the statutory functions carried out by the An Bord Altranais / Irish Nursing Board and the UK's Nursing and Midwifery Council, designated professionals are now required to register with a statutory professional body, adhere to a professional code of conduct and be denied the right to practise if they are deemed by their peers to be unfit. The Act ensures that those designated professionals will now have to demonstrate the same high level of professional accountability to the public as nurses and doctors.

While there have been numerous progressive legislative and policy

Box 12.1 Designated health and social care professions under the Health and Social Care Professionals Act

- Clinical biochemist
- Dietician
- Medical scientist
- Occupational therapist
- Orthoptist
- Physiotherapist
- Podiatrist
- Psychologist
- Radiographer
- Social care worker
- Social worker
- Speech and language therapist   *(GOI 2005b Part 4, Section 1, p9)*

developments in relation to people with intellectual disabilities, in recent years, areas requiring attention include legislative reform accompanied with a Code of Practice in the area of incapacity to give consent (The National Association of the Mentally Handicapped in Ireland 2003), this should be along similar lines to The Adults with Incapacity (Scotland) Act (2000). The NDA and the Department of Health and Children acknowledge that many of the principles and requirements of recent social policy have yet to be realised in practice (NDA 2006c; DOHC 2006). According to NDA (2006c), the major reform programme in health, the National Strategy *Quality and Fairness, A Health System for You* (DOHC 2001), provides opportunities to:

- Introduce routine health service mapping
- Develop management information systems
- Resource effective participation mechanisms so that people with disabilities are decision-makers at all levels of health care
- Ensuring equitable provision
- Mainstream non-health functions
- Implementing standards and systems of inspection
- Build networks for sharing good practice and building collaboration
- Promote equality proofing of health care policies and provision.

Intellectual disabilities in Éire Ireland

Demographic profile of people with intellectual disabilities

National Intellectual Disability Database (NIDD) figures published in April 2006 show there were 25,518 people registered as having an intellectual disability (i.e. 6.51 per 1,000 population). The ratio of male to female is 1.31 to 1. People with mild intellectual disability are registered as 2.18 per 1,000. However, *Vision for*

Change (DOHC 2006) disputes this figure, estimating that the NIDD datasets contain only one-third of the people with mild intellectual disability in Ireland. People with moderate, severe, and profound intellectual disability are 3.74 per 1,000, an increase of 30% since the first Irish Census of Mental Handicap 32 years ago. This increase is partly explained by the growth in the general population over the same timespan as a result of the baby booms in the 1960s and 1970s, and in the increased lifespan of people with intellectual disabilities. The number of people with moderate, severe, and profound intellectual disability aged 35 years and over has increased from 29% in 1974 to 38% in 1996 and to 47% in 2006. This changing age profile has major implications for service development and helps to explain the increased need for additional provision in the intellectual disability field (Barron & Kelly 2006, pp11–13).

HSE service provision for people with intellectual disabilities in 2006

Health and personal social service provision for people with intellectual disabilities has developed in the past decade with a greater emphasis on integration at school, work and in the community. (Commission on Nursing 1998; DOHC 2006; NDA 2002, 2003b & 2006b).

The HSE provided €1.4 billion for services for people with an intellectual disability in 2006, an increase of 7.15% from the previous year. The HSE have committed themselves to similar increases over the next few years (HSE 2006). Eighty-five per cent of intellectual disability services are provided through contractual service level agreements negotiated between the HSE and more than 300 voluntary and non-statutory sector organisations (examples include religious orders and parents' associations) (Minister's statement). According to *Vision for Change* (DOHC 2006) the development of intellectual disability services have largely been determined in the past by the voluntary providers. While multidisciplinary teams generally provide person-centred care focused on the social, vocational, educational and residential needs of the person with intellectual disabilities, the quality and extent of this varies nationally. The plethora of recent social policy is likely to address many of these issues and enhance the consistency and quality of services for people with intellectual disabilities over time.

According to the NIDD (Barron & Kelly 2006, pp11–13):

- 24,556 people (96%) receive services. This is the highest number of people recorded since the Irish National Database was established in 1995
- 313 people (1%) currently receive no services at present but will require appropriate services in the period 2007–2011
- 649 people (3%) are not using services and have no identified need for services during the planning period 2007–2011. Almost 60% of this cohort (373 people) are in the mild or 'not verified' range of intellectual disability
- Of the 24,556 people receiving services in 2006, 16,245 (64%) live at home with parents, siblings, relatives, or foster parents
- 8,181 live in full-time residential services, the highest figure recorded on the

NIDD since 2001. This is the third consecutive year of data indicating that more people live in group homes in their communities than in residential centres

- The number of people accommodated in psychiatric hospitals has decreased by 48 since 2005, to 348
- 24,386 people use at least one day programme. Of this group, 8,044 are in full-time residential placements and 4,776 are in receipt of residential support services such as respite care
- 19,152 people use one or more multidisciplinary support service. The most commonly used services by adults are social work, medical services, and psychiatry. The most commonly used services by children are speech and language therapy, social work, and psychology

There has been significant growth in the level of provision of full-time residential services, residential support services, and day services in the past decade. This reflects the significant government investment programme in the intellectual disability sector. Key developments during the period 1996 to 2006 noted in their report include:

- A doubling of the number of people living in group homes following deinstitutionalisation
- A 64% reduction in the number of people with intellectual disability accommodated inappropriately, or no longer requiring care in psychiatric hospitals
- A continued expansion in the availability of residential support services, in particular planned or emergency centre-based respite services, which have grown by 387%; 4,242 people use this type of residential support service, allowing them to continue living with their families and in their communities
- Increased provision in almost all areas of adult day services and in the level of support services delivered as part of a package of day services to both children and adults

Since inception in 1996 the yearly NIDD results have provided robust data, which have identified trends in demographics and service development. As highlighted by Barron and Kelly (2006), one of these trends is that over a quarter of people with a moderate, severe, or profound intellectual disability who are aged 35 years or over are living in home settings. As their significant carers start to age beyond their caring capacity, formal supervised living arrangements will need to be provided. Because people with intellectual disability are living longer, the likelihood of their outliving their caregivers has increased substantially. The NIDD data highlight the need for services to develop provision for this group, and in what quantity to proactively avoid crisis situations, if resources allow.

Service requirements in 2006 and beyond

According to Barron and Kelly (2006) the needs of 2,371 people with intellectual disabilities are only partly being met or not met at all. This is an increase of 101, or

4%, since 2005. To address this, the following is required in 2007–2011 (though most service needs arise immediately):

- 2118 full-time residential placements
- 270 day programmes
- 233 individuals living in psychiatric hospitals in 2005 need to be resettled in more appropriate accommodation

In 2006 a further 11,818 people were receiving services but will require alternative, additional, or enhanced services in the next five years, an increase of 228, or 2%, since 2005.

The 2006 NIDD dataset, in line with data in recent years, suggests that, despite a threefold increase in the intellectual disability service budget, which has resulted in substantial levels of service provision in day, residential and multidisciplinary support services, there is significant ongoing demand for new intellectual disability services and a growing requirement to enhance existing services (Barron & Kelly 2006, DOHC 2006).

While the annual NIDD datasets provide the best available description of the current level of service provision and assist in the development of new services based on identified need at national and regional level, there is still much that they do not tell us. Examples include rich data on the needs of people with intellectual disabilities who have mental health, physical health, forensic and challenging behaviour needs and how, or if, these are being met.

While England and Scotland have developed national strategies for people with intellectual disabilities (Scottish Executive 2000; DH 2001), Ireland has focused on a broad disability agenda with a range of legislative and policy outcomes. It still remains to be seen if the 'disability' umbrella approach will sufficiently ensure that the specific needs of people with intellectual disabilities and their families/carers are not comprised in this larger grouping. The fact that the Disability Act (GOI 2005a) has a strong focus on person-centred needs may assist in reducing this affect.

What is required is a needs-based periodic review of intellectual disability needs and services at national and regional level, similar in scope to the recent Éire Ireland Mental Health Review A *Vision for Change* (DOHC 2006) and the Review of Mental Health and Learning Disability services in Northern Ireland *Equal Lives* (DHSSPS 2005). The review should:

- Identify the current range and quality of service provision, including skill mixes and the roles of each skills group and their scope for development
- Identify unmet need
- Identify current North-South initiatives and how these may be developed
- Recommend service development based on evidence- and research-based best practice

The periodic review of intellectual disability services could then be used as the foundation for the ongoing development of a national strategy for people with intellectual disabilities.

Mental health service provision

Following a two-year major review of Irish mental health services, the Expert Group on Mental Health Policy published *A Vision for Change* (DOHC 2006). The report acknowledged that the mental health needs, as well as the forensic and offending behavioural needs of people with intellectual disabilities have been poorly addressed (Murphy et al 2000; McKeon 2004;) and that many people with intellectual disabilities residing in mental health services are there by default rather than because of their needs. The key shortcomings include:

- Lack of specialised mental health services for people with intellectual disability
- The client group's difficulties and frustrations in accessing mental health services
- Poor interprofessional collaboration by mental health specialists with experts in the intellectual disabilities field

A Vision for Change (DOHC 2006) recommends:

- The development of an Intellectual Disability Mental Health Service (IDMHS) based on the same service principles as those for all mental health services proposed in the policy: citizenship, inclusion, access and community-based services (Irish College of Psychiatrists 2004; Department of Health 1996) (Figure 12.2).

Figure 12.2 Key service elements for the mental health needs of people with intellectual disability

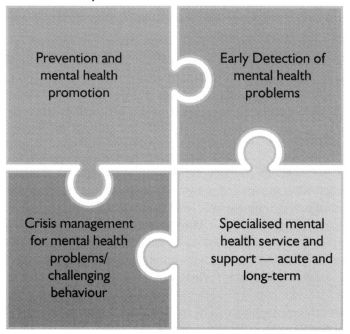

Prevention and mental health promotion

Early Detection of mental health problems

Crisis management for mental health problems/ challenging behaviour

Specialised mental health service and support — acute and long-term

(DOHC, 2006 p. 127 based on Mansell et al 1994)

Figure 12.3 Interface between mental health of intellectual disability (MHId) team and other services

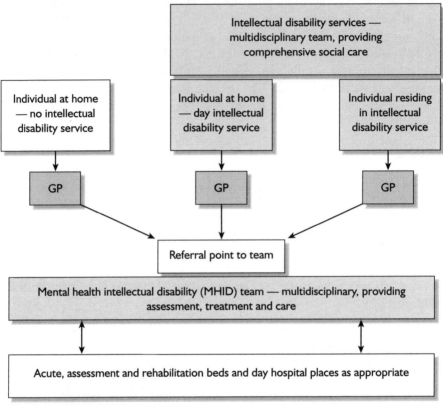

- That the IDMHS be based on the service model conceptualised for people with intellectual disabilities (Mansell et al 1994) (Figure 12.3) rather than a generic mental health model where one size does not always fit all
- That emphasis is placed on mental health promotion, early detection and promoting access to primary care by the generic intellectual disability services

A Vision for Change (DOHC 2006) fully recognises the uniqueness of intellectual disability nurses and views their expertise as central to the successful development of a new high quality IDMHS (Box 12.2).

A Vision for Change (DOHC 2006) should be viewed as a sound exemplar of an in-depth, honest and evidence-based best practice review for all health and personal social service provision aiming to meet the needs of people with intellectual disabilities. Three further areas requiring particular attention for review are:

- Services meeting or needing to be established to meet the physical health needs of people with intellectual disabilities,
- The needs of children with intellectual disabilities
- A complete review of all intellectual disability services, including skill mix

Box 12.2 *Vision for Change* recommendations

Intellectual disability mental health services
(DOHC 2006b, p74)

- Two multidisciplinary community mental health teams (CMHTs) for adults with intellectual disability per 300,000 population
- One multidisciplinary CMHT for children and adolescents with intellectual disability per 300,000 population
- Based in, and operating from, community mental health centres
- Providing individual multidisciplinary assessment, treatment and care, with an emphasis on home assessment and treatment if possible, either in the individual's family home or at a residence provided by an intellectual disability service
- Five acute beds in the acute inpatient unit
- One day hospital per 300,000 with ten places
- Ten rehabilitation beds in intellectual disability residential centres that have approved centre status

Forensic mental health services
(DOHC 2006b, p135)

- One national intellectual disability forensic mental health team and national unit to provide secure care to those with intellectual disability
- Inpatient care
- One acute inpatient unit per catchment area of 300,000 population with 50 beds, of which five beds for mental health services for people with intellectual disability (sub-unit)
- Ten rehabilitation beds in intellectual disability residential centres which have approved centre status
- Ten-bed national secure unit for those with intellectual disability

Intellectual disability nursing in Éire Ireland

An Bord Altranais (ABA) is the statutory body established by the Nurses Act (GOI 1950) and redeveloped following the Nurses Act (GOI 1985). Its primary concern is:

> '...to promote high standards of professional education and training and professional conduct among nurses'

(GOI 1985, Section 2 [1])

ABA's overall responsibility is in the interest of the public (ABA 2006). According to the Nurses Act (GOI 1985) the term 'nurse' means a person registered in the Live Register of Nurses as provided for in Section 27 of the Nurses Act (1985) and includes a midwife and nursing includes midwifery. The Board consists of 29 members, 17 of whom are elected by nurses and 12 of whom are appointed by the Minister for Health. Unlike the UK's Nursing and Midwifery Council (NMC) intellectual disability nurses have their own constituency, thus ensuring that one member of An Bord is a directly elected intellectual disability nurse. In my view this may help to address the wrongly assumed belief that there is universal hegemony for the dominant biomedical nursing discourse or other similar discourses, which have not always been in the best interests of the intellectual disability nurse or the person with intellectual disabilities over the past half century.

According to Sheerin (2000), political pressure in the 1950s from parent groups led the Irish Department of Health to ask An Bord Altranais to explore the possibility of providing specialised training for nurses working in the field of what was then termed 'mental subnormality'. A second influence may have also been the development in the UK of the mental subnormality nurse syllabus and acceptance of a new UK nurse registration 'Registered Nurse Mental Subnormality' (RNMS) in 1957. An Bord Altranais responded positively to the Irish Department of Health's request, and intellectual disability education and training commenced in 1959 at two newly opened schools: St Louise's, Clonsilla (County Dublin) and St Mary's Drumcar, County Louth. The first mental handicap nurses were registered in 1960 (Sheerin 2000; McCormack 2004).

The current preregistration intellectual disability nursing course in Ireland, based on recommendations contained in the Commission for Nursing Report *The Blueprint for the Future* (CON 1998), is a four-year degree programme leading to a Bachelor of Science degree in nursing. The first cohorts commenced in 2002. There are eight courses annually with a total of 240 places. Postregistration and postgraduate programmes offered to registered nurses in intellectual disability have increased in the last two years but are limited to certain geographical areas (DOHC 2006). For example, Trinity College Dublin, Ireland's Oxbridge, provides postgraduate degrees in nursing at masters and doctorate level, as well as providing opportunities for postdoctoral research in which registered intellectual disability nurses actively participate. A masters degree in intellectual disability nursing is under development.

Table 12.1 Nurses registered in Ireland in 2005

	Active	Inactive	Male	Female	Total
Total number of nurses	62,639	15,913	5,956	72,596	78,552
Nurses registered with an Intellectual Disability qualification	3,890	583	481	3,992	4,473

ABA/INB, 2006

Table 12.2 Irish intellectual disability nurse registrations in 2005

Ireland	EU	Others	Total
21	21	0	42

ABA/INB, 2006

According to the latest An Bord Altranais statistics, there were 78,552 nurses registered in Ireland in 2005 (Table 12.1). Of these, 4,473 were registered intellectual disability nurses, of which 3,890 were active; 481 were male and 3,992 were female (Table 12.2) (ABA/INB 2006). Similar to the UK, registered intellectual disability nurses in Éire Ireland work with all age ranges and all levels of intellectual disability including people with mild, moderate, severe, profound and multiple disabilities. The age range includes a growing population of older people. A wide range of services is provided, including:

- Daycare, including assessments, early intervention services, preschool and special education development
- Respite care, including community group houses and local centres
- Vocational training, sheltered and supported employment

(Report of The Commission on Nursing 1998; DOHC 2006)

However, community intellectual disability teams are sparse, so most people with intellectual disabilities not receiving the specialist support they require at home. There are 117 clinical nurse specialists (CNS) working in the intellectual disability services, and no advanced nurse practitioners (ANP), so there is a need to develop specialist and advanced nurse practitioner roles for nurses in intellectual disability based on assessed needs (DOHC 2006).

As in the UK, the role and value of the intellectual disability nurse has continually been under scrutiny in recent decades. On each occasion the unique identity and role of intellectual disability nursing has been seen as essential to the delivery of a high quality service to people with an intellectual disability and therefore worth preserving and enhancing (CON 1998; DOHC 2006). However, the intellectual disability nursing profession has, rightly or wrongly, felt undervalued and under threat over the past two decades. While it is not possible to explore in-depth all factors that may be contributing to this state, one stands out – the disparity in salaries between registered intellectual disability nurses and non-professionally registered social care workers employed in the same or similar intellectual disability services. For example, a recent advertisement in the *Irish Independent* (a national broadsheet newspaper) recruiting registered professionals and non-professions offered the following remuneration packages:

- Staff Nurse Point 1:   €28,877 to Point 13: €42,164 pro rata
- Social Care Worker Point 1: €32,862 to Point 12: €43,939 pro rata

(St Michael's House 2006, p19)

Intellectual disability nurses welcome the increase in community participation of people with intellectual disabilities. They are keen to collaborate with a wide range of skilled people who are not on a professional register or adhere to a professional code of conduct to enable this, because of the skills they offer to people with intellectual disabilities and because it goes some way to addressing the shortage of intellectual disability nurses in a rapidly expanding service. However, the remuneration anomaly, and poor recognition and use of their specialist skills, does not help to recruit and retain student nurses and those with valuable experience And it does little to enable the well being of people with intellectual disabilities in terms of health. Instead it reinforces the believe in the profession that there is increasing 'deprofessionalisation' of the service, as first highlighted in The Commission on Nursing Report (CON 1998). The Department of Health and Children is aware of this (Horan 2004) and was expected to address this in 2007.

The future

'It is in the grasp of the discipline...to identify its unique identity and place in the profession. The future of [Intellectual Disability] nursing is in the hands of [Intellectual Disability] nurses'

(Sherrin 2000, p174, author's words in brackets)

Every professional and profession needs to continually define, redefine and promote their role in the increasingly diverse, complex and changing field of intellectual disabilities. Intellectual disability nursing's core focus is on enabling the well-being of people with intellectual disabilities. We have demonstrated this since our birth in the late 1950s by our versatility and adaptability in addressing the needs of citizens with intellectual disabilities regardless of the setting, using a wide range of professional knowledge, practices and values that are grounded in evidence- and research-based best practice. Our future as a profession is based on continuing to achieve that core aim by seeking out opportunities for being at the forefront of developing and delivering quality practice. For example, as key members of the multidisciplinary team contributing to the assessment of needs and service statements under the Disability Act (GOI 2005a), there are opportunities for intellectual disability nurses to continue to seek out and promote what they can and do offer in terms of meeting individual needs.

The current national health strategy and related policies focus on improvements in health, quality assurance, evidence and research based best practice, yet intellectual disabilities and intellectual disability nursing are rarely mentioned. There is a need for the profession to be more politically active in the shaping of national policy and to clearly detail the valued and valuable contributions it makes in addressing need. Intellectual disability nurses may need to continue to think more broadly, and articulate the expertise that they are best placed to offer people with intellectual disabilities to enhance their quality of life. Two ways of achieving this may be for the profession to carry out a major review of itself and to produce and periodically update a public document that promotes the roles of the intellectual disability nurse in Ireland. This could be achieved using case studies that are exemplars of current best practice. This would enhance student nurses' understanding of the unique, diverse and necessary roles they are emerging into and promote to agencies and other professionals our expertise and scope of practice.

Because of the significant increase in service development, guided by key legislative and policy frameworks, the future for people with intellectual disabilities and experts to enable them to fulfil their lives looks increasingly positive.

References

(websites checked 21 May 2007)

Adults with Incapacity (Scotland) Act (2000). Edinburgh, The Stationery Office

An Bord Altranais /The Irish Nursing Board (ABA/IRB) (2006) *(www.nursingboard.ie)*

Barron S, Kelly C (2006) *National Intellectual Disability Database.* Annual Report of the National Intellectual Disability Database Committee 2006. Dublin, Health Research Board *(www.hrb.ie)*

Commission on the Status of People with Disabilities (1996) *A Strategy for Equality*: Report of the Commission on the Status of People with Disabilities. Dublin, Stationery Office

Commission on Nursing (1998) *A Blueprint for the Future:* The Report of the Commission on Nursing. Dublin, Stationery Office

Department of Health (1996) *Discussion Document on the Mental Health Needs of Persons with Mental Handicap* (Mulcahy Report). Dublin, Stationery Office

Department of Health (1990) National Health Service and Community Care Act. London, DH, London

Department of Health (2001) *Valuing People:* A New Strategy for Learning Disability for 21st Century. London, The Stationery Office

Department of Health and Children (DOHC) (2001) *Quality and Fairness: A Health System for You.* Dublin, DOHC

Department of Health and Children/Department of Health, Social Service and Public Safety, Northern Ireland (DOHC/DHSSPS) (2001) *A Nursing Vision of Public Health.* Dublin, DOHC; Belfast, DHSSPS

Department of Health and Children / Department of Health, Social Service and Public Safety, Northern Ireland (DOHC/DHSSPS) (2003) *From Vision to Action.* Dublin, DOHC; Belfast, DHSSPS

Department of Health and Children (2006) *A Vision for Change.* Report of the Expert Group on Mental Health Policy. Dublin, DOHC

Department of Health, Social Services and Public Safety (2005) *Equal Lives*: Draft Report of Learning Disability Committee. Belfast, DHSSPS

Government of Ireland (1937) Bunreacht na hÉireann. Dublin, Stationery Office

Government of Ireland (1945) Mental Treatment Act. Dublin, Stationery Office

Government of Ireland (1950) Nurses Act. Dublin, Stationery Office.

Government of Ireland (1984) National Social Service Board Act. Dublin, Stationery Office

Government of Ireland (1985) Nurses Act. Dublin, Stationery Office

Government of Ireland (1999a) Employment Equality Act. Dublin, Stationery Office

Government of Ireland (1999b) National Disability Authority Act. Dublin, Stationery Office

Government of Ireland (2000a) Comhairle Act. Dublin, Stationery Office

Government of Ireland (2000b) Equal Status Act. Dublin, Stationery Office

Government of Ireland (2001) Mental Health Act. Dublin, Stationery Office

Government of Ireland (2004a) Health Act. Dublin, Stationery Office

Government of Ireland (2004b) Education for Persons with Special Educational Needs Act. Dublin, Stationery Office

Government of Ireland (2005a) Disability Act. Dublin, Stationery Office

Government of Ireland (2005b) Health and Social Care Professionals Act. Dublin, Stationery Office

Government of Ireland (GOI) (1990) Health (Nursing Homes) Act. Dublin, Stationery Office

Government of Ireland (GOI) (2007a) Health Act. Dublin, Stationery Office

Government of Ireland (GOI) (2007b) Health (Nursing Homes) (Amendments) Act. Dublin, Stationery Office

Health Service Executive (HSE) (2006) An introduction to the HSE. Dublin, Health Service Executive. *www.hse.ie/en/*

Horan P (2004) Nursing people with intellectual disabilities: a profession under threat? *Frontline of Learning Disability* 58 p. 24–25 I

Irish College of Psychiatrists (2004) Proposed model for the delivery of a mental health service to people with intellectual disability. Occasional Paper OP58

Keenan P (2007a) A synopsis of the Republic of Ireland's Disability Act 2005. *The Frontline of Learning Disability* (in press)

Keenan, P (2007b) An exploration of the Republic of Ireland's Disability Act 2005. Part 1: A discussion of legal concepts and definitions. *Frontline of Learning Disability* (in press)

Keenan P (2007c) An exploration of the Republic of Ireland's Disability Act 2005. Part 2: The ASPR approach – potential advantages, disadvantages and opportunities. *Frontline of Learning Disability* (in press)

Keenan P (2007d) An exploration of the Republic of Ireland's Disability Act 2005. Part 3: ensuring service user involvement in the ASPR approach. *Frontline of Learning Disability* (in press)

Keenan P (2007e) An exploration of the Republic of Ireland's Disability Act 2005. Part 4: A synopsis of intellectual disability service requirements in the Republic of Ireland 2006–2010 *Frontline of Learning Disability* (in press)

Keenan P (2007f) An exploration of the Republic of Ireland's Disability Act 2005. Part 5: 'Detainees' with intellectual disabilities in relation to 21st century Irish mental health and disability legislation. *Frontline of Learning Disability* (in press)

Law Reform Commission (2005) Consultation Paper, *Vulnerable Adults and the Law: Capacity.* Dublin, The Law Reform Commission

Mansell J, McGill P, Emerson E (1994) Conceptualising service provision. In: Emerson E, McGill P, Mansell J (eds) Severe Learning Disabilities and Challenging Behaviour, Designing High Quality Services. London, Chapman Hall

McCormack B (2004) Trends in the development of Irish Disability Services. In Noonan Walsh, P, Gash H (eds) (2004) *Lives and Times: Practice, Policy and People with Disabilities.* Bray, Rathdown Press

McKeon M (2004) People with intellectual disability who cause offence in law. *Frontline of Learning Disability* **58**, 18–19

Mencap (2001) *A Guide to Community Care Law.* London, Mencap

Murphy M, Harrold M, Carey S Mulrooney M (2000) A survey of the level of learning disability among the prison population in ireland. Dublin, Department of Justice, Equality and Law Reform

National Association of the Mentally Handicapped in Ireland (namhi) (2003) *Who Decides and How?* People with Intellectual Disabilities – Legal Capacity and Decision Making: A Discussion Document. Dublin, namhi

National Disability Authority (2002) *Guidelines for the Inclusion of People with Disabilities in Research.* Dublin, NDA

National Disability Authority (NDA) (2002) *Disability Related Research in Ireland 1996–2001*. Dublin, NDA

National Disability Authority (NDA) (2003a) *Towards Best Practice in the Provision of Further Education, Employment and Training Services for People with Disabilities in Ireland*. Dublin, NDA

National Disability Authority (2003b) *Review of Access to Mental Health Services for People with Intellectual Disabilities*. Dublin, NDA

National Disability Authority (NDA) (2005a) *Promoting the Participation of People with Disabilities in Physical Activity and Sport in Ireland*. Dublin, NDA

National Disability Authority (NDA) (2005b) *Person-centred Planning for People in Ireland who have Disabilities – Plain English Version*. Dublin, NDA

National Disability Authority (NDA) (2006a) *A Short Guide to the National Disability Authority*. Dublin, NDA

National Disability Authority (NDA) (2006b) *Code of Practice on Accessibility of Public Services and Information Provided by Public Bodies*. Dublin, NDA

National Disability Authority (NDA) (2006c) *(www.nda.ie)*

Quinlivan S (2004) Law and disability in Ireland. In: Noonan Walsh P, Gash H (2004) *Lives and Times: Practice, Policy and People with Disabilities*. Bray, Rathdown Press

Quinn G (2002) Government needs to withdraw Disabilities Bill. *The Examiner*. 18 February 2002

Scottish Executive (2000) *The Same as You?* A Review of the Services for People with Learning Disabilities. Edinburgh, Scottish Executive

Sheerin F (2000) Mental handicap nursing. In: Robins J (2000) *Nursing and Midwifery in Ireland in the Twentieth Century – Fifty Years of (The Nursing Board) 1950 –2000*. Dublin, An Bord Altranais

Special Olympics Ireland (SOP) (2003) Strategy 2004–2007. Dublin, Special Olympics Ireland

Special Olympics Ireland (SOP) (2006) Mission Statement

St Michael's House (2006) Recruitment advertisement. Jobs and Careers. *Irish Independent* 21 December 2006, p19

Websites

(accessed 7 June 2007)

Government of Éire Ireland (all Éire Ireland's legislation and key social policy) *www.irlgov.ie*

An Bord Altranais /The Irish Nursing Board (ABA): *www.nursingboard.ie*

Department of Health and Children /An Roinn Sláinte Agus Leanaí (DOHC): *www.dohc.ie*

Health Research Board/An Bord Taighde Sláinte (HRB): *www.hrb.ie*

Health Service Executive/Feidhmeannacht na Seirbhise Sláinte (HSE): *www.hse.ie*

National Disability Authority: *www.nda.ie*

National Federation of Voluntary Bodies providing services to people with Intellectual Disability: *www.fedvol.ie*

Special Olympics Ireland: *www.specialolympics.ie/en*

Frontline of Learning Disability: *www.frontline-ireland.ie*

Citizens Information Board: *www.citizensinformationboard.ie*

Fundamental nursing concepts for person-centred care

CHAPTER 13

Fundamental nursing concepts

Leadership, self-awareness and reflective practice

Judi Thorley

Introduction

This chapter aims to demonstrate that reflective practice, self-awareness and leadership are important qualities for living up to the challenge of delivering and facilitating high quality services for people with learning disabilities. Different leadership qualities in person-centred approaches are pursued which can be adopted by learning disability nurses to support a democratic change management style.

The use of leadership skills in practice will be explored and reinforced with practice examples. Nurses have found themselves in a position where it is essential to understand the drivers for change for primary and secondary care, but to affect and effect change this knowledge is not enough to make changes to practice. Being aware of – and understanding – the 'culture' of organisations is essential if you are to impact on service delivery. The evidence that supports the continued issue of barriers to accessing healthcare for people with learning disabilities will be explored, as will the resulting policy documents. Current guidance and the potential potency of specific roles will be explored. The value of and need for reflection will be a theme that is visited throughout this chapter.

The way that people with learning disabilities live their lives has been changing in an ever-evolving process over the last 30 years. To support people with learning disabilities to live a full, valued and quality lifestyle, the role of the learning disability nurse has had to adapt and change.

This continuous need to change, transfer skills and have an innovative and diverse approach to meeting the needs of people with learning disabilities is challenging at best, and potentially destructive at worst. This chapter aims largely, through practice-based reflection, to encourage practitioners to:

- Develop increased confidence and aspiration
- Work in an ever-changing world to meet individual needs
- Enhance their level of understanding of self-awareness, reflection and leadership qualities

Leadership and self-awareness

In *A Vision for Learning Disability Nursing* (United Kingdom Learning Disability Consultant Nurse Network 2005) the apparent confusion of a social model of service provision and a social model of disability is discussed and clarified. In this document a social model of disability is identified as understanding that people with disabilities find themselves disabled not only by physical issues but also by social, economic, psychological and attitude barriers that impact on their capacity to engage fully in society (Prime Minister's Strategy Unit 2005). Learning disability nurses have a key role in providing leadership when working with people with learning disabilities, family carers and professionals in mainstream health care to ensure that health needs are recognised, accessed and delivered.

Leadership is a concept that nurses particularly require to bring about person-centred care (*The NHS Plan,* DH 2000). Every nurse practitioner will have a view as to what constitutes a good leader.

Crucially, one of the consistent and key messages from a plethora of literature on leadership is the importance of being self-aware. Understanding one's own feelings, values and strengths allows for a certain presence and confidence to be exhibited which all support the motivation of others.

Self-awareness is described by Goleman (2002) as one competence of being a good leader. Goleman refers to the competences that make a good leader as 'emotional intelligence.' And describes the four domains of emotional intelligence

- Self-awareness
- Self-management
- Social awareness
- Relationship management

The effective leader needs to understand his or her values and passion, articulating skillfully using all aspects of their personality but primarily their strengths. Using one's strengths will animate and project confidence, inspiring motivation and commitment in others.

A good leader understands his or her personal irritations, is willing to share personal detail and can modify their behaviour to elicit the best results (Goleman 2002).

When describing his personal leadership skills and management of the 9/11 disaster, Mayor Giuliani (2002) concentrates on the need to know and to understand oneself, and being clear in articulating values. Like Goleman, Guiliani (2002) emphasises the importance of self-awareness and relationships. Recognising the talents in individuals and nurturing those talents to give confidence and creating a vision is what learning disability nurses do to support people with learning disabilities to live a valued lifestyle. Being able to listen to others and consider alternative views are skills that the learning disability nurse has developed as part of using person-centred approaches.

A learning disability nurse is a skilled specialist, who is comfortable working in a person-centred way to understand what a person with learning disabilities wants and needs to live a fulfilled life. Being able to put others at the centre, focusing on their needs, supporting them to articulate their dreams is a crucial leadership skill. Leadership is an evolving process – experience, personality and personal values contribute to the way in which we respond when leadership skills are required.

Reflective practice

Learning disability nurses require qualities and skills in reflection to develop their practice through understanding their actions and the actions of others, coupled with understanding the dynamics of the situation, and the drivers for change.

As a learning disability nurse, awareness of policy/leadership initiatives in primary and secondary care is required, so that as a practitioner, one can identify the opportunities for meeting the needs of people with learning disabilities. For example, current targets in primary care around coronary heart disease, cancer and mental health all present the learning disability nurse with the opportunity to advise general practitioners, and other primary care professionals. They can promote health screening of people with learning disability, and advise that such illnesses and diseases have increased with differing patterns of health need (Kerr 1998), helping the primary care professionals to achieve their targets

There has been a steady development of learning from experience in professional practice over the past 20 years (Quinn 2000). Various authors espousing the value for both novice and expert of reflecting on practice have detailed models that encourage analysis of the situation and of the individual's role in the outcome to benefit future experiences (Quinn 2000). Contemporary practice has influenced me to adopt a structured model such as Gibbs (1988) (Figure 13.1) and Johns (1996) (Box 13.1).

Figure 13.1 Gibbs' (1988) model of reflection

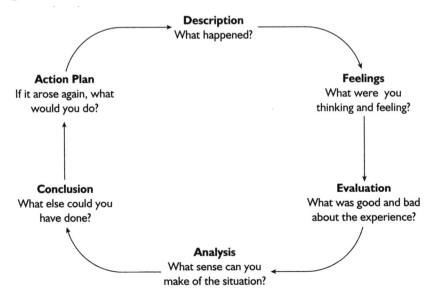

Box 13.1 Johns' (1996) model of reflection

The following cues are offered to help practitioners to access, make sense of, and learn through experience.

Description

- Write a description of the experience.
- What are the key issues within this description that I need to pay attention to?

Reflection

- What was I trying to achieve?
- Why did I act as I did?
- What are the consequences of my actions for the patient and family, myself and the people I work with?
- How did I feel about this experience when it was happening?
- How did the patient feel about it?
- How do I know how the patient felt about it?

Influencing factors

- What internal factors influenced my decision making and actions?
- What external factors influenced my decision making and actions?
- What sources of knowledge did or should have influenced my decision making?

Alternative strategies

- Could I have dealt better with the situation?
- What other choices did I have?
- What would be the consequences of these other choices?

Learning

- How can I make sense of this experience in light of past experience and future practice?
- How do I **now** feel about this experience?
- Have I taken effective action to support myself and others as a result of this experience?
- How has this experience changed my way of knowing in practice?

(Johns 1994)

These models require the practitioner to set out what happened, how I was thinking and feeling, what was good and bad about the experience. This separation of the content and process from the thoughts and feelings is useful to give the learning disability nurse time to be clear about motivation and mitigating factors. It promotes analysis of not only your own feelings and thoughts but of others involved in the situation. To demonstrate the benefits of this reflective approach and to explore the leadership role, two practice examples will be pursued (Boxes 13.2 and 13.3)

Reflection can be used to identify opportunities for change and development in practice. From a cognitive processing perspective, articulating the art of reflection

Box 13.2 Practice example

This example focuses on the issue of fair and equitable access to primary and secondary health services for people with learning disabilities. In 1996 I was seconded by my NHS trust to complete my postregistration adult nursing and diploma. As a trained learning disability nurse with more than seven years' experience, I was quite clear in my own mind of the issues faced by people with a learning disability when accessing 'ordinary' health services. These personal experiences included access to acute or secondary healthcare. I had experience of poor and often inequitable services which seemed to focus on the fact that the person whom I was supporting to attend Accident and Emergency (A&E), central outpatients or a ward had a learning disability and therefore experienced pain differently from the rest of society, or not at all. For example, when attending A&E with a gentleman who had a suspected ankle fracture and requesting analgesia, the doctor queried how I knew that this man was in pain when he was unable to verbalise this himself. I had to ask the gentleman to show the doctor where his pain was, and I described how changes in the gentleman's behaviour indicated that he may be experiencing pain.

McCaffery and Beebe (1989) maintain that pain is what the patient says it is. Unfortunately this view fails to support clinicians from a non-learning disability background to look further than the spoken word. Another gentleman had a large cyst (approximately the size of a 50p piece) on his right cheek, which due to its position drew a lot of attention from people. Following investigation to establish and rule out malignancy, the consultant met with the gentleman and myself, as the named nurse and advised that it was not malignant and therefore surgery would not be looked at. I found myself in the position of advocate, a familiar position for learning disability nurses (Mitchell 2004), questioning the decision of the consultant and urging consideration based on quality of life. Would the consultant be happy to live with such a visible, unsightly lump on his face?

Applying a reflective model of learning to the situation described enables me to think how the person with learning disabilities, the doctor and nurses may have felt in this situation. Gibbs (1988) and Johns (1996) ask the practitioner to separate the content, process and feelings of a situation and to examine their personal responses, feelings and consequences. My responses may have been guarded and negative due to feelings of frustration, anger and reduced expectation all based on previous experience.

The consequence of my behaviour and contribution to the situation could have been reluctance by doctors and nurses to build a relationship with the person with learning disabilities, a feeling of inadequacy and possibly hostility. Continuing with this reflective model I can view my experience in a different way and offer different approaches for future situations, which would have an impact on the experience of the person with learning disabilities. Reflecting on the experiences described from the viewpoint of a member of staff working in an acute or primary healthcare setting faced with someone who is possibly very ill, frightened and has difficulty in communicating can leave clinicians feeling disempowered and unsure of how to apply the skills that they have in meeting individual needs (Gibbs & Thorley 2003). Reflection from this viewpoint may lead to the realisation that learning disability nurses may put up many barriers and could appear to be not always supporting colleagues in different health settings to understand the possible needs of people with learning disabilities.

Activity

Think about an issue that you have experienced in practice. Using Gibbs (1988) (Figure 13.1) or Johns (1996) (Box 13.1) model of reflection, separate the content and the process, as described in Box 13.1:

- Think about what happened
- How did you feel?
- How do you think the others involved may have felt?
- What could have been different?
- How might this have changed the outcome?

supports the learning disability nurse to identify why something occurred as it did, what can be done differently and how to go about it.

The unpopular patient?

A consideration for learning disability nurses is the negative perception that some mainstream staff may have of people with learning disabilities. Felicity Stockwell published findings relating to the concept of the 'Unpopular patient' over 30 years ago (Allen 2003). Stockwell identified factors such as 'physical defects', which affected the nurses' care of individual patients. The patient who has a learning disability could fall into this 'unpopular patient' group, affecting the care they receive from nurses. Johnson (1995) identified differences in interactions based on perceived active contribution by patients in assisting nurses to carry out their role. As people with learning disabilities often have more dependant needs, this could perpetuate a negative view. Social needs and the concept of social problems are complex in their development and are based on shared experiences, impact on individuals, and size of the group (Manning 2003).

Barriers to access

With only 2–3% of the population in the UK having a learning disability this group is a minority and campaigning for equity and fair access has not always come high on the political agenda. All care needs were met in the institution, so the primary and secondary healthcare needs of people with learning disabilities when living in the community were highlighted and inequities in access and quality of service provision started to emerge. This increased need for access to primary healthcare in areas of resettlement from institutions is specifically highlighted in the publication *Once a Day* (DH 1999a) as is the fact that people with learning disabilities are two and half times more likely to have increased health needs that require medical intervention than the general population. The impact of moving service provision for people with learning disabilities into the community has been acknowledged and evidenced with an increase in demand. Unfortunately, acute and primary health service clinicians lacked experience and understanding of people with learning disabilities and experience of accessing

Box 13.3 Practice example

This example considers the particular cultural issues of working in an acute hospital setting, and the personal experiences and values that individuals might have in that setting, which led to the development of a successful rolling programme of learning for hospital staff.

Having trained as a postregistration student in general nursing, I was faced with a different perspective of people with learning disabilities going into hospital. I saw how difficult it could be to get vital information, how communication often failed due to a lack of different resources and how the awareness and understanding of general staff severely affected their confidence in supporting people with learning disabilities. Being aware of these issues and the culture and systems of the general hospital I was able to approach staff in the Accident & Emergency department, acknowledge how the department ran and encourage the staff to consider the service they were providing to people with learning disabilities.

I took the time to build relationships, calling in and making myself available if staff wanted a chat. Using this approach enabled an open discussion where the staff in the A&E department themselves identified that they did not provide a complete service. Not going to the staff with a list of what needed to change and how this could happen ensured that the dialogue was open and staff identified areas for improvement themselves.

The staff were very clear about their lack of awareness of learning disability and health needs. Together we planned teaching sessions, which used the handover period to deliver the half hour sessions. Building their trust, responding to and acknowledging their work commitments and stresses led to requests for more teaching, a resource file and the development of guidance for triage and the possible needs of people with learning disabilities.

services has been poor (Mencap 2004). This type of experience is far from unique – Langan et al (1993), Stein (2000) and Walmsley (2004) all describe the barriers to accessing services faced by people with learning disabilities. The government good practice guidance *Signposts for Success* (1998) and *Once a Day* (1999a) each have examples of experiences of people with learning disabilities, which range from:

> '*the doctor didn't know how to talk to me*' (DH 1998) to

> '*the trouble is that when you phone up for an appointment it takes ages to explain why she can't wait long and gets upset. Then they still keep you waiting ages and get cross with you if she disrupts the waiting room*' (DH 1999a)

The barriers faced by people with learning disabilities to accessing health services can be seen as multifaceted – not just physical access but also cognitive, emotional and social access (Langan et al 1993). *Facing the Facts* (DH 1999b) highlighted the specific issues faced by people with learning disabilities in accessing the help and support they require. Despite this recognition of the barriers and issues which have led to publications of good practice guidance and a white paper to address this, acceptance of the need to ensure a fair and equitable service for this group of patients is slow in coming. This may be due to the fact that to accept the issues means admitting that there is room for improvement and that clinicians have not got their practice exactly right.

Understanding the 'culture' of organisations

Culture is the 'buzz' word of today's healthcare setting, used extensively in policy documents and literature relating to individual organisations. Savage (2000) suggests that its use implies a quality service that values service users and staff and is ready to face the challenge of making changes to improve the service delivered. Culture is somehow assumed to be something that staff and patients in the NHS understand and in the context of policies and publications is used to symbolise the government commitment to ensure satisfaction and quality.

Brown (1998) suggests that culture is a manifest of shared values, beliefs, norms and shared understanding that create and sustain shared meaning. While acknowledging that as human beings we all have values, beliefs and norms, Batteau (2001) challenges the view that these beliefs, values, and norms are shared and facilitate shared understanding and meaning. Batteau suggests that culture is about individual interpretation of symbols, which resonate differently and demand a collective view that is fluid and responds to and creates change. The message for NHS staff in recent government publications such a *Making a Difference* (DH 1999c) and *The NHS Plan* (DH 2000) is empowerment of 'coalface staff', involvement of service users and the flexibility to offer a range of choices. Both of these publications capitalise on the current trend to consider culture as a potential avenue of change in organisations. If you as a learning disability nurse are to help people with learning disabilities capitalise on the 'culture change' and shift of power to frontline staff, patients and carers, you need to learn about the culture in the key stakeholder organisations in your area. Know who makes the decisions, use your self-awareness skills to build relationships and – most importantly – understand your own values, those of your organisation and people with a learning disability and family/carers. Wheatley and Kellner-Rogers (1995) highlight the fact that as human beings we bring unique experience, values, beliefs and, importantly, emotions, all of which make up a culture and influence an organisation. Remember that you **can** make a difference.

Making change happen

Felce et al (1998) identify that for fundamental change to happen for people with learning disabilities there needs to be joined-up thinking and action by all key stakeholders, including people with learning disabilities, family and carers, government, paid staff and local agencies and communities. Change will not happen by any one intervention or action alone. This statement of fact is crucial to the issues of leadership in delivering health services for people with learning disabilities, as access to healthcare impacts on many stakeholders and certainly is not the sole responsibility of specialist services.

Be aware of and understand the communication in:

- *The NHS Plan* (DH 2000)
- *Valuing People* (DH 2001a)
- *National Service Frameworks* for
  —*Older People* (DH 2001a)
  —*Mental Health* (DH 1999d)
  —*Long-term Conditions* (DH 2005a)
- *Choosing Health* (DH 2004a)
- *Self-Care* (DH 2005b)
- *Creating a Patient-led NHS* (DH 2005c)
- *Our Health, Our Care, Our Say* (DH 2006)

The critical leadership message is the same; support people to have choice and provide patient-focused services. To achieve the vision of a patient-led NHS (DH 2005c) requires partnership working between professionals and – possibly more importantly – with patients and the public. Identification or recognition of ill health is an area of concern for people with learning disabilities and even when health needs are identified, access to physical and cognitive services poses a challenge to people with learning disabilities and their family or carers.

How does this vision of self-care acknowledge and address the intrinsic issues related to learning disability and self-management to maintain health and wellbeing? *Self-Care* (DH 2005b) recognises that there is a continuum of need. Some patients will require very limited input to maintain their own health and that of family members. Different types of support are suggested, the first of which is appropriate and accessible advice and information. This issue is further emphasised in *Our Health, Our Care, Our Say* (DH 2006). 'Accessible' for people with learning disabilities may dictate a range of methods and interventions, all of which will require face-to-face support of a lesser or greater degree, depending on the degree of learning disability. As a learning disability nurse competent with communication using different formats you have a potential powerful, supportive role to play in supporting primary and secondary care to meet this challenge.

Suggestions to improve access for people with learning disabilities – such as waiting area environments with space and a calm atmosphere, visual and audible communication, and flexible procedures are made in the Disability Rights Commission communication (DH 2004b). These suggestions are echoed in *Treat me right!* (Mencap 2004) and *Assessment for Improvement: the annual healthcheck* (Healthcare Commission 2005), which concentrates on core and development standards such as collaborative working among health and social care organisations. These are to ensure that individual needs are met, discrimination is challenged, and that suitable accessible information is available.

When these standards are implemented, NHS trusts will be measured against them. Performing badly against these will affect a trust's status and is not an option. Your role is to be aware of the current direction of travel in government policy to enable you to capitalise on the opportunities.

Acknowledging the skill base of staff working in mainstream health services is essential (Gibbs & Thorley 2003). Williamson and Johnson (2004) support this view and describe staff in mainstream services as being the best equipped to meet individual needs with the support or collaboration of specialist services. *Creating a Patient-led NHS* (DH 2005c) acknowledges that this creates a requirement of frontline staff to consider the 'whole person', considering health and well being from the person's viewpoint, incorporating issues of health promotion and prevention to develop autonomy and not purely to respond to ill health. Williamson and Johnson (2004) suggest that the best way to meet individual need and ensure that people with learning disabilities receive the best service is to work in collaboration. Changing ways of working to put the patient at the centre requires a culture change in secondary and primary care (DH 2005c). Considering the person as a whole, taking account of physical, emotional *and* social needs is not a new concept for learning disability nurses. People with learning disabilities may present with behaviours and reactions that are not socially acceptable. The skill of the learning disability nurse is to work with the person to address some of these presentations, developing and maintaining the skills which individuals already have and identifying ways to overcome areas of need (Barr 1998). Your leadership challenge is to work collaboratively to support primary and secondary health staff to view the person with learning disabilities holistically. This will only be achieved through partnership and collaborative working.

Working together and learning from the skills of all staff in the NHS is explicit in *Creating A Patient-led NHS* (DH 2005c). Bureaucracy and inflexible ways of working and stifle development of patient-led services but working in partnership using a multidisciplinary approach supports creativity, innovation and flexibility and leads to autonomy and choice for patients (DH 2005c). Empowering patients and providing choice and information to create autonomy require creative and innovative leadership from frontline NHS staff.

Health facilitation and health action planning

The need to exercise rights, independence, choice and inclusion have been detailed in *Valuing People* (DH 2001a). This paper provides clear 'must-do's' for commissioners and providers of services. Specifically looking at unmet health needs as a result of inequity in access, this paper acknowledges the need for health facilitators to ease access to primary and secondary health services, ensuring delivery of a service designed around individual needs of a consistently high standard and with additional support where necessary. Providing individuals with the opportunity to develop health action plans – that clearly identify the health need action to be taken, by whom, and when – is the role of the professional most involved in that individual's care. Learning disability nurses have a leadership role to play in facilitating the development of the health action plan but may not necessarily be the most appropriate people to lead on its development. The practice nurse or diabetes nurse may be the most appropriate as they are more involved in meeting the health needs of the person with learning disabilities. Working with people with learning disabilities and providing their health action plan in an accessible format ensures that they are involved in the process and that they then take on some ownership and can exercise some autonomy with others involved in maintaining their health (Williamson & Johnson 2004). Guidance on what a health action plan might look like was provided by the Department of Health in 2002. Essentially this guidance was not prescriptive and provided a flexible framework to use for individuals, while suggesting ways in which the information could be shared with primary and secondary care services (DH 2002).

Health action planning is a tool that can help everyone caring for people with learning disabilities to reduce inequalities and ensure involvement of the person themselves. The drive to ensure that each person with learning disabilities has a health action plan is a key part of the role of health facilitators, as is training primary and secondary care staff as to the possible needs of people with learning disabilities. In raising primary and secondary care staff awareness it is essential to draw out the impact of national targets and show how screening and addressing the health needs of this group can contribute to meeting these national targets. Turner and Moss (1996) in their review of Health of the Nation targets and other health problems and people with a learning disability identified the need for training for primary and secondary care staff and noted the reliance of primary care on the individual recognising and taking steps to rectify ill health.

The challenge for everyone working with people with learning disabilities is that clients may lack the cognitive ability to recognise and react to their own health. Health facilitators can use critical leadership to support primary and secondary care professionals to overcome communication barriers and work together to promote individual levels of self-care.

Understanding unmet health needs

To impact on the services for people with learning disabilities you as a leader need to be aware of the unmet health needs experienced by people with learning disabilities, and the different solutions employed to overcome these. There has been extensive research over the past decade in identifying the barriers and issues faced by people with learning disabilities in accessing and receiving fair and equitable healthcare. Stein (2000) found that although, on the whole, GPs were positive and clear about their role in meeting the health needs of people with learning disabilities, many did not see it as part of their role, due to the perceived impact on their resources of possible special or additional needs. A study by Hunt et al (2001) found that the primary health care teams had little knowledge of the possible needs of people with learning disabilities, which leads to poor understanding of the barriers or issues, which affect the service received and delivered. Matthews (2002) summarises the findings of research into unmet health needs of people with learning disabilities in four categories:

- Poor communication skills
- Inability to use facilities properly

- Difficulties using public transport
- The primary health care team's lack of knowledge about learning disabilities

The issue of communication difficulties is a much-publicised area of concern. Langan et al (1993), Kerr (1998) and Stein (2000) all acknowledge the issues presented by people with learning disabilities and the impact of professionals' lack of insight or understanding. Addressing this issue of communication has led to several recommendations of good practice around the use of individual records. Curtice and Long (2002) describe the development of a 'health log' which is a framework to identify individual health needs and plan intervention based on health improvement. The use of individual records as a focus for understanding health need is not a new concept.

Kitt et al (1996), Matthews and Hegarty (1997) and *Signposts for Success* (DH 1998) all suggest a visible record of health needs. The OK Health Check (Matthews & Hegarty (1997) is based on a screening check. Such tools provide a health professional with a focus for health need and the potential for increased understanding. However, as Curtice and Long (2002) acknowledge, the level of understanding of health among the learning disabled population is limited, which can impact on quality of information and uptake of services. Despite having more health needs than of the general population, people with learning disabilities visit the doctor less often (DH 1998; 1999a). *Once a Day* (DH 1999a) and *Valuing People* (DH 2001a) highlight the need for training and raised awareness of the possible health needs of people with learning disabilities as a way to start to reduce inequity and fairness related to accessing health services.

Conclusion

Self-awareness, reflection and the leadership role are critical qualities for learning disability nurses to build relationships and work collaboratively and in partnership to facilitate understanding and promote raised awareness of the possible needs of people with learning disabilities.

From personal and professional experience in influencing roles as a learning disability nurse practitioner, I have been able, through undertaking relevant continuing professional development courses beyond initial registration, to explore the underpinning theories of such concepts and most importantly, to understand self.

Both the *Leadership at the point of care* course and the *RCN Clinical Leadership* programmes have offered me the opportunity to explore personal qualities and understand personality types. Both courses through taught modules has allowed me to understand:

- Myself as an individual
- How groups and teams work
- Culture and organisations
- Models of leadership
- Models of change management

Leadership courses offer the opportunity to have the time out to develop skills, exploring different healthcare systems and understanding the politics of an organisation that has been essential for professional and personal survival.

Learning disability nurses in the future will need to be able to:

- Spot opportunities in policy
- Recognise local drivers for change
- Build relationships
- Reflect on practice
- Understand yourself and others
- Understand your organisations

This chapter has shown how enhanced self-awareness, skills and qualities for reflection and leadership skills can support learning disability nurses to affect and effect change.

References

Allen D (2003) Popularity Stakes. *Nursing Standard* **17**, 42, 14–15

Brown A (1998) *Organisational Culture* (2nd edn). London, Financial Times Pitman Publishing

Barr O (1998) Responding to the health needs of people with learning disabilities. In: Thompson T, Mathias P (eds) *Standards and Learning Disability.* London, Baillière Tindall, pp 306–323

Batteau AW (2001) Negations and ambiguities in the cultures of organization. *American Anthropologist* **102**, 4, 726–740

Clarke D (1982) *Mentally Handicapped People Living and Learning.* Eastbourne, Baillière Tindall

Curtice L, Long L (2002) The Health Log: developing a health monitoring tool for people with learning disabilities in a community support agency *British Journal of Learning Disabilities* **30**, 2, 68–72

Department of Health (1998) *Signposts for Success – good practice guidance.* London, The Stationery Office

Department of Health (1999a) *Once a Day: a primary care handbook for people with learning disabilities.* London, The Stationery Office

Department of Health (1999b) *Facing the Facts: a policy impact study of social care and health services.* London, The Stationery Office

Department of Health (1999c) *Making a Difference: strengthening the nursing, midwifery and health visitor contribution to health and healthcare.* London, The Stationery Office

Department of Health (1999b) *National Service Framework for Mental Health.* London, The Stationery Office

Department of Health (2000) *The NHS Plan: a plan for investment, a plan for reform.* London, The Stationery Office

Department of Health (2001a) *Valuing People: a vision for the 21st century.* London, The Stationery Office

Department of Health (2001b) *National Service Framework for Older People.* London, The Stationery Office

Department of Health (2004a) *Choosing Health: making healthy choices easier.* London, The Stationery Office

Department of Health (2004b) *Improving Hospital Services for Disabled People: you can make a difference*. Disability Rights Commission. London, The Stationery Office

Department of Health (2005a) *National Service Framework for Long Term Conditions*. London, The Stationery Office

Department of Health (2005b) *Self-Care – A Real Choice: Self-Care Support – A Practical Option*. London, The Stationery Office

Department of Health (2005c) *Creating a Patient-led NHS: Delivering the NHS Improvement Plan*. London, The Stationery Office

Department of Health (2006) *Our Health, Our Care, Our Say: a new direction for community services*. London, The Stationery Office

Department of Health, Social Services and Public Safety (2004) *Equal Lives: Review of policy and services for people with a learning disability in Northern Ireland*. Belfast, Department of Health, Social Services and Public Safety

Felce D, Grant G, Todd S, Ramcharan P, Beyer S, McGrath M, Perry J, Shearn J, Kilsby M, Lowe K (1998) *Towards a Full Life: Researching policy innovation for people with learning disabilities*. Oxford, Butterworth–Heinemann

Gibbs G (1988) *Learning by Doing: a guide to teaching and learning methods*. Oxford, Oxford Brookes University, Further Education Unit

Gibbs M, Thorley J (2003) Vulnerable groups: individuals with learning disabilities. In: Wood I, Rhodes M (eds) *Medical Assessment Units: The initial management of acute medical patients*. London, Whurr pp 43–51

Giuliani RW, Kurson K (2002) *Leadership*. New York, Hyperion

Goleman D (1996) *Emotional Intelligence: why can it matter more than IQ*. USA, Bloomsbury Publications

Healthcare Commission (2006) *The Annual Health Check in 2006/2007*. London, Healthcare Commission

Hunt C, Wakefield S, Hunt G (2001) Community nurse learning disabilities: A case study of the use of an evidenced-based screening tool to identify and meet the health needs of people with learning disabilities. *Journal of Learning Disabilities* **5**, 1, 9–18

Johns C (1996) Visualizing and realizing caring in practice through guided reflection. *Journal of Advanced Nursing* **24**, 1135–1143

Johnson M (1995) Rediscovering unpopular patients: the concept of social judgment. *Journal of Advanced Nursing* **21**, 3, 466–475

Kerr M (1998) Primary health care and health gain for people with learning disability. *Tizard Learning Disability Review* **3**, 6–14

Kitt L, Flynn M, Rimmer M (1996) *Advocating for health: personal health record*. London, National Development Team

Langan J, Russell O, Whitfield M (1993) Community care and the general practitioner: primary health care for people with learning difficulties. *Summary of final report to the Department of Health*. Bristol, Norah Fry Research Centre

Levitt R, Wall A, Appleby J (1999) *The Reorganized National Health Service* (6th edn). Cheltenham, Stanley Thornes

Manley K (2000) Organisational culture and consultant nurse outcomes, Part 1: organisational culture. *Nursing Standard* **14**, 34–38

Manning N (2003) Social needs, social problems and social welfare In: Erskine A, May M (eds) *The Student's Companion to Social Policy*. Oxford, Blackwell 35–42

Matthews D, Hegarty J (1997) The OK Health Check: a health assessment checklist for people with learning disabilities. *British Journal of Learning Disabilities* **25**, 138–143

Matthews D (2002) Learning disabilities: the need for better health care. *Nursing Standard* **16**, 40–41

McCaffery M, Beebe A (1989) *Pain: Clinical Manual For Nursing Practice*. USA, CV Mosby

Mencap (2004) *Treat me right! Better healthcare for people with a learning disability*. London, Mencap

Mitchell D (2004) Learning disability nursing. *British Journal of Learning Disabilities* **32**, 115–118

Quinn F (2000) Reflection and reflective practice. In: Davies C, Finlay L, Bullman A (eds) *Changing Practice in Health and Social Care*. London, Sage, pp81–90

Savage J (2000) The culture of 'culture' in National Health Service policy implementation. *Nursing Inquiry* **7**, 230–238

Scottish Executive (2000) *The Same As You? A review of services for people with learning disabilities*. Edinburgh, The Stationery Office

Scottish Executive (2002) *Promoting Health, Supporting Inclusion: the national review of the contribution of all nurses and midwives to the care and support of people with learning disabilities*. Edinburgh, The Stationery Office

Stein K (2000) Caring for people with learning disability: a survey of general practitioners' attitudes in Southampton and South-west Hampshire. *British Journal of Learning Disabilities* **28**, 9–15

Turner S, Moss S (1996) The health needs of adults with learning disabilities and the Health of the Nation strategy. *Journal of Intellectual Disability Research* **40**, 5, 438–450

Walmsley J (2004) Involving users with learning difficulties in health improvement: lessons from inclusive learning disability research. *Nursing Inquiry* **11**, 1, 54–64

Welsh Assembly Government (2002) *Realising the Potential Briefing Paper 3: Inclusion, Partnership and Innovation: A Framework for Realising Potential of Learning Disability Nursing in Wales*. Cardiff, Welsh Assembly Government

Wheatley MJ, Kellner-Rogers M (1995) Breathing life into organizations. *Journal for Quality and Participation* **18**, 4, 1–5

Williamson A, Johnson J (2004) Improving services for people with learning disabilities. *Nursing Standard* **18**, 24, 43–53

CHAPTER 14

Fundamental nursing concepts

Managing change, innovation and leadership

Premchuniall Mohabeersingh and Mark Jukes

Introduction

Sarah Mullaly (2001) has suggested that effective nursing leadership is central to the success of *The NHS Plan* (DH 2000), where the aim is for a service to be designed around the client. This promotion of person-centred care is high on the national policy agenda across the broad spectrum of health care, and is regarded as the essence of individualised, high quality client-focused services. This means that more nurses require better leadership skills, which is considered a major factor in improving direct person-centred interventions.

In learning disability, *Valuing People* (DH 2001) in England, defines a context for person-centred planning which is comprehensive, systematic and challenging to current local and national practices (O'Brien 2004).

From a philosophical perspective, person-centred planning involves a substantial shift in thinking from paternalistic and service-led governed approaches to care. In the past, the needs of people with learning disability were predetermined, in many instances without reference to individuals, the assumption being that the needs of any particular user group were homogenous and universal rather than individually defined. This is in the process of changing – however, recent reports from the Healthcare Commission (2006; 2007) have found negligent and abusive practices towards people with a learning disability in Cornwall and Sutton and Merton Primary Health Care NHS Trusts.

In these reports, people were also found not to have individual needs identified, or met, through a person-centred assessment or plan of care. Staff were also found to have an absence in leadership skills to transform such archaic practices. These findings have fuelled the need for an extensive audit of learning disability services.

Person-centred approaches

For the purposes of this chapter the term person-centred approaches will be adopted to reflect the broad application towards achieving both person-centred *care* and person-centred *planning*. For implementation purposes, both approaches require significant leadership and change management skills, to enable practitioners to promote, integrate and sustain such concepts, so that they may become internalised in services. This book so far has demonstrated that person-centred approaches involve holistic assessments and plans of care that are inclusive of those people across a broad spectrum of complex needs in learning disability.

People with such complex needs require a professional such as a learning disability nurse to:

- Help them aspire towards the goal of independence
- Manage dependency more effectively
- Improve on personal individual quality of life and care

Embracing person-centred planning approaches also emphasises a citizen and rights dimension and is probably one of the biggest challenges across the field of learning disability since the publication of *Normalisation* (Wolfensberger 1971) and *Social Role Valorisation* (Wolfensberger 1983). This philosophy places the person at the centre, and deliberately shifts power towards them. It can help to reclaim some of the freedom which is mostly taken for granted by others in society.

As a philosophy that espouses notions of choice, independence and inclusion, ideas embedded in the concept of person-centred planning (PCP) inevitably influence the way that services should be designed. The philosophy is therefore inseparable and continually influential on the practical implementation of person-centred planning.

However, Swift acknowledges:

> '...that it is precisely at the point to which individual aspirations and organisational pragmatics intersect, that PCP is most likely to fail'

Swift (2005, p87)

Valuing People made significant strides forward in making person-centred planning a means for delivering the government's key principles – rights, independence, choice and inclusion – and available to people who wish to plan their lives in this way.

For facilitators and practitioners this ambitious goal demands a high priority for leadership and management attention with sufficient resources for its successful implementation. Given the importance of person-centred planning as a tool for achieving change:

> 'We will make supporting its implementation one of the priorities for the Learning Disability Fund and the Implementation Support Team'

(DH 2001, p50)

Implementation of person-centred planning relies heavily on a shift in thinking by managers and frontline staff about the way support is offered. Although 'planning' features in the terminology, the plan is simply a first step.

'The plan is not the outcome'   (Ritchie et al 2003)

The plan should not be regarded as fixed and immutable over time, and adhered to in changing situations, but simply a guide in the moment, which needs continual review and updating in respect to the needs, decisions and desires of the clients. There is a need to understand person-centred care as a life philosophy – an aspiration about being human, about pursuing meaning of self, respecting individual differences, valuing diversity and equality, facing the anxieties, threats in our own lives, emphasising strengths in others and our own 'personhood'. While person-centred planning is seen as visionary, it is also thought to be idealistic and potentially unrealisable, and for some, making PCP a prescription in national policy is unlikely to produce the changes wanted in the lives of individual people with learning disabilities (Black 2000). A passionate vision and a thorough evaluation of practitioners' belief systems that underpin are required for person-centred planning to become a reality. The people who care need to be authentic and need person-centred approaches themselves. Professionals' relationships with service users should change from:

> *'being the experts on the person' [to being] 'experts in the process of problem solving with others'*   (Sanderson 2000)

Management of change

The literature on the management of change identifies a number of principles that may increase success in implementing person-centred planning in large and complex organisations. The implementation of person-centred planning requires an innovative strategy – *The Need for Change*. There are two reasons why the implementation of person-centred planning requires a modern approach:

- The style of planning used cannot simply be imported without some modification
- Person-centred planning requires fundamental changes in relationships from practitioners with people who have a learning disability

Adaptable: The planning process needs to be adapted for each organisation. Person-centred planning has generated enthusiasm for an unquestioning, quick adoption. However, Smale (1998) has found – in both literature on the adoption of innovations and the experience of the Practice and Development Exchange project – that most innovations in human services need to be 'reinvented' to meet the particular circumstances of each different service. Adapting person-centred styles means learning from experience what it takes to successfully implement the process in the service. Person-centred planning is based on learning through shared action, about finding creative solutions rather than fitting people into boxes. It is about problem solving and working together over time to create a change in the person's life, in the community and in the organisations (Sanderson 2000).

When the system takes over the planning process, the activity loses its flexibility, power and responsiveness, quickly becoming one more intrusive, insensitive and ineffective activity. Facilitators should adapt the processes they use on an individual basis. A person-centred approach requires real changes in organisational culture.

Changes in key relationships: Implementing person-centred planning requires 'second order' change in key relationships. Smale (1998) distinguishes between 'first' and second order change'. First order change is a change in behaviour or procedure, and second order change requires a change in key relationships with people as well as different skills and knowledge. Second order change is required in the implementation of person-centred planning. Person-centred planning requires that staff show a flexible and responsive approach to meet people's changing circumstances, guided by principles of good planning. Staff need to be constantly problem solving in partnership with the person and their family and friends, sharing power and decision making. An essential cultural change is that support staff have been asked to have warm and lasting relationships with people, a contrast from the professional distance of the past.

Successful implementation can be achieved by forming implementation groups (DH 2002) to facilitate its sustainability in practice. A person-centred approach evolves through creative collaboration by challenging boundaries of practices and thinking. The themes of person-centred planning in particular are reasonably clear:

- Listen to the focus person or their representatives
- Identify the person's preferences and core values
- Address the issues that disability presents
- Develop a vision of a desirable future
- Mobilise community resources

Change agents

If person-centred approaches are to be adopted and internalised by practitioners they could also benefit from the influence of person-centred management of change theory, which originates from in the school of humanistic psychology. Humanistic theories emphasise social relations and psychological needs in the workplace (Mayo 1945).

Sanderson (2002) has also found that in person-centred teams, leadership, stability of staff with evidence and prior existence of person-centred approaches are associated with improved outcomes.

Theory of this nature and focus depends on collaboration, co-operation and motivation of employees, where an established relationship co-exists between job satisfaction, teamwork and the output of the quality of work achieved.

Lewin (1951) is recognised as one of the chief architects of management of change strategies and coined the phrase 'field-forces' to describe the process of group pressures on individuals as being fundamental as part of the dynamics involved for initiating group change processes.

Change agents require a strategy for facilitating change and is where Chin and Benne (1985) provide three well-known strategies for augmenting change:

- Empirical–Rational
- Normative–Re-educative
- Power–Coercive

Empirical–Rational

This is most frequently the strategy adopted by practitioners in health and social care where human beings:

- Are seen as rational
- Follow a pattern of self-interest – they will change when they are shown that the proposed change can be justified rationally and that they will ultimately benefit from such a change

Normative–Re-educative

In this strategic approach, what people do is determined by the norms to which they subscribe, and the degree of commitment they have to these norms. Norms come from one's society, culture, religion, family and other sources.

Change occurs when commitment to some present norms decreases to a point where new norms can be adopted. It is more than an increase in knowledge, but a modification of values and attitudes, as well as behaviour. It requires direct intervention by a change agent to aid in the unlearning and relearning process.

Power–Coercive

Here, use of legitimate power to force compliance with change is pursued. This change strategy is used by a person in a hierarchical position. The group is forced to comply without having any input. The nurse leader for example, as change agent must take into account his/her relationship with the group and target change. He/she will be most effective when the strategy adopted has consistency with the overall goals and does not sabotage his/her relationship with the group.

From a person-centred implementation perspective and the adoption of a change strategy, both Empirical–Rational and Normative–Re-educative approaches would appear to be most likely to succeed as change agents work with an implementation team. Good leaders of change should also contribute:

- A clear vision for the future
- A culture of change
- Dynamic management of the boundaries and development of an organisation as a learning community where skills are actively developed in tune with the emerging issues. (Bennis & Nanus (1985)

The role of implementation group change agents in person-centred planning has five key functions (Box 14.1).

Change is a process that needs to be managed. Like any successful journey, it needs to be deliberately planned and continuously monitored with a conscious allocation of competent, committed staff effort to complete essential tasks and

Box 14.1 Five key functions for change agents

- To implement person-centred planning throughout the service
- To learn from person-centred planning, how does the service need to change?
- To support facilitators and enable them to develop facilitative skills
- To communicate person-centred values/what is the group aiming to achieve through the service
- To evaluate the effectiveness of the planning. Is it changing people's lives?

achieve lean thinking, solving problems on the way. According to Smale (1998) an implementation group can lead an organisation through three key stages of development for person-centred care and planning:

- Gestation
- Initiation
- Development

Gestation

Who needs to be brought together to begin to discuss problems and to consider solutions and proposals? During this problem identification period, change managers are active in identifying problems and bringing people together. It is critical that they collaborate, gather a consensual view of what constitutes the 'problem' and that they avoid premature closure and solution formation. Once collaboration and consent have been approached, a proposal for change may be produced. When the stage of consent time has been reached, the initiation period begins.

Initiation

What activities need to be undertaken to turn good ideas into practical proposals for implementation? The initiation period requires time for interested staff to come together to sort out ideas and turn them into new approaches to practice. The implementation of policy changes from the top also requires time if staff are to work out how they are going to implement change. Engaging staff is essential in managing the activities.

Development

What action needs to be undertaken to adapt innovation to the particular circumstances of specific adoption sites? To bring about changes in practice, persistent effort over time is true for either changing management behaviour or actions of frontline staff. The processes involved in the development phase of innovations are rarely straightforward. Mistakes, setbacks and changes in circumstances in the environment cause revisions in the best-laid plans. Leadership is also required from senior management in the group.

Smale (1998) encourages framing of innovations as a problem solving process:

- What is the problem and for who is this a problem?
- Who wants to adopt person-centred care/planning ?
- What problems does it solve?

A danger is that person-centred care/planning may simply be pursued because it is fashionable, without spending time listening to people. According to Kotter (1996), this is crucial for developing a sense of urgency that will fuel the change. Kotter also makes the point that over 50% of the companies he has observed in an attempt to make changes do not create a sense of urgency that is communicated boldly enough to 'drive people out of comfort zones'. Handy (1981) also stresses this importance:

> 'Create an awareness of the need for change. Preferably not by argument or rationale but by exposure to objective fact'

Creating a sense of urgency does not preclude acknowledging good work that already exists. It is crucial that the change agent genuinely listens to others, and does not simply feign to do so while continuing to pursue his or her own agenda. The recurring cynicism of staff who believe that 'consultation' is an empty vessel and futile, and that senior health care managers have already made up their mind is all too often perpetuated by reality.

Open, straight and honest communications require a high degree of self-awareness in the change agent, so that unwitting self-deception, and incongruence between actions and words, are recognised and managed. This general capacity can be best understood as the need for the change agent to be authentic in his or her professional relationships. Perhaps the key to this relationship is unambiguous mutual expectations, more often achieved in theory than in practice.

Key to developing a clear set of mutual expectations is the development of trust – openness and candour seem to be the key to developing trust. Authenticity is not just applicable to the change agent. For the climate to be right to foster innovation, authenticity should run throughout the organisation. If senior managers do not 'practise what they preach' – that is, they are inauthentic – it will not be possible for the organisation to develop the trust required for good enough communication and clarification of expectations. Some of the complex ways in which managers of organisations fail to be authentic or practise what they preach have been identified.

> 'Participation is something the top orders the middle to do for the bottom...participative activities are initiated because someone at a high level directs others to get involved in task forces, set up teams, or treat their subordinates differently...it certainly appears that leaders are not modelling the behaviour they want others to adopt'

> (Kanter 1985, p244)

O'Brien suggests that failings and ignorance should be acknowledged:

> 'We promise to prevent, we promise to care, we promise to rehabilitate, we promise to make independence as if it were a charter

for the production of the latest Chevrolet, and our promises have been fruitful, up to a point. If we are to move beyond that point we need the courage and the grace to learn the lessons of our collective ignorance and fallibility...there is much to learn in close attention to our errors and failings as we work to share and improve the lives of people with a learning disability' (O'Brien 1987)

Organisations often have the manuals and the theory, application and genuineness are a problem. This is a potential nexus of conflict for person-centred approaches and is not about organisations – it is about people.

Mapping

A mapping activity requires an implementation group to identify the different roles, responsibilities and relationships that different individuals occupy in relation to change, for example:

- Who are the opinion leaders?
- Who are the enthusiasts?
- Who are the 'champions'?
- Who are the 'innovators'?

Mapping the territory includes the culture of the organisation as well as the key players. In mapping the people, the voice of those who disagree need to be considered. Are people able to influence? In many instances, the chances of managing change successfully are improved when the convergence or divergence of thinking is made more explicit. This means creating a climate where disagreements can be openly expressed so that all possible information available is put in the decision. In team participation, climate is a means to reduce resistance to change, encourage commitment, and produce a more 'human-oriented culture'. It incorporates three fundamental concepts:

- Influence over decision making
- Information sharing and interaction
- High task orientation is critical for team creativity and is characterised by
  —Reflexivity
  —Constructive controversy
  —Tolerance of minority ideas
  —A commitment to excellence

This is consistent with current thinking about 'learning' or 'innovative' organisations that stress the value of open communication to achieve a shared understanding and commitment to a vision and for effecting change (Box 14.2) (Senge 1990; Kotter 1995).

Person-centred approaches and assumptions are more likely to be understood and supported if employees can participate in a collaborative process in which this kind of message is heard:

- 'We want to go in this direction'
- 'We know it will not be easy'

Box 14.2 A model for creating effective change

- **Create a sense of urgency.** Examine the culture in which the organisation operates and the commissioning realities.
- **Create the guiding alliance.** Put together a group with enough power to lead the change and get it to work together as an effective team.
- **Develop vision and strategy.** Create a vision for a desired future state as a basis for directing the change effort. Develop strategies for achieving the vision.
- **Communicate the change.** Use every method to communicate constantly and explain the new vision and strategy and ensure the guiding alliance models the behaviour of employees.
- **Empower people for action.** There is a need for investment in learning that supports mutual adjustments and collaborative relationships, change structures and systems that will promote the vision, and encourage new ideas and innovative activities.
- **Generate short-term wins.** Plan and create visible improvements in performance. Visibly recognise and reward people who made the wins possible.
- **Consolidate gains and continue the change effort.** Use increased credibility to change all systems, structures, and policies that do not fit the vision and do not fit together. Recruit, promote and develop people who can implement the change vision. Reinvigorate the change process with new projects, themes and change agents.
- **Embed the new approaches in the culture.** Create better performance through user engagement and satisfaction. *(Adapted from Kotter 1995)*

- 'We also know that many of these ideas and practices conflict with what we have promoted in the past. Let us talk about those discrepancies and about how we can shift our course toward the new direction'

Steps in implementation

Some of the founders of person-centred planning approaches, John O'Brien and Beth Mount (1991) advocate the implementation of person-centred planning one person at a time.

> *'The assumption behind this is that to be effective a service needs to learn how to support people differently as a result of planning, rather than it becoming an "empty service" ritual'*

They argue that this is only possible 'one person at a time' (O'Brien & Lovett 1992).

Lindquest and Mauriel (1989) identify two approaches – a 'depth strategy' and a 'breadth strategy' – for adopting and implementing an innovation. These approaches have been cited by Swift (2005) as a result of the guidance document from *Valuing People* (DH 2001) and Robertson et al's (2005) large longitudinal evaluation project into the outcomes of person-centred planning. A depth strategy was to invest in high quality training and support for facilitators, while the breadth strategy was to offer larger numbers of people practical ways that they can start to improve how they listen and respond to people in ways that are consistent with *Valuing People*. With regard to the Robertson et al (2005) evaluation project, Sanderson et al (2006) posit that PCP can now be considered as evidence-based practice.

From a critical perspective, research bias could be cited in this study, as the four localities selected for the evaluation were primed in terms of training, at an average cost of £658 if calculated across all 93 participants, and that the claim for covering a broad perspective of people with a learning disability was limited as 73% lived in supported accommodation.

Sanderson et al (2006) identify from the research that PCP works better for some people than for others. If someone had a mental health, emotional or behavioural problems, autism, health problems or restricted mobility, they were less likely to get a plan. An additional challenge for PCP is making it work for people whom have profound and multiple disability.

Management of change through innovation as a 'rational model' for managing change is shown in Figure 14.1 as three interlocking triangles.

Each layer of a triangle represents a level of activity.

Triangle one: What changes should we make to make person-centred planning a reality? What stays the same?

Triangle two: Identify the people through mapping to understand the context and analyse the situation

Triangle three:
- Who needs to negotiate what with whom?
- Who needs what form of staff development?
- What organisational development needs to take place?

Figure 14.1 Innovation trinity

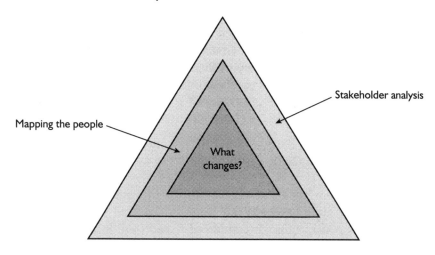

- Listen to positive and negative feedback
- Behaviour and actions.
- What are the consequences of change? Is innovation still right?

Seen in this way, each triangle represents a level of activity, not a stage of development. In practice, engagement in all of the levels of activity is essential. Action at each level causes the change agent to return to other levels of activity. Understanding the people involved in change, working with other people's ideas, and working with feelings and commitment, are central to using the innovation trinity to plan change and the whole management of change through innovation approach.

Implementing person-centred planning presents a challenge in doing this differently. Smull et al (1992) suggest that potential facilitators can be seen as 'naturals', 'learners' or people who are unlikely to have any talent for facilitation. The naturals in an organisation are those who clearly demonstrate person-centred values and continually seek ways to improve how they translate these into practice. Learners are people who broadly share the values but need extra support in finding ways to put these into practice. The rationale for training the naturals first as facilitators are that these are the people who will be most able to begin to put planning into practice, begin to create learning for the organisation and generate positive stories that can inspire and enthuse others.

In her study of innovative leaders in successful organisations, Rosabeth Moss-Kanter (1989) found that:

> *'The issue is to create the conditions that enable companies to take advantage of the good ideas which already exist, by taking better advantage of the talents of the people. By encouraging innovation and entrepreneurship at all levels, by building an environment in which more people feel involved, and empowered to take initiative, companies as well as individuals can be masters of change instead of its victims'*

What can we do to harness the talents of these facilitators? Firstly, these people should be enabled to see themselves as leaders, to develop their confidence, skills to make their own individual difference to person-centred planning. Secondly, challenging the systems and behaviours that repress individuality and force staff to retreat into their relative safety of their hierarchical job titles is vital. Thirdly, leaders are needed at all levels to recognise what they can learn from one another.

Leadership

According to the NHS Executive and King's Fund (2000), the future leader will have the certain characteristics and qualities to assist in reshaping services that are person-centred (Box 14.3).

In discussing the basic steps in the process of managing change, most of the successful innovators have a clear vision of the kind of service they want to offer. There is considerable discussion of 'leadership' in relation to innovation,

Box 14.3 Qualities and characteristics of a leader

Depth and breadth of vision
- Understands the importance of relationships and interaction at all levels
- Has the ability to look towards the future and facilitate change based on a comprehension of the whole health and health care system
- **Strategic thinking:** Able to comprehend the diversity of influencing factors in a situation and base decisions based on strategic thinking.

Awareness
- **Political:** Awareness of your profession's potential role in influencing and addressing local and national health and healthcare priorities.
- **Environmental:** Awareness of the range and diversity of organisations with the health service and their influence and impact on each other.
- **Personal confidence:** Ability to be flexible, recognise potential in others and influence rather than control.
- **Development:** Self-motivation, enthusiasm and energy. Commitment to lifelong learning and learning beyond registration.

NHS Executive and King's Fund (2000)

and in this there is frequent emphasis between 'visionary' and 'transformational' leadership.

Transformational leadership
Transformational leadership is particularly effective when organisations are in the process of renewal, development or innovation. Leaders' qualities engage with other people in a way that raises each other's levels of motivation, commitment and ethical moral practice.

Transformational leadership is where the leader:
- Establishes himself or herself as a role model by gaining the trust and confidence of followers
- Innovates
- Inspires vision, mentors and empowers followers to develop their potential and contribute more to the service
- Assists in having a long-term focus articulating future goals and plans for achieving them
- Rewards informally and personally
- Is emotional, turbulent
- Mixes home and work
- Simplifies   Bass (1998)

These qualities are in opposition to *transactional* leadership where the leader appeals to subordinates' self-interest, establishing specific exchange relationships with them by:

- Being task-centred
- Bargaining
- Separating home from work
- Having a short-term/medium-term focus
- Coaching sheltered learning
- Rewarding formally
- Being comfortable and orderly
- Complicating   Burns (1978)

This approach and style of leadership promotes clear lines of responsibility and accountability so that the system, service and status quo are maintained, and creates little room for thinking outside the box.

Conceptual applications of transformational leadership imply that those exercising such leadership have the vision of how things should be. A changemaster skill identified by Kanter is:

> '...the ability to articulate and communicate visions...people leading other people in untried directions are the true shapers of change...this second changemaster skill can be called "leadership"...this kind of leadership involves communication plus conviction, both energised through commitment'   (Kanter 1989)

For practitioners to implement lasting change towards person-centred approaches, an acknowledgement of the following points will aid success:

- Look for opportunities to start with success
- Start where the people who are doing the work are
- Listen and observe to see where organisations and people are in practice
  – what they do, their organisational culture, and their styles of management
  – directive and/or facilitative

What should be done in practice? The change agent should be looking for opportunities to initiate and support efforts to change organisational culture. Look towards those leaders and managers who consistently view all problems 'through the lens' of helping people get the lives they want, therefore traditional organisational habits/culture must be challenged. Understanding that changing a ritual/habit requires consistent effort and a minority influence strategy should be used. It is important to change the planning process and create a learning culture. Six change strategies as identified in Box 14.4 would enhance this process.

Turning the learning wheel is crucial in implementing person-centred approaches by providing protected learning time through reflective practice and clinical supervision. Continuously teaching person-centred thinking helps to build respect and partnership. To do this there are some key strategies:

- **Select** the right person with the right facilitative, interpersonal, communication skills, leadership and teamworking qualities
- **Identify** and measure the strength of the workplace for opportunities for change, and rate the opportunities rated accordingly: the effort required (organisational readiness, ease of change), talents of those who would lead

Box 14.4 Six change strategies

1. Identify the need for change
2. Create ownership and involvement
3. Create a positive environment for change
4. Work with staff to devise an action plan
5. Communicate the changes
6. Anticipate conflict and deal with resistance

the effort (naturals, learning, untalented and opposed), potential benefits (lean thinking).

- **Establish a forum** where managers can reflect on what is being learned and develop interventions and supports to overcome obstacles and sustain change, those involved in the change should meet regularly, have an agenda, devise an action, use the time to reflect and problem solve, (and not a time for crisis management).
- **Encourage regular reflection** on successes and difficulties, with suggestions from each member.
- **Welcome** issues or conflicts with policies, structures, organisational culture and change

Self-interest and shifts from group members with power positions hinder change implementation and change efforts fail for a variety of reasons (Box 14.5)

Lack of commitment is demonstrated through objections, an unwillingness to consider options or to look at process issues coupled with the use of personal 'hidden agendas.' Lack of authentic leadership behaviour may come from

- Top management
- Poor planning and co-ordination
- Inconsistent human resource policies or systems, such as inappropriate individual performance appraisal
- Inappropriate continuous professional development courses
- The way in which people are rewarded and developed

Box 14.5 Why change fails

- Lack of consistency and clear vision
- Lack of authentic leadership behaviour
- Lack of consistent messages
- Lack of communication
- Lack of commitment
- Lack of compelling evidence for the benefits of change – based on unrealistic expectations for the change

These approaches could be more representative of a transactional style of leadership than a preferred transformational style.

If services focus on changing language without changing actions, relationships, finances and structures, person-centred approaches may be lost in a mire of organisational cognitive dissonance and professional interests. New names and phrases always risk becoming euphemisms. It is essential to gather qualitative (people stories, narratives) and quantitative (research outcome measures, audit) information to see whether person-centred approaches are being applied in ways that make a difference to people.

Both these research methods have their benefits and disadvantages, but when combined, such data and personal stories can help professionals and managers reflect, learn and communicate a myriad of ways in listening and doing.

Several factors need to be in place to make person-centred approaches work for people and make a difference. These include:

- Adherence to the underlying principles of person-centred care
- Identifying sufficient financial provision and focused human resources
- A competent, committed and an excellent team
- Management from an empowering organisation that institutes clear planning and direction for the future

Achieving person-centred care needs sufficient time to spread its virtues and is sustained before policy makers, practitioners and users become tired of waiting and a new raft of policy initiatives emerges.

For achieving effective PCP, services will need to invest in leadership in PCP, to build the capacity of firstline managers to use person-centred thinking and planning, and find effective ways to support facilitators and link learning from planning to organisational change (Robertson et al 2005).

Transformational leadership competencies

For modern people management skills for the 21st century, transformational leadership competencies that reflect person-centred themes could be an approach to integrate into continuing professional development courses and programmes for key practitioners and first-line managers (Figure 14.2).

Five sets of competencies are identified which the authors deem essential for mapping modern people management skills for the 21st century. They are core themes in person-centred thinking and services and continuing professional development programmes.

Harnessing information and knowledge

- Critical analysis skills for purposes in understanding and the application of research findings.
- Audit and outcome measures.
- Skills for continuous networking and alliance building

Figure 14.2 Transformational leadership competencies

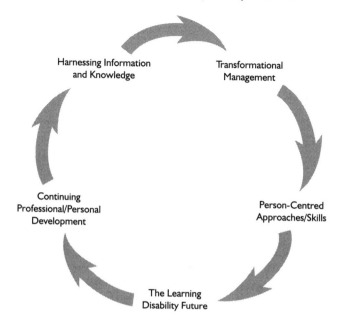

Transformational management
- Strategic vision and alliances for innovation
- Management of collaborative relationships on the boundaries of health, social care, education, leisure, work and housing
- Organisational dynamics
- Human resource development
- Marketing

Person-centred approaches and process skills
- Individual and group facilitation.
- Communication and negotiation skills
- Conflict management resolve
- Mapping people and organisational skills
- Vision–innovation–creativity for thinking outside the box
- Networking

The learning disability future
Influencing service design using:
- Citizenship model, individualised thinking, rights
- People's stories, experiences, narratives, life-story work
- Evidence-based practice
- Interagency perspectives
- User, family and carers outcomes

Continuing professional and personal development

- Vision and goals
- Leadership styles and theories
- Personal values and beliefs
- Safety planning and risk taking
- Resilience work
- Change management theories and skills

Conclusion

Person-centred care approaches further empower people with a learning disability, and enable practitioners to plan, implement and manage change in practice in support of this aspired goal.

For practitioners, person-centred approaches involve a substantial shift in thinking from paternalistic governed approaches to care. Person-centredness is founded on a rights-based approach and embraces principles of choice, independence, inclusion and empowerment.

As a philosophy, person-centredness is based on learning through shared action, finding innovative solutions to problem solving and engaging professionals and users effectively to ensure that ideas, experience and support flow freely with no gatekeeping of these attempts.

To sustain and build on the development of person-centredness is to think strategically, otherwise there is a danger of falling back into traditional policy and practice implementation methods and achieving only superficial and fragile change.

Strategies for leadership require strategic approaches in such renewing services so that person-centred approaches can cascade throughout the service to become an internalised concept for all involved in such an individualised philosophy.

Practitioners in key positions of influence are required to embrace the process of managing change, so that the success of person-centred approaches becomes a reality and not contrived, distorted or embarked on in a tokenistic manner.

Implementation is reliant on those practitioners who can influence change through a structured and well-thought out strategy – not left to chance.

References

(websites accessed 7 June 2007)

Bass BM (1998) *Transformational Leadership: industry, military and educational impact.* Mahwah, New Jersey, Lawrence Erlbaum

Bennis W, Nanus B (1985) *Leaders: the strategies for taking charge.* New York, Harper & Row

Black P (2000) Why aren't person-centred approaches and planning happening for as many people and as well as we would like? *(www.pardigm-uk.org/pdf/Articles/patblackpaper.pdf)*

Burns JM (1978) *Leadership.* London, Harper & Row

Chin R, Benne KD (1985) General strategies for effecting changes in human systems. In:

Bennis WG, Benne KD, Chin R (eds) The Planning of Change (4th edn). New York, Holt, Rinehart & Winston, pp22–45.

Department of Health (2000) *The NHS Plan*. London, The Stationery Office

Department of Health (2001) *Valuing People: a new strategy for learning disability for the 21st century*. London, The Stationery Office*(www. dh.gov.uk/learningdisabilities)*

Department of Health (2002) *Planning with People: towards person-centred approaches* London, The Stationery Office *(www. dh.gov.uk/learningdisabilities)*

Handy C (1981) *Understanding Organisations*. London, Penguin

Healthcare Commission and Commission for Social Care Inspection (2006) *Joint investigation into services for people with learning disabilities at Cornwall Partnership NHS Trust*. London, Commission for Healthcare Audit and Inspection

Healthcare Commission (2007) *Investigation into the service for people with learning disabilities provided by Sutton and Merton Primary Care Trust*. London, Commission for Healthcare Audit and Inspection

Kanter RM (1983) *The Change Master*. London, Allen & Unwin

Kotter JP (1995) *Leading Change*. Boston, Harvard Business School Press

Kotter JP (1996) *Leading Change*. Boston, Harvard Business School Press

Lewin K (1951) *Field Theory in Social Science*. New York, Harper & Row

Lindquest KM, Mauriel JJ (1989) Depth and breadth in innovation. In: *Research on the Management of Innovation: The Minnesota Studies*. Grand Rapids, Ballinger/Harper & Row for the University of Minnesota

Mayo E (1945) *The Social Problems of an Industrial Civilization*. New York, Andover Press

Mullaly S (2001) Leadership and Politics. *Nursing Management*. **8**, 4, 21–27

National Health Service Executive and King's Fund (2000) *Strategic Leadership*

O'Brien J (1987) A guide to lifestyle planning. In: Wilcox B, Bellamy GT (eds) *A Comprehensive Guide to the Activities Catalogue: an alternative curriculum for youth and adults with severe disabilities*. Baltimore, Paul H Brookes

O'Brien J (2004) If person-centred planning did not exist, *Valuing People* would require its invention. *Journal of Applied Research in Intellectual Disabilities* **17**, 11–15

O'Brien J, Lovett H (1992) Finding a way toward everyday lives: the contribution of person-centred planning. In: O'Brien J and CL (eds) *A Little Book About Person-centred Planning*. Toronto, Inclusion Press, pp113–132

O'Brien J, Mount B (1991) Telling new stories: The search for capacity among people with severe handicaps. In: Peck L, Brown L (Eds) *Critical Issues in the Lives of People with Severe Disabilities*. Baltimore, Paul H Brookes

Robertson J, Emerson E, Hatton C, Elliott J, McIntosh B, Swift P, Krinjen-Kemp E, Towers C, Romeo R, Knapp M, Sanderson H, Routledge M, Oakes P, Joyce T (2005) The impact of person-centred planning. Lancaster University, Institute for Health Research

Ritchie P, Sanderson H, Kilbane J, Routledge M (2003) *People, Plans and Possibilities: Exploring person-centred planning:* Edinburgh, SHS Ltd

Sanderson H (2000) Person-centred teams. In: O'Brien J, O'Brien CL (eds) *Implementing Person-centred Planning*. Toronto, Inclusion Press

Sanderson H (2002) A plan is not enough: exploring the development of person-centred teams. In: Holburn S, Vietze P. *Person-Centred Planning: research, practice and future directions*. Baltimore, Paul Brookes Publishing, pp 97–126

Sanderson H, Thompson J, Kilbane J (2006) The emergence of person-centred planning as evidence-based practice. *Journal of Integrated Care* **14**, 2, 18–25

Senge PM (1990) *The Fifth Discipline: The Art and Practice of the Learning Organisation.* New York, Doubleday

Smale G (1998) *Managing Change Through Innovation.* London, The Stationery Office

Smull MW, Burke Harrison S (1992) *People with severe reputations in the community.* Alexandria, Virginia, National Association of State Mental Retardation, Program Directors

Smull M, Sanderson H (2005) *Essential Lifestyle Planning for Everyone*, Manchester, Helen Sanderson Associates

Swift P (2005) Organisational factors influencing the effectiveness of person-centred planning. In: Robertson et al (2005) *The Impact of Person-centred Planning.* Lancaster University, Institute for Health Research, pp 87–102

Wolfensberger W (1972) *The Principle of Normalisation in Human Services.* Toronto, National Institute on Mental Retardation

Wolfensberger W (1983) Social Role Valorisation: proposed new term for the Principle of Normalisation. *Mental Retardation* **21**, 6, 234–239

CHAPTER 15

Fundamental nursing concepts

Risk assessment, risk management and safety planning

John Aldridge

Introduction

Over the last 10 years or so, the subject of risk has grown in importance in health and social care for people with learning disabilities. In health care particularly, this increased emphasis has been driven by policy factors, such as the public safety agenda, clinical governance (DH 1998) and the Nursing and Midwifery Council *Code of Professional Conduct* (NMC 2002). Additionally, increased awareness of professional accountability and 'litigation culture' seem to have combined to produce an overly cautious and bureaucratic approach to risk in the care of people who have learning disabilities.

A small minority of people who have learning disabilities have behaviours that challenge and they may have an additional mental illness. The care of this group of people brings in much of the legislation and policy drivers directed at mental health services, such as the Care Programme Approach (DH 1999) or the Mental Health Act (1983). An internet search using a search engine such as Google Scholar produces results suggesting that services are obsessed with the risks posed *by* learning-disabled offenders (especially sex offenders). However, Lindsay (2002) suggests that there is little reliable evidence to suggest that sex offending is over- or under-represented in the learning-disabled population.

Valuing People (DH 2001a) takes the stance that people with learning disabilities are more likely to be *at risk*, particularly from harassment, attack or abuse. Jenkins and Davies (2004) explore the phenomenon of abuse of adults with learning disabilities and offer some evidence that the incidence is relatively high, though there appears to be insufficient systematic data to give an authoritative picture.

The picture that emerges is that providing support for people with learning disabilities often involves the consideration of risk in some way or another. Services appear to perceive risk as a negative thing, something to be avoided at all costs. However, Morgan (1999) points out that risk is an essential component of everyday living and that we all take risks. She proposes that risk can be positive if seen as an opportunity for personal development and growth. We may need to balance the positive and negative aspects of risk to achieve the best outcomes for all involved.

Morgan and Wetherall (2004) suggest that services may be more concerned with 'covering their own back' and that (in a mental health context):

> *'Seldom do we find a serious attempt to engage the service user's personal agenda'*

However, the National Patient Safety Agency has made an effort to consult with people with learning disabilities and to identify risks from their viewpoint (NPSA 2004). Although this document does identify safety issues from clients' viewpoints, it does not suggest how we might manage those risks using a person-centred approach. In the context of post-*Valuing People* services, the challenge seems to be about attempting to develop support systems and strategies that meet the needs of both service user and service provider.

What is risk?

Many services and practitioners seem to treat risk as one-dimensional – 'something might go wrong' and do not look beyond their concern about a possible negative outcome. However, an exploration of the literature suggests that risk has at least two dimensions. The New Zealand Ministry of Health (1998) defines risk as:

> *'...the likelihood of an adverse event or outcome'*

Any assessment of risk therefore needs to consider not only 'what might go wrong?' but also 'how likely is it to happen?' As we will see, the second question is a difficult one to answer definitively, but is an essential part of deciding what to do about the risk.

For instance, if I leave my house I might be knocked down by a passing car. If I thought no further than that, I probably wouldn't go out. I also need to think about how realistically likely it is that I would be knocked down and then try to balance this likelihood against my need to get on with my life.

Morgan (2000) adds further dimensions by defining risk as:

> *'...the likelihood of an event happening with potentially harmful or beneficial outcomes for self and/or others'*

This definition reminds us that events, as well as having possible negative outcomes (I might be run over) also have potential positive outcomes (I can go to the shops). The outcomes may affect more than one person – there are several 'stakeholders' involved.

Any debate about risk also involves a consideration of the concept of safety. Safety can be seen as the antithesis of risk. If I am safe, then I am not at risk. However, safety is something of an illusion; arguably, I can't completely guarantee my own safety or that of others. What is perhaps more important is whether I *feel* safe, or believe myself to be safe.

Risk and people with learning disabilities

People with learning disabilities as a threat

Much of the concern about risk and people with learning disabilities is that they present a risk, or threat, to others. Much of this concern could be seen to be rooted in the eugenics movement of the early 20th century (Tredgold 1909) that led to the building of large institutions aimed at protecting society from 'mental defectives'. However, we do need to acknowledge that a very small number of people with learning disabilities do present a threat to others because of challenging behaviour, some forms of mental illness or offending behaviour. This is not the place to enter into a debate about the nature of challenging behaviour, but using aggression may be one of a limited number of ways that an individual has to cope with stressful demands and situations.

People with learning disabilities as vulnerable people

Equally, we need to consider that some people with learning disabilities may be vulnerable. Northway (2002) warns us to be cautious not to equate learning disability with vulnerability, as this may lead to misguided attempts to 'protect' them by treating them as perpetual children. However, some people with learning disabilities (especially severe or profound disabilities) do have some characteristics that make them ideal victims. Such characteristics include:

- **Intellectual impairment:** someone who does not recognise a situation as abuse and doesn't realise that it is wrong
- **Mental illness:** someone whose thoughts and emotions are temporarily disturbed and who may not be able to make rational decisions
- **Physical impairment:** someone who physically cannot protect themselves, run away or retaliate
- **Communication impairment:** someone who cannot tell others what has happened, or mobilise protection because of communication difficulties
- **Devaluation:** someone about whom the abuser (and perhaps society as a whole) might say (or think), 'they don't matter so much, anyway'
- **Social isolation:** someone who lives apart from the mainstream of society and who has a very small social network of people who might help to protect them.
- **Disempowerment:** someone who is subject to the legitimate (e.g. Mental Health Act) or implicit (e.g. a person receiving care) power of another person.

Threat and vulnerability are not mutually exclusive – it is not an 'either-or' thing. It is quite possible that, in different situations, some people with learning disabilities may be both a threat and vulnerable at the same time. Emerson et al (1988) point out that people whose behaviour is a challenge are most likely to 'lose out' on community services and have fewer options for supportive services.

This phenomenon can be described by a two-dimensional matrix, in which a person broadly fits into one of the four categories according to their level of vulnerability and threat (Figure 15.1).

Figure 15.1 The Threat–Vulnerability matrix

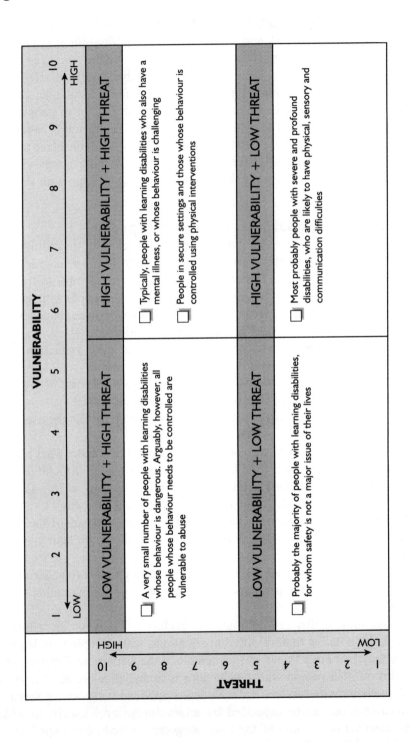

The NPSA (2004) identifies five areas of risk for people with learning disabilities:

- Inappropriate or unsafe use of physical interventions (control and restraint)
- Vulnerability in general hospitals, poorer standards of care and treatment
- Swallowing difficulties and dysphagia
- Lack of accessible information, impairing peoples' ability to make informed decisions
- Illness or disease (physical and mental) being misdiagnosed or undiagnosed (diagnostic overshadowing)

The dichotomy between threat and vulnerability can be extended to incorporate a further dimension that relates to people and the environment. This presents us with a two dimensional matrix with four possible situations (Figure 15.2):

- People with a learning disability as a threat to other people
- People with a learning disability vulnerable from other people
- People with a learning disability as a threat to the environment
- People with a learning disability vulnerable from the environment

Figure 15.2 The nature of risk

	PERSON	ENVIRONMENT AND POSSESSIONS
THREAT	Threat posed by the individual to self and others	Threat posed by the individual to the environment and possessions
	☐ Aggression and violence to others ☐ Abuse and exploitation of others ☐ Deliberate self-harm ☐ Sexual offending ☐ Promiscuity	☐ Damage to property, buildings, public environment ☐ Theft of others' property ☐ Damage to own possessions
VULNERABILITY	Vulnerability of the individual from others	Vulnerability of the individual from the environment (which incorporates their systems of support)
	☐ Aggression and violence by others ☐ Abuse and exploitation by others ☐ Irrational decision-making ☐ Sexual vulnerability ☐ Financial vulnerability ☐ Non-consensual care & treatment ☐ Ineffective or inappropriate care & treatment ☐ Vulnerability of the individual posed by the nature of their condition (e.g. dysphagia due to cerebral palsy)	☐ Environmental hazards ☐ Damage by others to possessions & property ☐ Theft of property ☐ Unsafe or inappropriate living & care arrangements

Who needs to feel safe?

One of the basic tenets of Protective Behaviours is that :

'We all have the right to feel safe all of the time' (PBUK, on line)

This is a deceptively deep statement that contains a number of important elements:

All means all. There are no exceptions to this belief. Everybody, including people whose behaviour is challenging, or who have committed offences, have the right to feel safe.

Feeling safe is a right. The ability to feel safe is not something that needs to be earned by 'good behaviour' or by 'being normal'. It is a basic moral and human right, underpinned by the Human Rights Act (1998).

Feeling safe. We might ask, 'Why do we not have the right to *be* safe?' The problem with this is that it might be used as a reason for others to restrict our freedom in order to make us safe for our own good. Sometimes we 'risk on purpose' but usually we *feel* reasonably safe and confident in doing so because the three key elements of choice, time limit and control are present. Feeling safe is broadly about feeling happy, comfortable and confident.

All of the time. Again, there are no exceptions. We are not saying that people have the right to feel safe some of the time. There are no 'special circumstances' in which it is acceptable for people not to feel safe. If it is necessary to use physical interventions with people, *everyone* has the right to feel safe in that.

When considering risk and safety in the context of learning disabilities services, we need to balance the needs of three groups of people.

People with learning disabilities. Person-centred care places the client at the centre of decision-making and the care process. Clearly, if the person feels vulnerable, it is important that services respond appropriately and help them to feel safe. Equally, if we are working with a person who is perceived as posing a threat to others, they still have the right and a need to feel safe. There is a growing awareness (NPSA 2004; Hawkins et al 2005) that the use of physical interventions is a frightening and unsafe experience for service users. Therefore, when we carry out safety planning, it is imperative that we look at things from the service-user's viewpoint.

Other service users, family members and the general public. These people have a right to feel safe and we have a duty of care to them to protect their safety. We also need to recognise that, although family members do not have the power of veto over decisions made regarding their adult children, they expect us to act responsibly and not to take unnecessary risks.

Service professionals. It is important to realise that there are a number of ways in which we need to feel safe. If we are working with people whose behaviour is challenging we may need to take action that ensures our own safety if we are attacked. Less apparent is our need to feel safe in the decisions that we make. We need to feel confident that things are not going to go wrong, that people will not be harmed and that we will not be held accountable for neglect of our duty of care. This is one of the main reasons why professionals are often very cautious about taking risks.

Clearly we need to balance the views, needs and wishes of these three groups when planning for safety. It is quite likely that people may have conflicting ideas that need to be worked through. Safety planning may involve a compromise in the positive sense, in that the needs of all parties are recognised and incorporated into any strategies, so that everyone feels confident. The question that everyone asks themselves is *'Do I feel happy about this?'* Kinsella (2000) offers a structure that we might use to balance happiness and safety (Figure 15.3).

Figure 15.3 Balancing safety and happiness

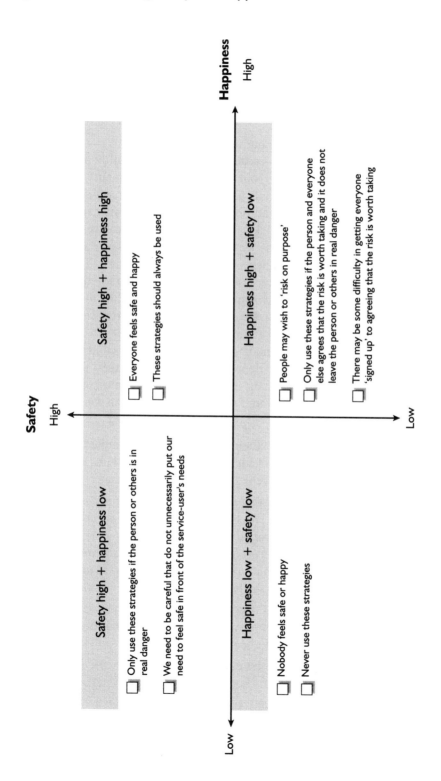

Safety

High

Safety high + happiness high

☐ Everyone feels safe and happy

☐ These strategies should always be used

Safety high + happiness low

☐ Only use these strategies if the person or others is in real danger

☐ We need to be careful that do not unnecessarily put our need to feel safe in front of the service-user's needs

Happiness

High

Happiness high + safety low

☐ People may wish to 'risk on purpose'

☐ Only use these strategies if the person and everyone else agrees that the risk is worth taking and it does not leave the person or others in real danger

☐ There may be some difficulty in getting everyone 'signed up' to agreeing that the risk is worth taking

Low

Happiness low + safety low

☐ Nobody feels safe or happy

☐ Never use these strategies

Low

Risk assessment

Safety planning needs to begin with an assessment of risk, but this is rather more complicated than merely thinking about 'How likely is it that something may go wrong?'

The New Zealand Ministry of Health (1998) comment that:

> 'Risk assessment is an estimation of the likelihood of particular
> adverse events occurring under particular circumstances within a
> specified period of time'

This adds a number of factors to our original definition.

Estimation. Risk assessment is an *estimation* of likelihood. Civil and constructional engineers can carry out precise risk assessments because they can calculate the strength of materials and the stresses under which they will be placed. A new bridge should not fall down if the engineer has carried out their calculations accurately. However, risk assessment in human services is something more of an art than a science because we cannot precisely measure all of the many influencing factors and we are not necessarily in control of these. If a person has a history of 'risk behaviours' we can use this to estimate the likelihood of them behaving in this way in the future. However, if they are intending to do something new, such as going to the shops on their own, we might be reduced to educated guesswork in deciding how risky that might be.

Circumstances. We need to think about the *circumstances* and the context of the risk. Peoples' safety may alter depending on how well they feel, how well supported they are, who is supporting them, how other people behave, whether they are at home or at work and so on. Prinns (1986) comments that:

> 'It is wiser to think of dangerous situations rather than dangerous people'

Time. Risk assessments are, by their very nature, time-limited. Because the circumstances and the person may change, we need to revisit any risk assessment regularly. The Royal College of Psychiatrists (1996) remark that:

> 'Risk is dynamic and may depend on circumstances which can alter
> often over brief time periods. Therefore risk assessment needs a
> short-term time perspective and must be subject to frequent review...
> adequate risk assessment can rarely be done by one person alone.
> Wider information is needed and it is almost always helpful to discuss
> the assessment and the management plan with a peer or supervisor'

I would go further than that and suggest that risk assessment is a team effort and there is no reason why a person-centred process should not be used. Indeed, the Department of Health (2001b) indicates that:

> 'Before you examine, treat or care for competent adults you must
> obtain their consent'

This statement clearly includes any risk assessment. If the person cannot give informed consent, a rigorous Best Interests checklist from the Mental Capacity Act (2005) Code of Practice should be used. Additionally, the latest judgement in the 'Bournewood Case' given by the European Court of Human Rights suggests that we would be acting illegally if we did anything involved in a person's care without either attempting to gain consent or by using Best Interests. A plea that 'it is necessary in order to protect people' is not acceptable if the care contravenes the person's human rights (Hewitt 2004).

Morgan and Wetherall (2004) indicate that risk assessments using numerical scoring are problematic and may be limited in their ability to inform decision-making. However, we are still left with the question 'how big a risk are we talking about?'.

The risk assessment matrix (Plate 15.1) offers a tool that helps us to decide how serious the risk is, and how likely it is that a negative outcome will result. Both likelihood and outcome are represented as the two axes on a nominal 10-point scale. The matrix simply multiplies the seriousness of outcome by the likelihood of it happening to give an overall risk score. The risk scores are banded, using a 'traffic light' system to denote the overall level of risk.

- **Condition Green.** Risks that are minor or unlikely to happen are unlikely to require the full weight of safety planning. If a safety issue is in this category, I recommend that you don't go any further.

- **Condition Amber.** At this level of risk, it is appropriate to write a simple safety action plan

- **Condition Red.** Risks at this level are serious and require a full risk reduction plan

- **Condition Double Red.** Risks at this level are extremely serious and will require an urgent Risk Reduction Plan.

It is important that the matrix is used transparently; using a team approach, by all stakeholders – including the client – and that it forms the focus for debate. Debate is healthy, but it is important that everyone reaches a consensus eventually.

Risk management or safety planning?

Risk assessment and risk management historically have been used in bureaucratic and service-led ways that run contrary to the precepts and beliefs of person-centred planning. Traditional approaches to risk management view things entirely from the organisation's point of view and often fail to recognise the need to take risks if people are to develop and grow as individuals. The aim of much risk management is to eliminate risk. As we have seen, we can reduce risk, but it is impossible and unethical to attempt to eliminate it entirely.

The New Zealand Ministry of Health (1998) observes that:

> 'Risk management aims to minimise the likelihood of adverse events occurring within the context of the overall management of an individual, to achieve the best possible outcome and deliver safe, appropriate, effective care' [my emphasis]

The key elements here are that any safety plan needs to:

- Balance the best possible outcome for *everybody*. It is not acceptable for one person to suffer merely because it meets other peoples' safety needs.
- Be safe and effective. Clearly, a safety plan that fails to promote peoples' safety is of no use to anyone.
- Be appropriate. We should not be using a 'sledge hammer to crack a walnut'. We need to acknowledge and work with the belief that people have a need and a right to take risks and to use a sense of proportion.

Arguably, if we recognise the dignity of risk this humanises and enables service users, rather than demonising and disabling them. There is a wealth of difference between 'taking a risk' and being neglectful or foolhardy. Taking a risk implies that we have weighed up the positive and negative issues, the possible outcomes and likelihood of them happening. A transparent team approach that involves all the stakeholders is more likely to result in a strategy in which most people are happy for most of the time.

The three elements of effective safety planning

To be effective, safety planning needs to use three mutually supportive elements (Figure 15.4):

- Effective training and skill
- Effective method
- Effective teamwork

If any of these is absent, the whole strategy collapses and becomes ineffective. (Figure 15.5).

Figure 15.4 Effective safety planning

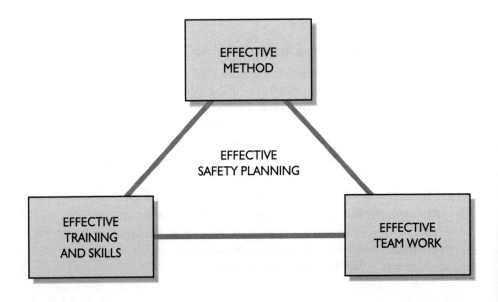

Figure 15.5 Ineffective safety planning

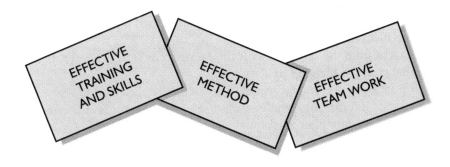

Effective training and skill. Support staff need to be trained in strategies that help to enable service users, while promoting their safety. If physical interventions are used, staff need to be properly trained in their use. Training and skill also extends to service users, who may need help to express their safety needs, as well as perhaps becoming more emotionally literate, having more coping strategies at their disposal so that they don't need to behave in unsafe ways.

Effective method. We need to use person-centred processes throughout and to use appropriate structures and systems. If staff uses physical interventions, they need to use them appropriately and correctly. The process of developing a safety plan needs to be transparent and democratic, so that people are encouraged to put their point of view (which might differ from others').

Effective teamwork. All support staff, service users and family members need to be 'singing from the same hymn sheet'. It only takes one dissenter to jeopardise the effectiveness of a whole plan and the efforts of everyone else involved. The process of developing a safety plan needs to be a team process, with all stakeholders involved. In that way, if people are given a chance to have their say, they are less likely later on to work to their own private agenda.

Ten steps to safety planning

Part A: Person-centred risk assessment
Step 1: Describe the risk and identify the level of risk
- Who or what is at risk?
- What is the 'untoward event' that people are concerned about? Try to be as precise as possible
- Who or what poses the threat?
- What does the service user think or feel about the risk?
- What do we know about the history of the risk? Has it happened before?
- Decide on the level of risk, using a team process

Step 2: Involve and inform all the stakeholders throughout the process

In practice, it is difficult to separate steps 1 and 2 and these are most likely to be worked through in parallel.

- Try to involve the service user as much as possible, or if this is not possible, at least keep them fully informed
- Gain consent from the service user (or use a rigorous Best Interests checklist in keeping with the Mental Capacity Act))
- If appropriate, involve and inform the client's family and/or advocate
- Involve and inform the whole multidisciplinary team (consistent with completing the safety plan quickly)

Step 3: Describe the setting conditions or context of the risk

- In what situations does the risk tend to occur?
- Who might be involved?
- Are there any patterns or trends that people have noticed?

Step 4: Describe the triggers or antagonising factors

- What increases the likelihood of the risk happening?
- Are there any things that make it worse and make things escalate?

Step 5: Describe the helpful or protagonising factors

- What decreases the likelihood of the risk happening?
- What helps to ease the situation and prevent things getting worse?

Step 6: Identify the advantages and disadvantages of taking the risk

- What does the service user stand to gain by taking the risk?
- What do others stand to gain by not taking the risk?
- What does the service user stand to lose if we take no risk at all?

Part B: Developing a person-centred safety plan

Step 7: Identify the aim of the safety plan

Do you want to:

- Reduce the likelihood of the risk? or/and
- Reduce the severity of the risk?

If we want to retain an acceptable quality of life for everyone, it will probably be undesirable and unrealistic to try to reduce the likelihood to zero. It is generally a good idea to try to shift the risk into the Green band if possible, though in some cases the strategy may be one of 'damage limitation'.

Step 8: Explore the options for reducing the level of risk

- What kinds of things might people do to reduce the risk?
- Think creatively about the approaches and strategies that people (including the client) might use

Step 9: Decide on the least restrictive, effective alternative from your list of options

- Use the principles of the 'least restrictive alternative' (Turnbull 1981; LaVigna

& Donnellan 1986). Try to choose an option that gives the greatest freedom to the individual, while protecting everyone's safety.

- Consider what the service user thinks and whether they consent to the plan. This is particularly important if the safety plan is about protecting the client – they might want to take a risk.
- Try to balance the needs of everyone involved, perhaps by making positive compromises (Figure 15.6).

Figure 15.6 An options matrix

NEGATIVE FOR SERVICE USER POSITIVE FOR OTHERS	NEGATIVE FOR EVERYBODY
Try to avoid this option	Never use this option
☐ Can you justify putting other peoples' needs above the service user's	☐ Nobody feels safe or happy
☐ Are you trying to use a sledge hammer to crack a walnut?	☐ Avoid using this option merely because it keeps everyone safe - there is likely to be a more positive option
☐ Does this unnecessarily infringe the service user's legal and human rights?	
☐ Is there a better compromise?	
POSITIVE FOR EVERYBODY	**POSITIVE FOR SERVICE USER NEGATIVE FOR OTHERS**
Try to use this option where possible	Try to avoid this option
☐ Does this safely balance everyone's needs?	☐ Can you justify putting the service user's needs above those of others?
☐ Is everyone happy and in agreement	☐ Does this compromise your duty of care to other people?

Step 10: Write the safety action plan or a full risk reduction plan

The safety action plan (Figure 15.7) is similar to a health action plan, with which, it is hoped, service users will be familiar. It is a 'shortcut' to a full risk reduction plan and can be used when the level of risks are generally relatively low and when the client does not pose a threat to others.

The risk reduction plan (Figure 15.8) is a much more detailed plan that is more appropriate to risks that are more serious, and especially when a client presents a threat to other people. Although it is more prescriptive, there is no reason why the client should not be involved in its development. They should certainly be aware of its content and they should have given their consent to it, unless they are detained under a Section of the Mental Health Act (1983).

The risk reduction plan is similar in format to a conventional care plan, in that it details exactly what people will do, how, and when to reduce the risk. The emphasis here is on *reducing* the risk, while promoting as much freedom as possible. The principle of the least restrictive alternative should be used. However,

Figure 15.7 Safety action plan

SAFETY ACTION PLAN			
Service user's name	Date of assessment	Date for evaluation	Key worker
What is the risk about?	Level	How we will reduce the risk	How successful were we?

Sheet number............of............

SAFETY ACTION PLAN

Sheet number............of............

Figure 15.8 Risk reduction plan

RISK REDUCTION PLAN

FOR (client's name)

The risk is:

| We plan to reduce the risk to: | DOUBLE RED | RED | AMBER | GREEN |

Date set: Key person responsible:

The aim of this risk reduction plan:

The strategy for this risk reduction plan:

Who will be involved:

This is exactly what we will do to reduce the risk:

We will use this plan when:

The safety net:

If the untoward event happens or seriously threatens to happen we will do this:

We will know if our plan is working if:

We will review and evaluate our plan on:

Signature of key person responsible

Evaluation

How successful has this strategy been? Use recorded data to help you make this decision

Future action

Does this strategy need to be used in the future? Does it need to be modified?

Signature of key person responsible | Date of evaluation

it also contains a section for a safety net, which describes what people will do if things look realistically as though they are going to go wrong. This is very much part of the process of 'taking a risk'. What we are saying here is: 'Yes, we will take a calculated risk, but if things go wrong we do have a fall back position.' It is very important to have thought out the safety net beforehand, rather than having to think in an emergency how to deal with a potentially hazardous situation.

Plate 15.2 shows a flowchart that shows the steps through the process of safety planning and shows the shortcuts that can be safely made.

Conclusion

Safety planning with people who have learning disabilities is relatively complex and difficult, not least because of the diversity of peoples' needs. We are not simply caring for people who might be dangerous – we are also attempting to recognise the needs of people who might be vulnerable. The post-*Valuing People* agenda of person-centredness, set within a framework of independence, choice, inclusion and rights presents a number of dilemmas and problems to professionals, service users and family members. Whose rights should we be serving? How do we balance the needs of the service user against those of everyone else who might be involved? Issues derived from mental health services and the public safety agenda further complicate much of the work of professionals in challenging behaviour services. One is often left struggling to find a way through the maze of legislation, agendas and ideologies. What happened to social role valorisation and does that all go out of the window when we are working with people who can behave in threatening and dangerous ways?

There are no easy answers to these questions but I hope that this chapter has presented some useful ideas that might help services work towards a more person-centred approach to safety planning.

References

(all websites accessed 4 June 2007)

Department of Health (1998) *A First Class Service:* quality in the new NHS, London, The Stationery Office

Department of Health (1999) *Effective Care Coordination in Mental Health Services: modernising the care programme approach.* London, The Stationery Office

Department of Health (2001a) *Valuing People*: a new strategy for learning disability in the 21st century. London, The Stationery Office

Department of Health (2001b) *12 Key Points on Consent: the law in England.* London, The Stationery Office

Emerson E, Cummings R, Barrett S et al (1988) Challenging behaviour and community services: 2. Who are the people who challenge services? *Mental Handicap* **16**, 16–19

Hawkins S, Allen D, Jenkins R (2005) The use of physical interventions with people with intellectual disabilities and challenging behaviour – the experiences of service users and staff members. *Journal of Applied Research in Intellectual Disabilities* **18**, 1, 19–23

Hewitt D (2004) Hempsons News Flash, October 2004, *Bournewood patients: The common law is not enough* [on line] *(www.hempsons.co.uk)*

Jenkins R, Davies R (2004) The abuse of adults with learning disabilities and the role of the learning disability nurse. *Learning Disability Practice.* **7**, 2, 30–38

Kinsella P (2000) *Person-centred Risk Assessment (http://valuingpeople.gov.uk/dynamic/ valuingpeople126.jsp)*

LaVigna G, Donnellan A (1986) *Alternatives to Punishment: solving behaviour problems with non-aversive strategies.* New York, Irvington

Lindsay W (2002) Research and literature on sex offenders with intellectual and developmental disabilities, *Journal of Intellectual Disability Research.* **46**, Suppl 1, 74–85

Mental Capacity Act (2005) Draft Code of Practice, London, The Stationery Office *(www. dca.gov.uk/menincap/mcbdraftcode.pdf)*

Ministry of Health (New Zealand) (1998) *Guidelines for Clinical Risk Assessment and Management in Mental Health Services.* Wellington, New Zealand, MoH. *(www.moh. govt.nz/moh.nsf/Files/mentalra/$file/mentalra.pdf)*

Morgan H (1999) Supporting people with learning disabilities – it's a risky business. *www. learningdisabilities.org.uk/page.cfm?pagecode=PRARSP*

Morgan S (2000) *Clinical Risk Management: a clinical tool and practitioner manual.* London, Sainsbury Centre for Mental Health

Morgan S, Wetherall A (2004) Assessing and managing risk. In: Norman I, Ryrie I (eds) *The Art and Science of Mental Health Nursing.* Maidenhead, Open University Press

National Patient Safety Agency (2004) *Understanding the Patient Safety Issues for People with Learning Disabilities.* London, NPSA

Northway R (2002) The nature of vulnerability. *Learning Disability Practice* **5**, 6, 26

Nursing and Midwifery Council (2002) *Code of Professional Conduct.* London, NMC

Prinns H (1986) *Dangerous Behaviour, The Law and Mental Disorder* London, Tavistock

Protective Behaviours UK *(www.protectivebehaviours.co.uk)*

Royal College of Psychiatrists Special Working Party on Clinical Assessment and Management of Risk (1998) *Assessment and Clinical Management of Risk of Harm to Other People*, Council Report CR53. London, RCP

Tredgold AF (1909) The feebleminded – a social danger. *Eugenics Review* **1**, 97–104

Turnbull H (1981) *The Least Restrictive Alternative: Principles and Practices.* Washington, American Association on Mental Deficiency